Introduction to Hospital Accounting

Third Edition

Introduction to Hospital Accounting

L. Vann Seawell, DBA, CPA
Professor of Accounting
Indiana University

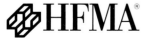HFMA® HEALTHCARE FINANCIAL MANAGEMENT ASSOCIATION

TWO WESTBROOK CORPORATE CENTER
SUITE 700
WESTCHESTER, ILLINOIS 60154

KENDALL/HUNT PUBLISHING COMPANY
2460 Kerper Boulevard P.O. Box 539 Dubuque, Iowa 52004-0539

Printed in the United States of America
10 9 8 7 6 5 4 3 2 1

Library of Congress Cataloging-in-Publication Data
Seawell, L. Vann (Lloyd Vann), 1930–
   Introduction to hospital accounting / L. Vann Seawell.—3rd ed.
      p.   cm.
   Includes bibliographical references and index.
   ISBN 0-8403-6310-9 : $60.65
   1. Hospitals—Accounting.   I. Title.
HF5686.H7S4   1992
657′ .832—dc20
                                                                      91-22305
                                                                        CIP

To Stan. Beloved teacher and mentor.

To Jack and Sam. True friends and admired colleagues.

To Bingo and Priss. Gone but not forgotten.

To Joy. She lights up my life.

Contents

Foreword

This third edition of Dr. Seawell's *Introduction to Hospital Accounting* marks another milestone in the progress of the profession of healthcare financial management and in the services of the Healthcare Financial Management Association. The development of the profession and the Association both evidence dedication to managing our nation's hospitals in a conscientious, cost-effective manner.

External influences on the financial management of hospitals have grown significantly in the years since Dr. Seawell began writing for the specialty of healthcare financial management. Generally accepted accounting principles applicable to health care now reflect the work of the Financial Accounting Standards Board, and the recently updated specialty audit guide issued by the American Institute of Certified Public Accountants. Those who pay for healthcare services and provide financing for the industry are increasing their search for and scrutiny of information. Health care is a major focus of public policy debate, and an aging population, technological advances, and increasing public interest in good health have significantly expandced the role and complexity of hospital operations. There also has been significant change in the organizational relationship between hospitals and other healthcare organizations. All of these changes have placed new demands on the financial information systems and the financial management of healthcare institutions. In this publication, Dr. Seawell has carefully balanced this growing sophistication of the financial management profession with the objective of providing an introduction.

Since the last edition of Dr. Seawell's book, the Association has also grown and changed. During this time, the Association changed its name, substituting the word *Healthcare* for *Hospital*. The change recognizes the changing nature of the industry and the role of the financial managers whom the Association serves. The

Association has met the challenges of the profession through expansion and modification of traditional services and products and introduction of new services, including data services, career services, and new opportunities for member interaction.

This will not be the last edition of this text, and HFMA will also continue to evolve to meet changing member needs. There will be a continuing flow of individuals entering the profession who will find this book an invaluable resource. Dr. Seawell's other books and the broad array of Association services and products will provide the additional assistance needed by these professionals to meet the ever-growing demands and opportunities of the profession. This book by Dr. Seawell continues to be a crucial cornerstone of that process.

R. R. Kovener

Preface

The origins of this book may be traced back more than 35 years to when Professor Stanley A. Pressler of the Indiana University Graduate School of Business urged one of his students to take a serious interest in the accounting and financial management practices employed by hospitals. I was that fortunate student. With Stan's guidance, I wrote a mimeographed booklet for use in connection with a correspondence study course on the fundamentals of hospital accounting. That course, the first its kind, was cosponsored by the Indiana University Graduate School of Business and the American Association of Hospital Accountants (later to become the Healthcare Financial Management Association).

The success of the course, along with the encouragement of Sister Mary Gerald and Robert M. Shelton, led me to write *Principles of Hospital Accounting* (Physicians' Record Company, 1960). This book was subsequently revised and retitled *Introduction to Hospital Accounting* for publication by HFMA in 1971, 1977, and 1986.

Historically, then, the present volume is the result of a number of efforts extending over three decades. While still introductory in nature, much of the discussion within these pages is at a level of sophistication appropriate to the considerable progress that hospitals have made in accounting and financial management in recent years. Several chapters have new materials, and the book includes revised and expanded end-of-chapter assignment exercises. The glossary includes many additional accounting and financial terms not found in earlier editions. A number of other changes have been made, largely in response to helpful comments received from users of the previous edition. I am grateful for their interest and assistance, and I welcome criticisms and suggestions from readers of this edition.

The publication of this book is yet another indication of the dedication of the HFMA board of directors, officers, committees, and staff to an ongoing educational program in the healthcare field. I deeply appreciate this opportunity to contribute again to that program, hoping that my writing may prove worthy of the trust and support given to me by so many people over so many years.

While I dare not attempt to list the names of all who have assisted me in this undertaking, I must recognize the following persons to whom I owe a special debt of gratitude:

Richard L. Clarke
President, HFMA

James C. Patton
Partner, Ernst & Young

Ronald R. Kovener
Vice President, HFMA

Alice M. McCart
Manager, HFMA Editorial
Development

Ronald E. Keener
Vice President, HFMA

Lynn J. Brown
Brown Editorial Service

None of these individuals, however, has any responsibility for whatever errors of commission or omission may appear in this book. That responsibility is entirely mine.

L. Vann Seawell
Bloomington, Indiana
May 28, 1991

Nature and Function of Hospital Accounting

Accounting is an essential service activity found in all economic entities and organizations, regardless of type or size. The primary purpose of accounting is to provide useful financial information about an organization's activities and affairs. This information is intended to be used for purposes of intelligent decision making by the organization's management and by interested external groups such as investors, creditors, other resource providers, governmental agencies, and the general public. Because such decisions directly affect the manner in which limited resources are allocated and employed in our economy, the information generated by the accounting process plays a significant role in determining the types and quantities of products and services that are produced and consumed. With this in mind, the recording and reporting of adequate and reliable financial information relevant to users' needs clearly must be viewed as a function of extreme importance in our economic system.

The economic entity with which this book is specifically concerned is the hospital enterprise organized and operated either on a not-for-profit or profit-seeking basis. This emphasis on accounting as related to the hospital organization in particular seems warranted because, although the basic principles of accounting are substantially the same for all types of organizations, hospital enterprises have many unique characteristics that require specialized applications of accounting principles and procedures. In addition, the healthcare business has grown to have massive economic and social significance, demanding an increasingly higher order of accounting and financial reporting practices. It seems reasonable to assume that this requirement will be realized most effectively and quickly through educational materials and programs dealing specifically with the particular accounting and financial reporting problems of hospitals and other healthcare entities. Healthcare organizations of all types can benefit greatly from the use of time-proven accounting techniques, reporting practices, and business methods that have been developed by commercial enterprises. It also should be noted that, although this book is focused largely on hospitals, the principles and practices described generally are applicable to most other entities composing the healthcare industry.

In seeking solutions to the serious problems being encountered currently in the provision of health care at reasonable costs, hospital managers and other interested groups are more heavily dependent than ever before on the information provided by highly sophisticated accounting systems. The effectiveness of hospital managers at all levels is directly related to the quality of the information developed by accountants, including business office personnel engaged in the least glamorous bookkeeping tasks. A similar dependency on, and need for, more and better financial information about hospitals also exists with respect to third-party payers, planning agencies, and other external groups.

Purpose of This Book Your interest in hospital accounting may arise from a desire to become a hospital accountant or auditor, or from a need to increase your capabilities in these areas. On the other hand, you may be preparing yourself for a career in hospital administration as a nonaccounting executive, recognizing that your preparation would not be adequate or complete without a study of accounting principles. In each case, this book is intended to serve as an introductory course emphasizing the methodology of hospital accounting but also providing an understanding of the meaning and managerial uses of accounting information. The broad coverage of subjects enables this book to be used as a complete course for those having no interest in an accounting career. The depth of coverage, however, is sufficient to permit others to continue their accounting education at an intermediate level.

This chapter examines some of the characteristics of the hospital enterprise, the economic environment in which it pursues its objectives, and the role of accounting in hospital management. You will see that there is a critical and continuous need for financial information about hospital activities and affairs, that this information is required for internal management purposes and also by external users, and that the accounting process provides that information. Then, in introductory fashion, the chapter explores the nature and content of financial statements developed by the accounting process. Your concern will be to obtain a general knowledge of the hospital business and a basic understanding of the end product of accounting—the financial statements—before you get involved in the details of accounting methodology beginning with the next chapter.

The importance of the healthcare business in this country is indicated in part by its size and rate of growth. Health care is said to be the second largest American industry (after construction) with annual expenditures in excess of $500 billion. No other nation spends so much (well over 10 percent) of its gross national product for health care as does the United States. In addition, with expenditures increasing by more than 10 percent annually, health care has been one of the nation's fastest growing industries. It is generally agreed that this trend is not likely to change significantly in the near future. An even greater emphasis, however, will be placed on efforts to ensure maximum returns from this huge investment in terms of the quality and accessibility of healthcare services.

The single largest component of the American healthcare industry is the network of over 7,000 hospitals whose annual expenses represent about 40 percent of total annual healthcare expenditures. Approximately 97 percent of these hospitals are registered with the American Hospital Association (AHA). The Hospital Data Center of the AHA conducts an Annual Survey of Hospitals to obtain information pertaining to (among other things) the utilization, personnel, and finances of hospitals. Survey results are published annually by the AHA. The publication is known as the *American Hospital Association Guide to the Health Care Field,* with a separate statistical supplement entitled *Hospital Statistics.* Much of the following information is drawn from the 1988 Edition of *Hospital Statistics.* (You are urged to refer to these AHA publications for more detailed and complete information.)

Figure 1–1 presents selected information relating to the utilization, personnel, and finances of all AHA-registered hospitals in the United States. This information is provided for 1987 and 1972 to highlight some of the important changes that have taken place over this 16-year period. Note, for example, the decreases in number of hospitals, beds, average daily census, and occupancy percentage. Also observe the increases in expenses and outpatient visits.

In 1946, there were 6,125 AHA-registered hospitals with a total of 1,436,000 beds. Average daily census was 1,142,000, and occupancy was nearly 80 percent. Total full-time equivalent personnel numbered only 830,000, and total expenses were less than $2 billion.

The Economic Environment

Hospital Statistics

	1987	1972
Number of hospitals:		
Federal	342	401
Nonfederal psychiatric	684	543
Nonfederal respiratory diseases	5	72
Nonfederal long-term	131	216
Nongovernment not-for-profit short-term	3,289	3,326
Investor-owned short-term	828	738
State and local government short-term	1,542	1,779
Total number of hospitals	6,821	7,075
Number of beds (in thousands)	1,267	1,550
Admissions (in thousands)	34,439	33,265
Average daily census (in thousands)	873	1,209
Occupancy percentage	68.9	78.0
Outpatient visits (in thousands)	310,707	219,182
Full-time equivalent personnel (in thousands)	3,742	2,671
Expenses (in millions of $):		
Labor	99,096	21,455
Total expenses	178,662	32,667

Breakdown of Hospitals by
Ownership

Of the 6,821 hospitals included in Figure 1–1 for 1987, 5,611 (82 percent) are referred to as *community hospitals.* The AHA defines such hospitals as all nonfederal short-term general and other special hospitals whose facilities and services are available to the public. Of these 5,611 hospitals, 3,274 (58 percent) are nongovernmental not-for-profit hospitals, 1,509 (27 percent) are state and local governmental hospitals, and 828 (15 percent) are investor-owned hospitals. In 1987, the expenses of community hospitals were about 85 percent of the total expenses of all hospitals.

Figure 1–2 presents selected information relating to the utilization, personnel, and finances of community hospitals for 1987 and 1972. Note the changes that have occurred over this 16-year period.

Another statistic of interest is the average salary of employees in community hospitals. The average salary was $14,250 in 1981 and $21,938 in 1987. As shown in Figure 1–2, labor costs account for more than half of total hospital costs (53 percent in 1987 versus 63 percent in 1972).

Contributing Factors to
Increased Healthcare Costs

Aside from inflation, the rather dramatic rise in hospital expenses since World War II can be attributed in part to a vastly greater demand for an increasingly wide range of hospital services. Expanded hospital services required an increase in hospital personnel. The average earnings of hospital employees also have risen

	1987	1972
Number of beds (in thousands)	958	879
Admissions (in thousands)	31,601	30,709
Average daily census (in thousands)	776	734
Occupancy percentage	64.9	75.4
Average length of stay (days)	7.2	7.9
Outpatient visits (in thousands)	245,524	182,668
Full-time equivalent personnel (in thousands)	3,114	2,051
Expenses (in millions of $):		
Labor	80,992	15,930
Nonlabor	71,593	9,532
Total expenses	152,585	25,462
Total expenses (dollars):		
Per inpatient stay	3,850.16	749.47
Per inpatient day	538.96	94.87

Figure 1-2 Selected Information, Community Hospitals in the United States

substantially because of unionization, the application of minimum wage laws to hospitals, and an increasing competition for the available labor force. In addition, the last several decades have produced technological changes requiring the use of extremely sophisticated and expensive equipment operated by skilled and highly paid technicians.

One of the most important environmental influences on hospital operations is, of course, the third-party reimbursement system. Whereas most commercial businesses are paid directly by their customers for services and products sold to them, hospitals receive payment for a large majority of their services through reimbursement from third-party payers, including governmental agencies, Blue Cross plans, and commercial insurers. For many years, most reimbursements were made on a retrospective actual cost basis or on the basis of the rates hospitals charged for their services. In the 1980s, however, most cost-based and charge-based payment mechanisms were discarded in favor of prospective payment systems (PPS) based on a predetermined fixed price per case. Medicare reimbursement, for example, consists of predetermined amounts geared to diagnosis related groups (DRGs). These innovations in payment systems were designed to reduce the utilization of inpatient services and encourage greater utilization of less expensive alternative services (such as outpatient care), to promote cost efficiency in the healthcare system.

The full financial needs of many hospitals generally have not been met under either previous or existing reimbursement systems. Hospitals, facing increasing competition for patients, have found themselves in a price war. Greater attention has been given to marketing and public relations programs. The number of hospital acquisitions and mergers has increased, and many hospitals that were not cost efficient have been forced to close.

As a result, hospital managers are engaged in a desperate struggle to maintain the financial integrity of their institutions. Individual philanthropy and community fund-raising drives have declined in importance as sources of supplementary funds, and hospitals generally are now financing their long-term capital needs through bond issues and other forms of debt.

Hospital Organization

The largest category of American hospitals comprises short-term, general hospitals usually referred to as *community hospitals.* Most of them are voluntary, not-for-profit enterprises operated under corporate charters granted by the various states. Other community hospitals are governmental institutions or investor-owned businesses conducted on a for-profit basis. Although major emphasis in this book is given to nongovernmental, not-for-profit community hospitals, much of the discussion is relevant to all types of hospitals and to other healthcare entities.

Objective and Purpose of the Hospital

Regardless of the type of ownership, the essential function and primary mission of all hospitals is patient care. This is the basic objective and purpose of the hospital: the provision of quality service at reasonable costs to persons needing medical attention and hospital care. In addition, hospitals also perform vital roles in the areas of healthcare research and education.

In carrying out these tasks, hospitals employ many different types of physical, financial, and human resources. These resources, if they are to be used economically and effectively, must be segregated into manageable organizational units in which authority is centralized and responsibility is clearly assigned for each function. The duties of each employee should be carefully defined, and interrelationships among individuals and organizational units should be soundly structured so that all personnel may work together in a coordinated, cooperative effort. Only through a well-conceived plan of organization can the hospital achieve its service and financial objectives.

Organization of Hospital Management

A hospital's organizational pattern generally is expressed in a formal organization chart such as the one shown in Figure 1–3. You should understand that this chart is illustrative only; there is no single plan of organization applicable to all hospitals. Different organizational structures arise because of differences in hospital size,

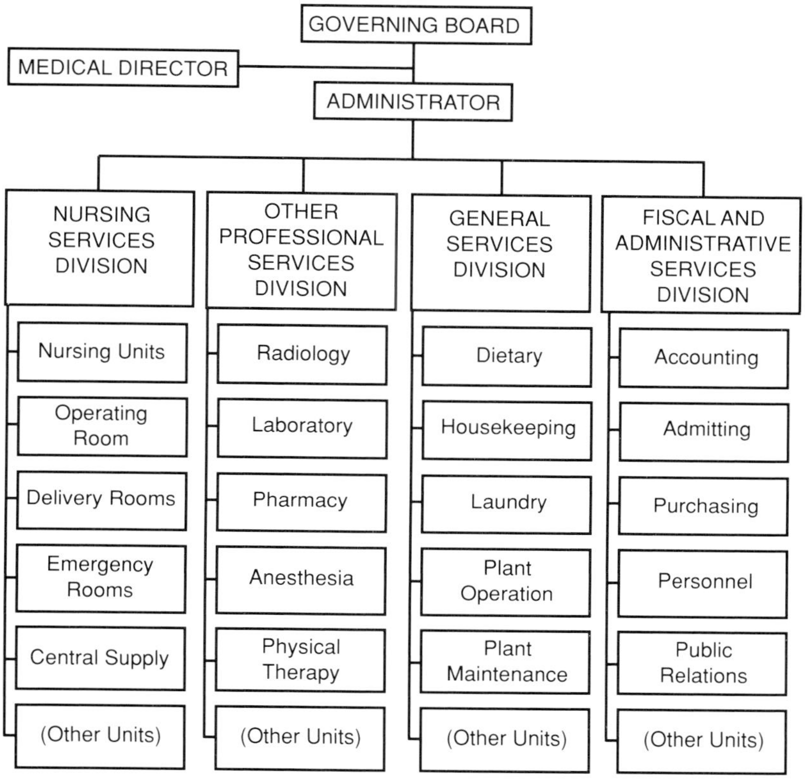

Figure 1-3 Hypothetical Hospital Organization Chart

range of services, personnel capabilities, management style, and other characteristics.

At the top of the organizational structure is the hospital's governing board, which often is called the *board of directors* or *board of trustees.* The ultimate authority and responsibility for the proper and prudent management of the hospital's affairs rests with this group. Typically, the board carries out its function through a number of standing committees, such as finance, medical affairs, and public relations. The board members, however, do not directly manage the day-to-day operations of the hospital; this authority is delegated to the hospital's chief executive officer (often having the title of *president* or *administrator*). Similarly, authority and responsibility for the medical aspects of hospital activity are assigned to a physician known as the *medical director* or *chief of staff.* The administrator and medical director, because their responsibilities are interdependent, must work always in close cooperation.

It is not possible, even in small hospitals, for the administrator to exercise continuous and direct personal supervision of all hospital activities. As indicated in Figure 1–3, hospital activities necessarily must be organized into major divisional units such as nursing services, other professional services, general services, and fiscal and administrative services. Each of the divisional units is headed by a manager or director who has authority and clearly assigned responsibility for its operations. Each division head is responsible to the administrator who, in turn, is responsible to the governing board.

The nursing services division, headed by the director of nursing, is responsible for daily patient-care activities. Employees of the division include nurses, nurses' aides, surgical technicians, ward clerks, and orderlies. The division comprises many departments, including nursing units generally organized by medical service classifications, operating rooms, delivery rooms, emergency rooms, and central supply.

The other professional services division provides ancillary services to patients. This division is subdivided into several professional departments, such as laboratory, radiology, pharmacy, EEG, EKG, and physical therapy. These departments, some of which are headed by physicians, provide essential diagnostic and therapeutic services.

The general services division is responsible for various support services necessary to patient care and to the operation of various other departments of the hospital. Departments organized within this division generally include dietary, laundry and linen, housekeeping, and plant operation and maintenance. Some hospitals have contracted with outside firms to perform certain of these support functions.

A fourth division of the hospital is that of fiscal and administrative services. This division includes such departments as admitting, accounting, purchasing, personnel, and public relations. The accounting department itself is divided into subordinate organizational units, including payroll, accounts receivable, accounts payable, budgets, and general accounting. The division is headed either by a director of fiscal services (affairs) or the hospital controller.

Need for Statistical and Financial Information

Within any enterprise, there is an imperative need for statistical and financial information. This is particularly true of hospitals because of the large number of individual, yet interdependent, organizational units whose operations must be planned, coordinated, and supervised. Effective management of the hospital requires that definite objectives be established by each organized area of responsibility. These objectives initially are expressed in statistical terms such as days of patient service, hours of nursing care, number of laboratory examinations, and pounds of laundry. These measurements of expected service volume then are translated into monetary terms, such as required dollars of expenditures and anticipated revenues. The service and financial objectives of each organizational unit are coordinated into an overall operating plan (budget) for the hospital as a whole. Such plans typically are developed for a period of one year, broken down into monthly segments. Personnel at all levels in the hospital should participate in the development of the plan.

As the year progresses, each month's actual results are compared with the budgeted objectives so that the performance of each organizational unit of the hospital can be evaluated by department heads, by divisional directors, by the hospital administrator, and by the governing board. Variances from the budgeted objectives are watched closely, and tough questions must be answered when significant deviations are noted. Where, within the hospital, do material variations exist? Why have these variances occurred? Who is responsible? What can be done about them? Answers to these questions permit intelligent decisions to be made so that off-target operating units are redirected onto the planned and proper course.

Thus, hospital managers perform their function effectively through the use of statistical and financial information, both historical and projected. This information is essential to the manager in planning the hospital's operations, in evaluating the actual performance of hospital personnel, and in taking corrective action to overcome unfavorable conditions and trends. Of course, the information must be timely, adequate, relevant, and reliable, or the manager's decisions are likely to be unsound and ill-advised.

Internal Uses of Financial Information

In addition to the internal use of statistical and financial data by management, groups external to the hospital also use much of the same information. These external groups include third-party payers, banks, suppliers, planning agencies, investors, and donors. Hard economic decisions are made by all these groups, and they have a direct impact on the ability of the hospital to pay its expenses, borrow money, obtain credit, acquire new plant and equipment, add new services, and pursue research and educational programs. You can be sure that these decisions will not favor the hospital that is unable or unwilling to supply the kinds of statistical and financial information required by these various external groups.

External Uses of Financial Information

The hospital accounting function, simply stated, is to provide useful information about the hospital's activities and affairs. This information is of a statistical and financial character; it is both historical and

The Accounting Function

projected in nature. As you have seen, this information has vitally important uses in the internal management of the hospital and equally important uses in the decisions made by parties external to the hospital. In short, accounting is an *information* system; it is the source of information absolutely essential to the management of the individual hospital and to the functioning of the hospital industry.

Hospital Accounting Defined

Hospital accounting can be defined as the accumulation, communication, and interpretation of historical and projected economic data relating to the financial position and operating results of a hospital enterprise, for purposes of decision making by its management and other interested parties. Take a moment to examine the parts of this definition.

The term *accumulation* refers to the process of recording and classifying the business transactions and financial events that occur in the economic life of the hospital. This, if you wish, is the "bookkeeping" aspect of the accounting function. It consists of several procedural operations that you will discover in subsequent chapters.

By *communication* is meant the process of reporting recorded information to those who use it. There are many types of accounting reports, and they contain different kinds of information. The content of these reports generally depends on the particular needs of users, but there is a substantial body of information that is believed to serve certain common interests of all users. So this general-purpose information is routinely reported in financial statements such as balance sheets and income statements. There are other basic, required reports, but you will not need to concern yourself with them at this time.

The word *interpretation* refers to the effort made by accountants to analyze and evaluate reported information so that it may be better understood and more easily used by decision makers. It is not enough for the accountant merely to record and report; the accountant's responsibility extends to the function of assisting users in the interpretation of reported data. This is necessary if users are to comprehend fully the significance of the information and use it in an intelligent manner. More will be said about this matter at various points later in this book.

Much of the information recorded and reported through the accounting process, of course, is historical in nature. Historical economic data can serve many purposes, including substantiation of revenues and expenses for reimbursement and payroll tax reports. At least an equal share of the accountant's time, however, is spent developing annual budgets, long-range plans, and other projections of data into the future. Financial forecasting is a significant part of the accounting task.

The information generated by the accounting process is of two basic types. *Balance sheets* report financial position information; *income statements* report information relating to operating results. The financial position of a hospital at a particular point in time is measured in terms of the hospital's resources (assets), obligations (liabilities), and equity. The operating results of a hospital for a given period of time are measured in terms of revenues earned and expenses incurred during that period. These terms—*assets, liabilities, equity, revenues,* and *expenses*—are defined and described fully later in this chapter.

Finally, the definition of *accounting* indicates that the financial statements developed in the accounting process are intended to be useful for decision-making purposes. If accounting information were not useful, there would be no need for accounting and no demand for accountants.

Types of Information
Produced by Accounting

As you have learned, hospital accounting is a service activity whose primary function is the provision of useful quantitative information about the financial position and operating results of the hospital enterprise. Financial statements are the product of the accounting process. They are the means by which the information developed by the accounting process is communicated to hospital managements, creditors, third-party payers, and others who use the information as a basis for economic decision making. Your understanding of the accounting process will be considerably enhanced by briefly examining two of the basic financial statements before you deal with the procedures through which financial information is accumulated by accountants.

The several types of financial statements usually prepared by accountants are illustrated and described at appropriate points in this book. For the present, however, you should be concerned only with two: the balance sheet and the income statement. These statements are presented in Figures 1–4 and 1–5 for a hypothetical facility, Happy Valley Hospital. Certain simplifications and condensations of the data have been made to facilitate an introductory discussion of the essential elements and features involved. More detailed and real-world illustrations appear in subsequent chapters.

To be useful, accounting information must be not only relevant but accurate and reliable. The accuracy and reliability of the monetary and statistical data provided in accounting reports is

Financial Statements

Illustrative Balance Sheet
and Income Statement

dependent on an effective system of internal control. This system was defined well many years ago, and the definition remains valid and useful: *Internal control* comprises the plan of organization and all of the coordinated methods and measures adopted within a business to safeguard its assets, check the accuracy and reliability of its accounting data, promote operational efficiency, and encourage adherence to prescribed managerial policies.[1]

Such a system greatly reduces the possibility of serious errors in the accumulation and communication processes of accounting, thereby giving the hospital manager more confidence in accounting information and in decisions based on such information. The hospital accountant is responsible for the development and operation of the internal control system as an integral part of the accounting process. Specific internal control methods and procedures are discussed at various points throughout this book.

The Balance Sheet

A *balance sheet* is a presentation of the financial position of a hospital at a particular point in time. It also may be referred to as a *statement of financial condition* (or *position*). Financial position is measured in terms of resources (assets) owned and obligations (liabilities) owed by the hospital at a given date. The difference between these resources and obligations is the hospital's net assets, variously called *equity, capital,* or *net worth.* Thus, in the simplest terms, a balance sheet indicates how "well off" a hospital is on a particular date by listing the things of value the hospital owns in relation to its debts to suppliers, employees, and other creditors. The excess of things owned over things owed is the hospital's equity on that date.

The Accounting Equation

The balance sheet, a sample of which is shown in Figure 1–4, gets its name from the fact that it depicts a balance (an equality) between total assets, on one side, and the total of liabilities and equity, on the other side. This equality is known as the accounting equation:

$$\text{Assets} = \text{Liabilities} + \text{Equity}$$
or
$$\text{Assets} - \text{Liabilities} = \text{Equity}$$

To put it in personal terms, say that today you have $25,000 of assets (cash and other property) and $10,000 of liabilities (unpaid bills and other debts). By subtracting your liabilities from your assets, you determine that your equity (net worth) is $15,000. You

[1]Committee on Auditing Procedure, *Internal Control* (New York: American Institute of Certified Public Accountants, 1949), p. 6.

ASSETS			LIABILITIES AND EQUITY	
Cash		$ 540	Accounts payable	$ 300
Accounts receivable		2,500	Notes payable	275
Inventory		200	Accrued expenses payable	795
Prepaid expenses		60	Deferred income	30
Total current assets		3,300	Total current liabilities	1,400
Long-term investments		400	Long-term liabilities	3,200
Land, buildings, and equipment	$7,200		Total liabilities	4,600
Less accumulated depreciation	2,100	5,100	Hospital equity	4,200
Total assets		$8,800	Total liabilities and equity	$8,800

Figure 1–4 Happy Valley Hospital Balance Sheet, December 31, 19X1

could, of course, prepare a personal balance sheet for yourself, listing $25,000 of assets on the left and reporting $25,000 of liabilities and equity on the right side. This relationship of total assets to total liabilities and equity is fundamental to the debit-and-credit methodology employed in accounting operations, as you shall see in the next chapter.

The dollar amounts included in Figure 1–4 are not intended to be realistic. Obviously, no hospital is as small as the balance sheet in Figure 1–4 suggests. The magnitude of the dollar amounts is purposely minimized for clarity and ease of exposition. It is easier to read, discuss, and otherwise work with small numbers than with large numbers, and this practice will be followed throughout this book. If you wish, assume that the numbers in Figure 1–4 are stated in thousands (or millions) of dollars.

Statement Heading. Figure 1–4 presents the balance sheet of Happy Valley Hospital at December 31, 19X1. Notice that the heading of the statement consists of (1) the name of the accounting entity, (2) the name of the statement, and (3) the date of the statement. These three elements should always be included in the heading of the balance sheet.

Elements of Balance Sheets

The accounting entity in this case is Happy Valley Hospital. This is one of the most important and basic accounting concepts. Under this concept, the hospital itself is personified as an entity (being) separate and distinct from its governing board, management, and employees. The hospital is regarded as a "person" capable of owning property, incurring debts, buying and selling, rendering services, and taking other economic actions. Thus, you can say that "the hospital purchased equipment," that "the hospital borrowed $100,000 from the local bank," or that "the hospital paid $160,000 of salaries and wages to its employees last month." The accountant thinks of the hospital as an entity for whose economic activity a financial record must be kept. The object of the accountant's attention and effort is the hospital itself, not the personal affairs of board members, managers, and employees. Activity recorded in the hospital accounting records is limited to the financial affairs and business transactions of the hospital itself as an economic unit or entity in its own right.

As noted earlier, the name of this financial statement is *balance sheet,* but you should be aware of alternate titles such as *statement of financial position.* The name most widely used, however, is *balance sheet,* and this term will be used throughout this book.

The date of the Happy Valley Hospital balance sheet is December 31, 19X1, a specific point in time. A balance sheet is analogous to a snapshot that portrays a situation existing at a given moment. It is a "picture" of the financial position of Happy Valley Hospital on December 31, 19X1, only. The picture likely was somewhat different on December 30 and probably will be different again on January 1, 19X2. This is true because business transactions occur every day, and consequently the dollar amounts of assets and liabilities also change daily.

Generally Accepted Accounting Principles (GAAP)

The particular assets and liabilities to be included in balance sheets, and the dollar amounts at which they are stated, are determined by the application of a body of rules, conventions, concepts, and standards known as *generally accepted accounting principles (GAAP).* Special attention is given to this very important matter in the author's *Hospital Financial Accounting—Theory and Practice.*[2] For the present purpose, it is enough that you understand that there is an authoritative body of GAAP that accountants must observe in reporting financial information.

The primary source of GAAP is an independent organization called the Financial Accounting Standards Board (FASB). Since its formation in 1973, the board has issued more than 100 pronouncements referred to as *Statements of Financial Accounting Standards (SFAS),* several *Statements of Financial Accounting Concepts,* numerous *Interpretations,* and many other documents. Various other groups also have made significant contributions to the development of GAAP. The Accounting Standards Executive Committee (AcSEC) of the American Institute of Certified Public Accountants (AICPA),

---

[2]L. Vann Seawell, *Hospital Financial Accounting—Theory and Practice,* Second Edition (Chicago: Healthcare Financial Management Association, 1987).

for example, has issued a large number of *Statements of Position.* The AICPA Committee on Health Care regularly revises and publishes the *Hospital Audit Guide,* which includes GAAP as well as auditing standards. The work of the Healthcare Financial Management Association (HFMA) through its Principles and Practices Board (P&PB) also should be noted. To date, the P&PB has issued more than 10 *Statements* relating to financial accounting and reporting practices of hospitals and other healthcare entities.

Assets.   *Assets* may be defined as the economic resources of the hospital that are recognized and measured in conformity with GAAP. As indicated in Figure 1–4, the assets of Happy Valley Hospital total $8,800 at December 31, 19X1. Following is a brief explanation of each of the assets included in that balance sheet:

1. *Cash* is the amount of money on hand and in bank checking accounts maintained by the hospital.   Types of Assets
2. *Accounts receivable* represent the amount of money due the hospital from patients and their third-party sponsors for services provided to them but for which the hospital has not yet been paid.
3. *Inventory* is the cost of foodstuffs, fuel, drugs, and other supplies purchased by the hospital but not yet used or consumed.
4. *Prepaid expenses* include expense items such as insurance, interest, and rent that have been paid in advance. These items are assets in the sense that their prepayment will provide future benefits (insurance protection, use of borrowed money, and use of space or leased equipment) to the hospital.
5. *Long-term investments* represent the cost of governmental and corporate securities that the hospital owns and intends to hold for a period of time in excess of one year.
6. *Land, buildings, and equipment* consist of the original acquisition costs of tangible plant assets used in hospital operations.
7. *Accumulated depreciation* reflects the amount of plant asset costs consumed by the use of the assets and treated as operating expense of the hospital during the time that has elapsed since the assets were acquired. Notice that accumulated depreciation is deducted from the cost of the plant assets and that only the remaining "undepreciated" balance of cost is included in the total assets reported in the balance sheet.

Items 1 through 4 are totaled and presented in the balance sheet as total current assets. For the present, think of *current assets* as consisting of cash plus other assets that will be converted into cash or consumed by operations within one year from the balance sheet date. All other assets (items 5 through 7) are referred to as noncurrent (long-term) assets.

You have noticed that most assets are reported in the balance sheet at historical acquisition costs rather than current market values. Valuation of assets at cost is a basic accounting principle. This basis of valuation generally is employed in accounting because it is a permanent and objective measurement and because accountants assume that the monetary unit is reasonably stable; that is, that the purchasing power of money does not change materially over time. This assumption, because of earlier inflationary trends, naturally has been challenged by various groups who argue that assets should be presented in balance sheets at either current fair values or estimated replacement costs. Others have advocated the adjustment of historical costs (using the consumer price index) to reflect changes in the purchasing power of the dollar. In extended periods of sustained high rates of inflation, these proposals have considerable merit. This is, however, a topic beyond the scope of this book.

Sequencing of Assets

Another point worth noting at this time concerns the sequence in which the assets are listed on the balance sheet. Observe that the sequence is generally in the order of liquidity. The most-liquid asset (cash) is listed first; the least-liquid assets (land, buildings, and equipment) are last in sequence. This is standard practice in financial reporting.

Finally, you should understand that certain economic resources of the hospital are not included as assets in the balance sheet. A hospital may enjoy good public relations and high employee morale, but although these things may be regarded as resources of great value, they are not formally recognized as assets in hospital accounting. These items are excluded from reported assets because of the great difficulty involved in making an objective measurement of them in monetary terms. This problem is being studied, and perhaps someday a satisfactory solution will be forthcoming.

Liabilities. *Liabilities* may be defined as the economic obligations of the hospital that are recognized and measured in conformity with GAAP. Following is a brief description of the liabilities presented in the Happy Valley Hospital balance sheet:

Types of Liabilities

1. *Accounts payable* are amounts owed by the hospital to suppliers and other trade creditors for merchandise and services purchased from them but for which the hospital has not yet paid.
2. *Notes payable* generally consist of short-term borrowings by the hospital from banks and other financial institutions. These debts

usually are in the form of promissory notes issued by the hospital to the lender.

3. *Accrued expenses payable* are liabilities for expenses (employee salaries and wages, for example) that have been incurred by the hospital but for which the hospital has not yet paid.

4. *Deferred income* represents income (nursing school tuition, for example) that has been received in cash by the hospital but that the hospital has not yet earned and for which it is obligated to provide some specific service in the future.

5. *Long-term liabilities* typically are mortgage loans or hospital bond issues that will not be retired by the hospital in the near future (usually well beyond one year from the date of the balance sheet).

As you can see in Figure 1–4, items 1 through 4 are totaled and reported as total current liabilities; that is, obligations that will be paid by the use of current assets within one year from the balance sheet date. The other liabilities of the hospital therefore are referred to as *noncurrent* or *long-term liabilities*. Liabilities, generally speaking, are measured in terms of the dollar amounts that will be required to discharge them. Long-term liabilities, however, generally are reported in the balance sheet at the present value of the future payments required for their liquidation; but again, a discussion of this matter is postponed until later in the book.

As was true of assets, recognition problems also exist for liabilities. When is an obligation a liability in the accounting sense? As you pursue your study of this book, you will discover items you may consider liabilities that are not so treated in accounting. Similarly, you may encounter accounting liabilities you have not previously regarded as such. This is but another example of the patience you must have in beginning your study of hospital accounting. Full explanations cannot be given of all matters in the first chapter; your complete comprehension of the various concepts and procedures mentioned in this chapter will eventually be achieved, but only through a gradual building-block process.

Liabilities are presented in the balance sheet more or less in the order in which they will be paid. The proper sequence, however, is not always easy to determine, and compromises often must be made. It is essential, however, that balance sheets report total current liabilities and total liabilities (current and noncurrent) as indicated in Figure 1–4. Users of the balance sheets of hospitals are entitled to this information.

Sequencing of Liabilities

Equity.   Hospital *equity* may be defined simply as the excess of hospital assets over hospital liabilities. It is the hospital's residual ownership interest in its own assets after the claims of creditors against these assets are satisfied. Hospital equity is increased by net income (excess of revenues over expenses); it is decreased by net loss (excess of expenses over revenues).

Later on in this book, the subject of *fund accounting* is introduced. Fund accounting is employed by many hospitals and consists basically of a segregation of assets, liabilities, and equity into self-balancing groups of "funds." When this accounting procedure is used, a separate balance sheet can be prepared for each fund; or a single balance sheet may be prepared in which assets, liabilities, and equity are classified and reported according to the particular fund with which they are associated. In a fund accounting system, the equity account of each "fund" generally is referred to as the "fund balance."

Income Statements

An *income statement* is a presentation of the operating results of a hospital for a specified period of time. It also may be referred to as the *statement of revenues and expenses,* the *profit-and-loss statement,* or simply the *operating statement.* In any event, this statement reports the revenues earned and the expenses incurred by the hospital during a given period of time, such as a month, a quarter, or one year. The difference between the revenues and expenses of the period is reported as net income (or net loss, if total expenses exceed total revenues).

Elements of Income Statements

Statement Heading.   Figure 1–5 presents the income statement of Happy Valley Hospital for the year ended December 31, 19X2 (the year following the hospital's balance sheet illustrated in Figure 1–4). The heading of the statement includes (1) the name of the accounting entity, (2) the name of the statement, and (3) the period of time encompassed by the statement. These elements should always appear in the heading of income statements.

The accounting entity is identified here, as in the balance sheet previously discussed, as Happy Valley Hospital. It is the economic unit or organization whose activities are reported in the financial statement. A careful identification of the entity is required to clearly distinguish it from other entities such as the Happy Valley college, church, nursing home, or manufacturing company. As stated before under the entity concept, the hospital is personified as an economic being separate and distinct from its governing board, management, and employees.

Gross patient service revenues:		
Daily patient services	$ 6,000	
Other professional services	4,000	
Total	10,000	
Less deductions from patient service revenues	1,000	
Net patient service revenues		$9,000
Other operating revenues		500
Total operating revenues		9,500
Less operating expenses:		
Nursing services	3,400	
Other professional services	2,700	
General services	1,800	
Fiscal and administrative services	1,400	
Total operating expenses		9,300
Operating income		200
Add nonoperating revenues (net)		130
Net income for the year		$ 330

Figure 1–5 Happy Valley Hospital Income Statement, Year Ended December 31, 19X2

The heading also includes the name of the statement—income statement. This indicates the nature and function of the statement.

Observe that the illustrative income statement is dated "year ended December 31, 19X2." This specifies the accounting period to which the income statement elements are related (that is, the 12 calendar months of 19X2). It is improper and misleading to date the statement "December 31, 19X2," as this would imply that the information relates to a single day or, at least, to an indeterminate period of time ending on that date. The income statement often is prepared for a period of one month or one quarter as well as annually, and it is essential that the particular time period covered be clearly disclosed in the statement heading. Balance sheets also are prepared on a monthly or quarterly basis as well as annually. When financial statements are issued during the course of a year, they are referred to as *interim statements*. For the present, however, you will be concerned only with annual financial statements.

Most hospitals and other healthcare entities employ a fiscal year ending June 30 or September 30 rather than a calendar-year accounting or reporting period ending December 31. For ease of exposition, however, a fiscal year ending December 31 is assumed throughout this text.

The previously discussed balance sheet presented the assets, liabilities, and equity of Happy Valley Hospital at December 31,

19X1. These resources and obligations, of course, became the opening balances for the 19X2 year. For example, the closing cash balance on December 31, 19X1, becomes the opening cash balance on January 1, 19X2. As the 19X2 year unfolds day by day, Happy Valley Hospital will complete thousands of individual business transactions. Services will be provided to patients, supplies will be purchased and used, employees will be paid salaries and wages, cash receipts will arise from billings to patients and third parties, and various other operating activities will take place.

At the end of 19X2, another balance sheet can be prepared, as shown in Figure 1–6. This statement presents the financial position of the hospital at December 31, 19X2. (A vertical, or report, format is used here simply to illustrate an alternative form of presentation; Figure 1–4 presented a balance sheet in a horizontal format.) The December 31, 19X2, balance sheet does not reveal the details of the operating results for 19X2. A 19X2 income statement therefore is needed to disclose exactly what happened during the 12–month interval between December 31, 19X1, and December 31, 19X2. In this way, income statements serve as connecting links between successive balance sheets.

Revenues. Hospital *revenues* consist primarily of economic values earned by the hospital through the provision of services, and sales of products, to patients. Revenues also include receipts of unrestricted gifts and certain other donor contributions. Revenues typically are evidenced by an increase in hospital assets, either cash or receivables in most instances.

The revenues of a hospital are determined by the application of GAAP. In conformity with these principles, some increases in assets are recognized as revenues; other asset increases are not revenues. Cash received from an outpatient for a laboratory examination, for example, is revenue. A billing made to an inpatient for a day's room and board is recorded as an increase in accounts receivable and is recognized as revenue. In each case, the revenue is recorded when it is earned (that is, at the time the related service is rendered and the hospital has either received cash or has a claim against the patient for the value of the service provided). On the other hand, the receipt of cash arising from the borrowing of money from a bank is not revenue.

Reporting Revenues on the Income Statement

Hospital revenues arising from patient-care services generally are recorded at the value of those services as evidenced by the hospital's full, established rates (prices) for those services. This is true whether the hospital actually collects its full charges, contracts to accept less than full charges from third-party payers, or collects

Assets		
Cash		$ 575
Accounts receivable		2,600
Inventory		420
Prepaid expenses		80
Total current assets		3,675
Long-term investments		380
Land, buildings, and equipment	$7,500	
Less accumulated depreciation	2,210	5,290
Total assets		$9,345
Liabilities and Equity		
Accounts payable		$ 360
Notes payable		200
Accrued expenses payable		831
Deferred income		24
Total current liabilities		1,415
Long-term liabilities		3,400
Total liabilities		4,815
Hospital equity		4,530
Total liabilities and equity		$9,345

Figure 1–6 Happy Valley Hospital Balance Sheet, December 31, 19X2

nothing for the services provided. Most third-party payers, for example, pay less than established rates because their economic power permits them to negotiate lower rates. Hospitals also provide a considerable amount of service to indigent patients at nominal rates or on a free (charity) basis. Also, certain patients who are financially able to meet their obligations simply fail to pay the hospital for services they have received, and bad debts are recorded by the hospital.

Nevertheless, all patient-care services rendered by the hospital are usually recorded as revenues measured in terms of full, established rates. Figure 1–5, for example, reports $10,000 of gross patient service revenues, of which $1,000 is estimated to be uncollectible for the reasons just indicated. This produces $9,000 of net patient service revenues or, if you prefer, "collectible" patient service revenues. You should understand, however, that much of this $9,000 has not yet been collected: the balance sheet at December 31, 19X2, reports $2,600 of accounts receivable!

There are two other categories of revenues in the illustrative income statement. "Other operating revenues" include cafeteria sales, television and parking lot fees, rentals received, tuition from educational programs, research grants, and similar items. "Non-operating revenues" consist mainly of unrestricted contributions from donors and income from investments, net of nonoperating expenses and losses.

Supplementary Schedules for Summary Income Statements

The income statement in Figure 1–5 presents the revenues of the hospital in condensed form. In actual practice, of course, much more detail would be required. Necessary details often are provided in supplementary schedules to accompany the summary income statement. The schedules supply detailed information about the revenues earned by each organizational unit (revenues of each nursing unit, laboratory revenues, pharmacy revenues, and so on). In addition, patient service revenues may be classified in various inpatient and outpatient categories. Detailed classifications of revenue deductions, other operating revenues, and nonoperating revenues also are provided in these supplementary schedules.

Reporting Expenses in the Income Statement

Expenses. Hospital *expenses* may be defined roughly as the costs of services, supplies, and other items purchased and consumed by the hospital in the provision of patient-care services during a given period of time. In accordance with GAAP, expenses are measured and recognized in the period in which they are incurred or consumed in the production of hospital revenues. This may or may not be the same time period in which they are paid. When supply items are purchased for cash, for example, their costs are considered to be assets (inventory). Only when supply items are used or consumed in hospital activities are their costs recognized and reported as expenses by the hospital. Like most assets, expenses generally are measured in terms of historical costs.

The operating expenses in Figure 1–5 are reported in a functional classification; that is, they appear according to the divisional organizational units of the hospital. In actual practice, these divisional expense totals usually are supported by supplementary schedules in which details, classified by individual department and type of expense, are provided. General services expenses of $1,800, for example, could be reported by department (dietary, housekeeping, plant operation, and so on) and by type of expense (salaries and wages, supplies, purchased services, and so on). Illustrations of such schedules appear at a later point in this book.

Rather than reporting expenses in a functional classification as shown in Figure 1–5, Happy Valley Hospital might report its expenses in an object-of-expenditure, or natural, classification in the manner indicated in the following:

Operating expenses:	
Salaries and wages	$5,080
Supplies	1,753
Purchased services	1,520
Depreciation	310
Interest	206
Other	431
Total operating expenses	$9,300

This natural classification of expense typically appears in the published financial statements of hospitals. In internal management reports, hospital expenses are classified primarily on a functional basis so as to associate the expenses with organizational units and individuals who are responsible for them. This procedure, known as *responsibility reporting,* is especially useful for managerial control purposes.

The 19X2 net income of Happy Valley Hospital is $330, as indicated in Figure 1–5. As noted earlier, a net income (profit) increases the equity of the hospital. So, by adding the 19X2 net income to the equity balance at December 31, 19X1, we obtain the hospital equity figure appearing in the balance sheet at December 31, 19X2:

Effect of Net Income on Equity Balance

Hospital equity, December 31, 19X1	
(Figure 1-4)	$4,200
Add net income for 19X2 (Figure 1-5)	330
Hospital equity, December 31, 19X2	
(Figure 1-6)	$4,530

Had there been an operating loss in 19X2, the loss would be deducted in this computation. Recognize, however, that this is a simplification, in that factors other than net income (or net loss) may at times affect the hospital equity balance. This point is discussed further at a later point in this book.

Recording an Operating Loss

You should now have a general understanding of two of the principal financial statements composing the end product of accounting. With this behind you, you can move on to a study of the accounting operations that produce the financial information contained in these statements.

Questions   Q1–1. What is the basic objective and purpose of the hospital enterprise?

Q1–2. Draw up a simple organization chart for a hypothetical hospital to indicate your understanding of the basic organizational structure generally found in hospitals.

Q1–3. State briefly the function of a hospital's (a) governing board, (b) medical director, and (c) administrator.

Q1–4. Why is there a need for information about a hospital's financial position and operating results?

Q1–5. Describe briefly some of the major characteristics of the economic environment in which today's hospitals are operated.

Q1–6. What is the primary function of hospital accounting?

Q1–7. State briefly the purpose of a balance sheet.

Q1–8. Define *assets*. List five examples of assets that appear in hospital balance sheets.

Q1–9. Distinguish between current and noncurrent assets. Give an example of each.

Q1–10. Define liabilities. List five examples of liabilities that appear in hospital balance sheets.

Q1–11. Distinguish between current and noncurrent liabilities. Give an example of each.

Q1–12. State the accounting equation in two alternative forms.

Q1–13. What is meant by GAAP? What are the sources of GAAP?

Q1–14. What information should be provided in the heading of a balance sheet?

Q1–15. State briefly the purpose of an income statement.

Q1–16. Define revenues. List four examples of revenues that appear in hospital income statements.

Q1–17. Define expenses. List four examples of expenses that appear in hospital income statements.

Q1–18. Distinguish between (a) a functional classification of expenses and (b) a natural classification of expenses.

Q1–19. What information should be provided in the heading of an income statement?

Q1–20. "In a hospital balance sheet, assets are reported at their fair market values." Do you agree? Explain.

Q1–21. "In a hospital income statement, revenues represent cash receipts, and expenses represent cash disbursements of the period." Do you agree? Explain.

Q1–22. What are interim financial statements?

Q1–23. In hospital accounting, when should revenues and expenses be recognized and recorded?

Q1–24. What is the accounting entity concept?

Q1–25. What are two of the major objectives of an effective system of internal control in hospitals?

Exercises

E1–1. Given the following:

	Assets	Liabilities	Equity
(a)	$90,000	$60,000	$?30,000
(b)	80,000	50,000	30,000
(c)	85,000	35,000	50,000

Required: What are the missing dollar amounts?

E1–2. Given the following:

Prepaid expenses	$ 150
Long-term investments	600
Cash	260
Deferred income	110
Inventory	320
Plant assets, at cost	8,400
Accounts receivable	2,900
Accumulated depreciation	3,300

Required: What is the total amount of current assets? 3630

E1–3. Given the following:

Current liabilities	$1,500
Current assets	3,400
Plant assets, net of accumulated depreciation	5,200
Hospital equity	4,300
Long-term investments	400

Required: What is the amount of long-term (noncurrent) liabilities?

E1–4. Given the following:

Total operating expenses	$ 9,500
Gross patient service revenues	10,300
Nonoperating revenues (net)	140
Deductions from patient service revenues	1,100
Other operating revenues	600

Required: What is the net income for the year?

E1–5. Dippel Hospital's December 31, 19X2, balance sheet reported hospital equity of $8,645. Dippel's 19X2 net income was $714.

Required: What was reported as hospital equity in Dippel's balance sheet at December 31, 19X1?

Problems

P1–1. Keener Hospital provides you with the following information that relates to its financial position at September 30, 19X1:

Accrued expenses payable	$ 760
Inventory	480
Accumulated depreciation	2,800
Accounts payable	420
Prepaid expenses	90
Cash	600
Deferred income	15
Land, buildings, and equipment	8,800
Accounts receivable	2,450
Notes payable	150
Long-term investments	400
Bonds payable (due 19X9)	3,500

Required: Prepare in good form a September 30, 19X1, balance sheet for Keener Hospital.

P1–2. Alice Hospital provides you with the following information that relates to its operating results for the year ended December 31, 19X1:

Nursing service expenses	$3,900
Deductions from patient service revenues	1,200
Other professional service revenues	4,800
General service expenses	1,700
Nonoperating revenues	140
Fiscal and administrative service expenses	1,200
Daily patient service revenues	6,320

Other professional service expenses	$2,610
Other operating revenues	450

Required: Prepare in good form an income statement for Alice Hospital for the year ended December 31, 19X1.

P1–3. McCart Hospital provides you with the following information that relates to its financial position at August 31, 19X2, and its operating results for the year then ended:

Accounts payable	$ 430
Nonoperating revenues	190
Accounts receivable	2,950
Deferred income	60
Long-term investments	590
Nursing service expenses	4,300
Bonds payable (due 19X9)	4,100
Daily patient service revenues	6,830
Fiscal and administrative service expenses	1,600
Cash	340
Notes payable	180
Land, buildings, and equipment	8,600
Deductions from patient service revenues	970
Prepaid expenses	70
Other professional service expenses	2,900
Other professional service revenues	4,560
Accrued expenses payable	820
Accumulated depreciation	3,200
Inventory	240
Hospital equity, August 31, 19X1	3,660
Other operating revenues	630
General service expenses	2,100

Required: Prepare in good form (1) an income statement for McCart Hospital for the year ended August 31, 19X2, and (2) a balance sheet for McCart Hospital at August 31, 19X2.

P1–4. Clarke Hospital provides you with the following information that relates to its financial position at October 31, 19X1, and its operating results for the month then ended:

Bonds payable (due 19X6)	$2,500
Salaries and wages expense	5,260
Prepaid expenses	40
Hospital equity, September 30, 19X1	2,330
Daily patient service revenues	4,630
Interest expense	120

Nonoperating revenues	$ 110
Cash	170
Deferred income	20
Deductions from patient service revenues	420
Accounts payable	170
Land	250
Utilities expense	980
Other operating revenues	380
Notes payable	200
Accounts receivable	1,930
Accumulated depreciation	1,580
Accrued expenses payable	490
Other professional service revenues	3,470
Supplies expense	1,210
Building and equipment	5,000
Inventory	190
Depreciation expense	240
Other operating expenses	70

Required: Prepare in good form for Clarke Hospital (1) an income statement for the month ended October 31, 19X1, and (2) a balance sheet at October 31, 19X1.

Analysis of Business Transactions

2

The economic life of a hospital consists of a continuous stream of business transactions. At frequent intervals, for example, a hospital purchases medical and surgical supplies for its inventory. An invoice is received in due course from the supplier, and a check is written in payment of the billing. As required, the supplies are issued from inventory for use in the provision of patient-care services. Certain supplies may not be itemized on the patient's bill separately; other supplies are directly chargeable. Eventually, patients' accounts will be collected, and the cash receipts are deposited in the hospital's bank accounts. The cycle then begins anew.

Transactions of many different types occur daily in large numbers. Over a period of a few months, a hospital may complete thousands of individual transactions. Certainly, there must be a system by which this mass of activity can be efficiently processed and recorded so that the desired information about the hospital's business transactions can be produced on a timely and accurate basis. That system, of course, is the transaction segment of the hospital's accounting system. This chapter and several of the chapters immediately following describe the basic elements and operations found in all accounting systems.

In addition to making certain simplifying assumptions, we also will assume that the accounting records involved are manually maintained in handwritten or typewritten form. It is true, of course, that virtually all hospitals today necessarily employ various types of accounting equipment ranging from a simple bookkeeping machine to sophisticated data processing devices. Nevertheless, an exposition of the accounting process is greatly facilitated, and the procedural operations are more easily learned and clearly understood, when a manual system is assumed. You also should be aware that accounting principles are not altered by the employment of

Learning Accounting Techniques with Manual Systems

29

accounting equipment or computers; the principles are the same for manual systems as for mechanized and electronic systems. You can better comprehend what various types of accounting equipment and computers do if you learn first how manual records are maintained. How to program and operate such mechanized and electronic equipment, however, is beyond the scope of this book.

Documentary Evidence of Transactions

In creating records of business transactions, accountants must first be made aware that transactions have occurred. A system must be devised to document all business transactions as they occur, or at the earliest practicable point after their occurrence. It is of critical importance that no transaction be overlooked and go unrecorded. A failure to recognize and record all transactions results in lost revenues and incomplete financial information.

Documentary evidences of transactions include purchase requisitions, purchase orders, receiving reports, invoices, checks written and checks received, patient service requisitions, charge tickets, cash register tapes, cash receipt slips, deeds and contracts, bank deposit slips, correspondence with patients and creditors, intrahospital memoranda, and many other forms and business papers. This is the "red tape" for which accountants often are blamed. Although these documents are vital to the accounting process, they often have primary purposes and supplemental uses that are not directly related to accounting.

The documentation should provide all essential facts involved in the transaction. Accountants are particularly interested in authorizations; dates; accurate identification of the services, supplies, and other items involved; quantities; and dollar amounts. Without this information, the integrity of the accounting records is subject to question.

Thus, accountants require verifiable and objective evidence of the occurrence of bona fide transactions and of all essential facts involved. Not everything recorded in the accounting records, however, can be documented, or documented to the same degree. A certain amount of the information recorded and reported by accountants consists of approximations and estimates based on professional judgment and experienced opinion. This is one aspect of accounting that makes it interesting and challenging.

The Accounting Equation

The accounting equation, or model, was introduced briefly in Chapter 1. This equation, you may remember, was expressed as follows:

$$\text{Assets} = \text{Liabilities} + \text{Equity}$$

The left side of the equation represents assets, the things of value owned by the hospital (cash, receivables, inventory, plant assets, and so on). The right side of the equation consists of liabilities and equity, or claims against the assets of the hospital. These claims consist of the amount of assets owed to creditors (accounts payable, wages payable to employees, loans payable to banks, and other economic obligations) and the residual ownership interest in assets accruing to the hospital itself (equity). The equation must always balance; it expresses an equality that exists throughout the accounting process.

When a business transaction occurs, the accountant must analyze the transaction in terms of its effect on the accounting equation. A determination is made of the increase and/or decrease effects of each transaction on each element of the equation. Each transaction is analyzed to determine the amounts by which it increased and/or decreased assets, liabilities, or equity. The amounts are measured in terms of dollars. Documentary evidence provides the information needed to make this analysis.

Let us assume, as a starting point, that a hospital has $5,000 of assets, $2,000 of liabilities, and $3,000 of equity. The equation is as follows:

The Initial Accounting Equation

$$\text{Assets} = \text{Liabilities} + \text{Equity}$$
$$\$5,000 = \quad \$2,000 \quad + \$3,000$$

Now assume that the hospital borrows $600 from a bank. What effects does this transaction have on the accounting equation? Which of the elements of the equation were increased or decreased? The following shows the answer:

Effect of Borrowing on the Accounting Equation

Assets	=	Liabilities	+	Equity	
$5,000	=	$2,000	+	$3,000	(previous balances)
+600		+600			(effect of transaction)
$5,600	=	$2,600	+	$3,000	(resulting balances)

As a result of the bank loan, the hospital has $600 more assets (cash received from the bank) and $600 more liabilities (the debt owed to the bank that must be paid in the future). The receipt of a cash loan has no effect on the hospital's equity, nor is the cash receipt regarded as revenue.

Assume that the hospital repays $100 (disregarding interest) of the principal amount of the bank loan. The analysis is as follows:

Effect of Repaying a Loan on the Accounting Equation

Assets	=	Liabilities	+	Equity	
$5,600	=	$2,600	+	$3,000	(previous balances)
−100		−100			(effect of transaction)
$5,500	=	$2,500	+	$3,000	(resulting balances)

The hospital disbursed $100 cash, thereby reducing its assets and its liability to the bank (from $600 to $500). Repayment of the bank loan (disregarding interest) has no effect on the hospital's equity, nor does this expenditure constitute expense.

Effect of Purchases on the Accounting Equation

Assume that the hospital purchases $300 of supplies on account (on credit). In this transaction the hospital obtains a new asset (inventory) and incurs a liability (accounts payable) to pay the supplier at an agreed future date. The analysis then becomes the following:

$$
\begin{array}{rclcl}
\text{Assets} & = & \text{Liabilities} & + & \text{Equity} \\
\$5,500 & = & \$2,500 & + & \$3,000 \ \text{(previous balances)} \\
+300 & & +300 & & \ \text{(effect of transaction)} \\
\hline
\$5,800 & = & \$2,800 & + & \$3,000 \ \text{(resulting balances)}
\end{array}
$$

This transaction has no effect on the hospital's equity; neither is it a transaction that requires the recognition of revenue or expense.

Assume that the hospital purchases a new item of equipment for $400 cash. The analysis is the following:

$$
\begin{array}{rclcl}
\text{Assets} & = & \text{Liabilities} & + & \text{Equity} \\
\$5,800 & = & \$2,800 & + & \$3,000 \ \text{(previous balances)} \\
+400 & & & & \ \text{(effect of transaction)} \\
-400 & & & & \\
\hline
\$5,800 & = & \$2,800 & + & \$3,000 \ \text{(resulting balances)}
\end{array}
$$

The effect of this transaction is to increase one asset (equipment) and decrease another asset (cash). There is no effect on liabilities or equity, nor is there any revenue or expense to recognize.

Effect of Revenue Transaction on the Accounting Equation

Now let us consider a transaction that affects the hospital's revenue and therefore its equity. Assume that the supplies previously purchased in one of the transactions above are sold to patients for $350 and charged to their accounts (no cash is yet received from them). The analysis now becomes this:

$$
\begin{array}{rclcl}
\text{Assets} & = & \text{Liabilities} & + & \text{Equity} \\
\$5,800 & = & \$2,800 & + & \$3,000 \ \text{(previous balances)} \\
+350 & & & & +350 \ \text{(effect of transaction)} \\
\hline
\$6,150 & = & \$2,800 & + & \$3,350 \ \text{(resulting balances)}
\end{array}
$$

This transaction produces an increase in the hospital's assets (patients' accounts receivable). Every business transaction, however, has at least two effects. What is the other effect? Because liabilities are unaffected by the transaction, the other effect must be an increase in the hospital's equity. The principle is this: Revenues, evidenced by increases in net assets, are recognized as increases in the hospital's equity.

But you are probably wondering about the cost of the supplies that were sold and are no longer in the hospital's inventory! Yes, in addition to the revenue, the accountant must recognize the related expense:

Assets = Liabilities + Equity
$6,150 = $2,800   + $3,350 (previous balances)
−300   −300 (effect of transaction)
$5,850 = $2,800   + $3,050 (resulting balances)

Here, assets (inventory) are decreased by the cost of the supplies removed from inventory and sold to patients. The cost of supplies sold (or used) is treated as a reduction of the hospital's equity. The principle is this: Decreases in net assets are expenses, and expenses are recognized as decreases in hospital equity.

We could have recorded the revenue transaction and the expense transaction simultaneously. The analysis would have been

Assets = Liabilities + Equity
$5,800 = $2,800   + $3,000 (previous balances)
+350   +350 (effect of transactions)
−300   −300
$5,850 = $2,800   + $3,050 (resulting balances)

A point made in Chapter 1 was that net income (profit) increases hospital equity. This is because revenues increase equity and expenses decrease equity, and net income is the excess of revenues over expenses. As you can see in the simultaneous transactions just shown, hospital equity increased by $50, the profit made on the sale of supplies ($350 − $300 = $50).

Hospitals, however, have so many revenue and expense transactions that it is not feasible to attempt to record them individually as direct additions to, and deductions from, hospital equity. Instead, we expand the accounting equation to include two additional elements: revenues and expenses. The expanded equation is

Assets = Liabilities + Equity + Revenues − Expenses

Here, equity represents the equity balance at the beginning of the period. This extension of the equation simply expresses the principle that the equity balance at the beginning of the period is increased by revenues earned and is decreased by expenses incurred during the period. It also allows revenues and expenses to be treated

Expanding the Accounting Equation for Revenues and Expenses

as separate elements of the equation rather than as direct changes in the equity balance.

The expanded equation will be easier to work with if we add expenses to each side to produce this equation:

$$\text{Assets} + \text{Expenses} = \text{Liabilities} + \text{Equity} + \text{Revenues}$$

This avoids having positive and negative elements on the right side of the equation. Here, again, equity represents the equity balance at the beginning of the period. Subsequent expressions won't mention that equity means the equity balance at the beginning of the period (year, for example), but keep this fact in mind.

Now, using the expanded equation, let us analyze a new set of transactions for a different hospital with assumed opening balances including $300,000 of assets, $100,000 of liabilities, and $200,000 of equity. The assumed transactions are as follows:

1. The hospital borrowed $25,000 from a bank.
2. The hospital purchased supplies on account for $12,000.
3. Half of the supplies were issued from inventory and used in patient care. Patients were billed for $7,500.
4. The hospital paid $14,000 of salaries and wages to its employees.
5. Patients were billed (charged) for $15,300 of other services.
6. The bank loan was paid by a disbursement of $26,000, including interest of $1,000.
7. The hospital paid $9,000 on its accounts payable.
8. The hospital collected $18,400 on patients' accounts receivable.

Figure 2–1 analyzes the effects of these transactions on the expanded equation. Observe that each transaction has at least two effects and that the equation balances (left equals right) after each of the transactions are recorded.

Obtaining the Closing Equity Balance   At the bottom of Figure 2–1, you see that a closing entry has been made to eliminate the accumulated totals of revenues and expenses from the equation and to add the excess of revenues over expenses (the net income, or profit) to the opening equity balance. This produces the closing equity balance:

Equity, beginning of period		$200,000
Revenues of the period	$22,800	
Less expenses of the period	21,000	
Net income (profit) for the period		+1,800
Equity, end of period		$201,800

	Assets	+	Expenses	=	Liabilities	+	Equity	+	Revenues
Opening balances	$300,000	+	$ -0-	=	$100,000	+	$200,000	+	$ -0-
Transaction 1	+25,000				+25,000				
Resulting balances	325,000	+	-0-	=	125,000	+	200,000	+	-0-
Transaction 2	+12,000				+12,000				
Resulting balances	337,000	+	-0-	=	137,000	+	200,000	+	-0-
Transaction 3	{ −6,000		+ 6,000						
	{ + 7,500							+	+ 7,500
Resulting balances	338,500	+	6,000	=	137,000	+	200,000	+	7,500
Transaction 4	−14,000		+14,000						
Resulting balances	324,500	+	20,000	=	137,000	+	200,000	+	7,500
Transaction 5	+15,300								+15,300
Resulting balances	339,800	+	20,000	=	137,000	+	200,000	+	22,800
Transaction 6	−26,000		+ 1,000		−25,000				
Resulting balances	313,800	+	21,000	=	112,000	+	200,000	+	22,800
Transaction 7	−9,000				−9,000				
Resulting balances	304,800	+	21,000	=	103,000	+	200,000	+	22,800
Transaction 8	{ +18,400								
	{ −18,400								
Resulting balances	304,800	+	21,000	=	103,000	+	200,000	+	22,800
Closing entry									
(profit)			−21,000				+ 1,800		−22,800
Closing balances	$304,800	+	$ -0-	=	$103,000	+	$201,800	+	$ -0-

Figure 2–1 Transaction Analysis

In actual practice, closing entries are made at the end of each annual period as a part of the procedure known as "closing the books." Extensive attention is given to this matter in Chapter 4.

After the closing entry has been made, the accounting equation consists only of the closing balances for assets, liabilities, and equity. These balances are carried forward into the next accounting period and become the opening balances of that period. A new accounting cycle then begins.

Debit-and-Credit Methodology

In analyzing and recording the effects of business transactions, accountants employ a special method involving debits and credits. This method was first described in writing in a book published in 1494 by an Italian monk named Paciolo. Today, nearly 500 years later, the system described by Paciolo is still being used by accountants throughout the world.

Let us assume, for the moment, that only five types of accounts are employed in accounting: (1) assets, (2) expenses, (3) liabilities, (4) equity, and (5) revenues. The relationship among these accounts can be expressed by the basic accounting equation previously discussed:

$$\text{Assets} + \text{Expenses} = \text{Liabilities} + \text{Equity} + \text{Revenues}$$

Paciolo suggested that we refer to the left-hand side of the equation as the *debit side*. The elements of the left-hand side—assets and expenses—are therefore debit items (or debit balances). So, if the accountant makes an addition to the left-hand side of the equation, the entry is a debit. In other words, increases in assets and expenses are recorded by making debits to those accounts.

Similarly, Paciolo indicated that the right-hand side of the equation is called the *credit side*. The elements of this side—liabilities, equity, and revenues—are therefore credit items (or credit balances). So, if the accountant makes an addition to the right-hand side of the equation, the entry is a credit. In other words, increases in liabilities, equity, and revenues are recorded by making credits to those accounts.

Thus, increases in assets and expenses are debits; increases in liabilities, equity, and revenues are credits. It logically follows that decreases in assets and expenses are credits, and that decreases in liabilities, equity, and revenues are debits. In summary, the rules of debit and credit are as follows:

1. With respect to asset and expense accounts:
   a. Debit to increase.
   b. Credit to decrease.
2. With respect to liability, equity, and revenue accounts:
   a. Credit to increase.
   b. Debit to decrease.

Most introductory accounting students at first memorize these rules. As they gain experience by applying the rules to business transactions, however, debit-and-credit analysis becomes almost second nature.

Real Meaning of Debits
and Credits

Many persons begin a study of accounting with certain preconceived (and incorrect) notions about debits and credits. It is widely believed, for example, that a debit is something "bad" and that a credit is something "good." There also exists an erroneous idea that the term debit always means "decrease," and that credits always "increase" a balance. These notions are incorrect and, if not discarded, impair the study of accounting. The word *debit*, standing alone, simply means an entry or balance on the left-hand side of an accounting record. A debit means increase only with respect to assets and expenses; a debit to any other type of account is a decrease. Similarly, the word *credit* means nothing more than an entry or balance on the right-hand side of an accounting record. Whether a debit or a credit is an increase or a decrease, then, depends on the type of account to which it is related.

Use of Accounts

Accountants have devised a standard way to record debits and credits in accounts. An account form is basically a *T* shape:

(Account Name or Title)	
(left) Debit side	(right) Credit side

The name or title of the account appears at the top of the form above the horizontal rule. (For the purpose here, the terms *assets, expenses, liabilities, equity,* and *revenues* serve as the account names. More specific account titles are introduced in Chapter 3.) A vertical rule divides the account equally into a left side and a right side.

The Basic T Account

No matter what the account name, however, the left-hand side of a T account is the debit side; the right-hand side is the credit side. With respect to assets and expenses, entries made on the left (debit) side are increases ($+$), and entries made on the right (credit) side are decreases ($-$). The opposite is true in accounts for liabilities, equity, and revenues. These debit and credit rules are presented here in account form:

Assets		+	Expenses		=	Liabilities		+	Equity		+	Revenues	
Dr.	Cr.		Dr.	Cr.		Dr.	Cr.		Dr.	Cr.		Dr.	Cr.
$(+)$	$(-)$		$(+)$	$(-)$		$(-)$	$(+)$		$(-)$	$(+)$		$(-)$	$(+)$

Note that the word *debit* is abbreviated *Dr.* and the word credit is abbreviated *Cr.* These abbreviations are derived from equivalent words of the Latin language in which Paciolo wrote. They are not English abbreviations.

Figure 2–1 analyzed eight transactions in terms of the basic accounting equation. These same eight transactions now will be analyzed in T-account form, using debits and credits. You should recall the assumed balances, labeled (B), at the beginning of the period:

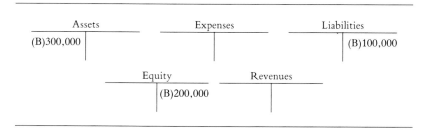

The five T accounts, as a group, are referred to as the ledger. As you can see, the ledger is "in balance"; that is, total debits equal total credits.

The first transaction to be analyzed and entered in this ledger is one in which the hospital borrows $25,000 from a bank. This transaction creates $25,000 of additional assets (cash) and $25,000 of additional liabilities (the amount now owed to the bank). The entry, numbered (1), is as follows:

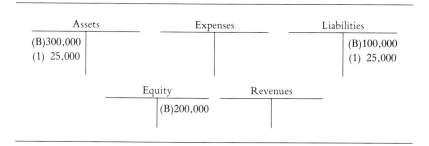

Thus, the required entry is a $25,000 debit to assets and a $25,000 credit to liabilities. The entry increases assets to a balance of

$325,000 and increases the liabilities to a balance of $125,000, and the ledger remains in balance.

The second transaction is the purchase of supplies (inventory) on account for $12,000. The entry, numbered (2), is as follows:

Assets		Expenses		Liabilities	
(B)300,000				(B)100,000	
(1) 25,000				(1) 25,000	
(2) 12,000				(2) 12,000	

Equity		Revenues	
(B)200,000			

This transaction, which produces a new asset (inventory) and a new liability (accounts payable) is recorded as a $12,000 debit to assets and a $12,000 credit to liabilities. Every transaction entry will have at least two effects; every entry will include at least one debit and one credit.

Do not fall into the trap of assuming that a transaction entry is always an increase in one account and a decrease in another. Each of the two entries made in the preceding accounts was an increase in one account and an increase in another. No decreases at all were recorded. Other types of transactions are recorded by a decrease in one account and a decrease in another (or the same) account, with no increase in any account. Still other transactions require an increase in one account and a decrease in another. So, it is possible to have any combination of increases and decreases.

Notice that the ledger is still in balance. The debit total of assets, $337,000 ($300,000 + $25,000 + $12,000) equals the credit totals of liabilities, $137,000 ($100,000 + $25,000 + $12,000), and equity, $200,000. This equality of debit and credit balances must be maintained at all times.

The next transaction consists of the sale of half the supplies inventory to patients for $7,500. Because all the supplies purchased in transaction 2 cost $12,000 but only half of them were sold, the cost of the supplies sold is $6,000. This $6,000 must be removed from assets (inventory) and charged to expenses (supplies expense).

Maintaining a Balance in the Ledger

The $7,500 billing to patients must be charged to patients' accounts receivable (debited to assets) and recorded as revenues earned by the hospital. The entry, numbered (3), is as follows:

Assets		Expenses		Liabilities
(B)300,000	(3) 6,000	(3) 6,000		(B)100,000
(1) 25,000				(1) 25,000
(2) 12,000				(2) 12,000
(3) 7,500				

	Equity		Revenues
	(B)200,000		(3) 7,500

This entry includes two debits and two credits. Entries having more than one debit or credit are referred to as *compound entries.* You also will encounter compound entries having two or more debits but only one credit, and entries having two or more credits but only one debit.

In transaction 4, the hospital pays $14,000 of salaries and wages to its employees. The entry, numbered (4), is as follows:

Assets		Expenses		Liabilities
(B)300,000	(3) 6,000	(3) 6,000		(B)100,000
(1) 25,000	(4) 14,000	(4) 14,000		(1) 25,000
(2) 12,000				(2) 12,000
(3) 7,500				

	Equity		Revenues
	(B)200,000		(3) 7,500

This entry records a decrease in assets (cash) and an increase in expenses (employees' salaries and wages expense).

The fifth transaction is the billing of hospital patients for $15,300 of services (room and board, laboratory, pharmacy, and so on):

Assets		Expenses		Liabilities	
(B)300,000	(3) 6,000	(3) 6,000			(B)100,000
(1) 25,000	(4) 14,000	(4) 14,000			(1) 25,000
(2) 12,000					(2) 12,000
(3) 7,500					
(5) 15,300					

Equity		Revenues	
	(B)200,000		(3) 7,500
			(5) 15,300

This entry records an increase in hospital assets (accounts receivable) and an increase in hospital revenues (revenues from services to patients). A portion of the accounts receivable established in this entry will be collected in cash in the eighth transaction.

Transaction 6 consists of the repayment of the bank loan of $25,000 plus $1,000 of interest assumed to be due to the bank. The required entry, numbered (6), includes two debits and one credit:

Assets		Expenses		Liabilities	
(B)300,000	(3) 6,000	(3) 6,000		(6) 25,000	(B)100,000
(1) 25,000	(4) 14,000	(4) 14,000			(1) 25,000
(2) 12,000	(6) 26,000	(6) 1,000			(2) 12,000
(3) 7,500					
(5) 15,300					

Equity		Revenues	
	(B)200,000		(3) 7,500
			(5) 15,300

Of this $26,000 cash disbursement, $1,000 is interest expense, and the remaining $25,000 is a reduction of liabilities (elimination of the bank loan payable).

The seventh transaction is the payment by the hospital of $9,000 of accounts payable to its suppliers. The required entry, numbered (7), is as follows:

Assets		Expenses		Liabilities	
(B)300,000	(3) 6,000	(3) 6,000		(6) 25,000	(B)100,000
(1) 25,000	(4) 14,000	(4) 14,000		(7) 9,000	(1) 25,000
(2) 12,000	(6) 26,000	(6) 1,000			(2) 12,000
(3) 7,500	(7) 9,000				
(5) 15,300					

	Equity		Revenues	
	(B)200,000		(3) 7,500	
			(5) 15,300	

These accounts payable arose in transaction 2 when the liabilities account was credited for $12,000. Now, because $9,000 of the accounts payable is being paid, the liabilities account is debited. The difference of $3,000 remains unpaid as part of the credit balance in the liabilities account.

The last transaction is the receipt of $18,400 in payment of a portion of accounts receivable due from patients for supplies and services provided to them in previous transactions (transactions 3 and 5). The entry, numbered (8), is as follows:

Assets		Expenses		Liabilities	
(B)300,000	(3) 6,000	(3) 6,000		(6) 25,000	(B)100,000
(1) 25,000	(4) 14,000	(4) 14,000		(7) 9,000	(1) 25,000
(2) 12,000	(6) 26,000	(6) 1,000			(2) 12,000
(3) 7,500	(7) 9,000				
(5) 15,300	(8) 18,400				
(8) 18,400					

	Equity		Revenues	
	(B)200,000		(3) 7,500	
			(5) 15,300	

This transaction requires entering a debit and a credit to the assets account. The entry, in this case, debits (increases) one type of asset (cash) and credits (decreases) another type of asset (accounts receivable).

Now we should determine the balance of each account. Consider, for example, the assets account that consists of an opening balance at the beginning of the period, five debits for the increases in assets during the period, and five credits for the decreases in assets during the period. The balance of assets at the end of the period may be determined as follows:

	Assets	
	(B)300,000	(3) 6,000
	(1) 25,000	(4) 14,000
	(2) 12,000	(6) 26,000
	(3) 7,500	(7) 9,000
	(5) 15,300	(8) 18,400
	(8) 18,400	
(Totals)	378,200	73,400
(Less credit total)	73,400	
(Closing balance)	(B)304,800	

Notice that the opening balance of assets plus the debits (increases) during the period totals $378,200; the credits (decreases) during the period total $73,400. The difference between the debit and credit totals is the end-of-period balance of assets, that is, a debit balance of $304,800. It is a debit balance, because the debit total in the account exceeds the credit total.

A balance for each of the other accounts may be determined in a similar manner. To determine whether the ledger is in balance, the individual account balances may be arranged in a *trial balance,* as shown in Figure 2–2.

Generating a Trial Balance

Figure 2–2 Trial Balance

	Balances	
	Dr.	Cr.
Assets	$304,800	
Expenses	21,000	
Liabilities		$103,000
Equity		200,000
Revenues		22,800
Totals	$325,800	$325,800

Notice that the accounts for assets and expenses have debit balances, and that the accounts for liabilities, equity, and revenues have credit balances. This is the normal state of affairs. Elements on the left-hand side of the accounting equation are debit items; elements on the right-hand side are credit items.

To obtain the end-of-period equity balance (taking into account the net income for the period), a *closing entry* is required, as indicated in the following, labeled (C):

Assets			Expenses			Liabilities	
(B)300,000	(3) 6,000	(3) 6,000	(C) 21,000		(6) 25,000	(B)100,000	
(1) 25,000	(4) 14,000	(4) 14,000			(7) 9,000	(1) 25,000	
(2) 12,000	(6) 26,000	(6) 1,000				(2) 12,000	
(3) 7,500	(7) 9,000						
(5) 15,300	(8) 18,400						
(8) 18,400							

Equity		Revenues	
(B)200,000	(C) 22,800	(3) 7,500	
(C) 1,800		(5) 15,300	

The closing entry eliminates the balances of revenues and expenses, and records the $1,800 difference (net income) as an increase in the equity account. The double rules in the accounts for revenues and expenses indicate that these accounts have been closed and have no balance. In the account for expenses, for example, debits equal credits; the account balance is zero.

Need for More Detailed Information

If financial statements were prepared from the accounts developed in the previous discussion, the information in those statements would be highly condensed data. The income statement for the period and the balance sheet at the end of the period would contain the information shown in Figure 2–3.

Whereas these are the general types of information required by financial statement users, the categories are much too broad to be useful. Much more detailed information must be provided.

From what services and other sources did the hospital earn its revenues, and how much revenue was derived from each source? What are the functional and natural breakdowns of the hospital's

Income Statement	
Revenues	$ 22,800
Less expenses	21,000
Net income for the period	$ 1,800
Balance Sheet	
Assets	$304,800
Liabilities	$103,000
Equity	201,800
Total liabilities and equity	$304,800

Figure 2–3 Condensed Income Statement and Balance Sheet

expenses, and how much expense was incurred in each classification? What specific assets are owned by the hospital, and how much money is invested in each of them? What specific liabilities does the hospital have, and what is the monetary amount of each of them? Which of these assets and liabilities are current, and which are noncurrent?

The next chapter begins to develop the detailed information necessary to answer such questions.

Questions

Q2–1. Indicate briefly the need for documentary evidence in accounting. Give five examples of documentary evidence used in hospital accounting.

Q2–2. Define the term *debit*.

Q2–3. Define the term *credit*.

Q2–4. "In accounting, debits represent something 'bad' (undesirable), whereas credits represent something 'good' (desirable)." Do you agree? Explain your opinion.

Q2–5. State the rules of debit and credit with respect to asset and expense accounts.

Q2–6. State the rules of debit and credit with respect to liability, equity, and revenue accounts.

Q2–7. What are compound entries?

Q2–8. What is a trial balance? What is its purpose?

Q2–9. Which of the following types of accounts normally have debit balances?
   a. Assets
   b. Liabilities
   c. Equity

d. Revenues
e. Expenses

Q2–10. What is the purpose of a closing entry?

Exercises

E2–1. On March 31, Hopi Hospital had assets of $500,000, liabilities of $300,000, and equity of $200,000. During April, the following transactions were completed:
1. Services rendered to patients, $100,000.
2. Collections on patients' accounts, $85,000.
3. Supplies purchased on account, $20,000.
4. Payments on accounts payable to suppliers, $16,000.
5. Supplies consumed in patient-care services, $18,000.
6. Other expenses paid in cash, $54,000.
7. Purchased equipment for cash, $12,000.

Required: What were the amounts of Hopi Hospital's assets, liabilities, and equity on April 30?

E2–2. On August 31, Zebra Hospital had $800,000 of assets, $500,000 of liabilities, and $300,000 of equity. The following transactions were completed during September:
1. Borrowed $75,000 from a local bank.
2. Repaid $25,000 of the bank loan, plus $750 interest for the month of September.
3. Provided $186,000 of services to patients.
4. Collected $193,000 on patients' accounts.
5. Other September expenses paid in cash, $184,000.
6. Purchased equipment for $15,000 cash.

Required: What were the amounts of Zebra Hospital's assets, liabilities, and equity at September 30?

E2–3. At May 31, Tiger Hospital had $650,000 of assets, $350,000 of liabilities, and $300,000 of equity. The following transactions were completed during June:
1. Charged patients for $204,000 of services.
2. Collected $190,000 on patients' accounts.
3. Purchased $31,000 of supplies on account.
4. Used $28,000 of supplies in patient-care activities.
5. Paid $35,000 on accounts payable.
6. Paid employee salaries and wages of $99,000.
7. Paid other expenses of $60,000.

Required: What were the amounts of Tiger Hospital's assets, liabilities, and equity at June 30?

E2–4. Tarzan Hospital began operations on January 1, 19X1, with $10,000 of assets, $6,000 of liabilities, and $4,000 of equity. Following are the ledger accounts at December 31, 19X1:

Assets		Expenses		Liabilities	
10,000	500	1,100		500	6,000
1,500	1,100	3,200			1,500
5,000	3,200				
4,200	4,200				

Equity		Revenues	
	4,000		5,000

Required: Reconstruct the 19X1 transactions of Tarzan Hospital to the extent possible.

Problems

P2–1. Assume that Joy Hospital on May 1 had $29,000 of assets, $12,000 of liabilities, and $17,000 of equity. Subsequently, the following transactions were completed:
1. The hospital borrowed $2,500 from a local bank.
2. The hospital repaid $1,000 of the bank loan. Disregard interest.
3. Supplies costing $1,800 were purchased on account and placed in inventory.
4. A new item of equipment was purchased for $4,600 cash.
5. The hospital paid $800 on its accounts payable.
6. Supplies previously purchased for $700 were sold to patients for $960 cash.
7. Patients' accounts were charged for $1,770 of hospital services rendered to them.
8. Cash collections on patients' accounts amounted to $1,150.

Required: Taking into account the cumulative effects of the eight transactions and the May 1 balances, what are Joy Hospital's total assets, total liabilities, and total equity?

P2–2. On October 1, Taylor Hospital had $450,000 of assets, $150,000 of liabilities, and $300,000 of equity. Transactions completed during the month of October were as follows:
1. The hospital borrowed $50,000 from a bank.
2. The hospital purchased supplies on account for $20,000.

3. Seventy-five percent of the supplies were issued from inventory and used in patient care. Patients were billed for $21,000.
4. The hospital paid $45,000 of salaries and wages to employees.
5. Patients were billed for $48,500 of other services.
6. The hospital paid $30,400 (including $400 interest) on the bank loan.
7. The hospital paid $17,000 on its accounts payable.
8. The hospital collected $59,000 on patients' accounts.

Required: Prepare an analysis of these transactions using the format illustrated in Figure 2–1.

P2–3. On December 1, Todd Hospital had $380,000 of assets, $120,000 of liabilities, and $260,000 of equity. Transactions completed during the month of December were as follows:
1. The hospital borrowed $20,000 from a bank.
2. Supplies purchased on account amounted to $14,000.
3. Supplies issued from inventory and used in patient care amounted to $10,000. Patients were billed for $16,000.
4. Employees were paid $28,000 of salaries and wages.
5. New equipment was purchased for $4,000 cash.
6. Patients were billed for $26,000 of other services.
7. The bank loan was paid off with a disbursement of $20,300, including interest of $300.
8. Payments on accounts payable amounted to $11,000.
9. Collections on accounts receivable were $39,000.

Required: Prepare a debit and credit analysis of the nine transactions in T-account form, including a closing entry at December 31. Indicate the balance of each account at December 31.

P2–4. On October 31, Iowa Hospital had $710,000 of assets, $230,000 of liabilities, and $480,000 of equity. Transactions completed during the month of November were as follows:
1. Supplies purchased on account totaled $29,000.
2. Supplies that had cost $26,000 were issued from inventory and used in patient care. Patients were billed $31,000.
3. Employees were paid $84,000 of salaries and wages.

4. Patients were billed for November services as follows:

Daily patient services	$51,500
Other professional services	37,500
Total	$89,000

5. Other operating revenues received in cash amounted to $2,800.
6. Purchase of new equipment on account was for $12,000.
7. Payments on accounts payable amounted to $24,700.
8. Collections on accounts receivable totaled $102,600.
9. Miscellaneous other expenses paid in cash came to $14,300.

Required: (1) Prepare a debit and credit analysis of the above information in T-account form, including a closing entry at November 30. (2) Prepare an income statement for November that is as detailed as possible.

Journal, Ledger, and Trial Balance

3

The preceding chapter was concerned with analyzing business transactions in terms of how they increase and decrease the basic elements of the accounting equation. Only five accounts were used in the analysis: assets, expenses, liabilities, equity, and revenues. A much greater number of accounts is needed, however, to provide the detailed information required by hospital management and other financial statement users. Such information is developed by the use of a *chart of accounts,* sometimes called a *classification of accounts.* A relatively simple chart of accounts is introduced in this chapter; a more sophisticated set of accounts is presented in Chapter 10.

Also in the previous chapter, transaction entries were recorded directly in the accounts. This procedure is not feasible in actual accounting practice because of the large volume of transactions that must be recorded each day. Instead, the effects of business transactions are recorded initially in an accounting record known as a journal. The process of making records of transactions in a journal is called *journalizing.* Subsequently, the journalized information is transferred (by a process called *posting*) into the accounts in the hospital's ledger. The major part of this chapter is devoted to a discussion of these procedures.

Let us assume that Smalltown is a rapidly growing community but one without a hospital of its own. Because the nearest hospital is in a city some distance away, the citizens of Smalltown decide to build their own community hospital. A Civic Improvement Committee is established to raise the necessary money for construction, equipment, and initial operating needs (working capital). An extended fund-raising campaign is completed on December 31, 19X0, when a

Illustration Data

goal of $100,000 is achieved. The hospital is incorporated under the laws of the state, and a corporate charter is duly obtained.

On receipt of the not-for-profit charter, the Smalltown Hospital begins its corporate existence on January 1, 19X1. During the ensuing year, the following transactions are completed by the hospital:

1. On January 1, 19X1, the hospital receives its initial equity of $100,000 from the citizens of Smalltown through the Civic Improvement Committee.
2. On January 2, 19X1, the hospital issues $50,000 of 8 percent, 10-year bonds at face value. Interest on these bonds is payable annually on December 31.
3. On January 3, 19X1, the hospital purchases plant assets for cash as follows:

Land	$ 25,000
Building	67,000
Equipment	45,000
Total cost	$137,000

The cost of the building includes the alteration and remodeling of an existing structure previously operated as a hotel.

4. During the year, total purchases of supplies on account by the hospital amount to $28,200. These include dietary supplies, pharmaceuticals, and other medical and surgical supplies.
5. As the year passes, $21,500 of these supplies are issued from inventory for use in hospital patient-care activities.
6. Services rendered to patients over the course of the year total $120,300 and are billed to patients as follows:

Daily patient services	$ 72,180
Ancillary services	48,120
Total revenues	$120,300

Daily patient services include room, board, routine nursing care, and minor medications. Ancillary services are those provided by departments such as operating rooms, laboratory, radiology, and pharmacy.

7. During the year, collections on patients' accounts amount to $94,500. (We will assume no charity service, bad debts, or other deductions from revenues occur.)
8. Payments on accounts payable to suppliers are $22,600.
9. During 19X1, the hospital receives in cash $13,800 of revenues from other sources (including unrestricted contributions and gifts).
10. Over the course of 19X1, the hospital pays operating expenses as follows:

Salaries and wages	$76,400
Utilities	12,700
Insurance	3,600
Repairs	2,900
Other expenses	1,300
Total	$96,900

11. On October 1, 19X1, the hospital obtains a short-term, 10 percent loan of $12,000 from a local bank.
12. On December 31, 19X1, the hospital pays interest expense on the bonds and bank loan as follows:

Interest on bonds	$4,000
Interest on bank loan	300
Total	$4,300

You should understand that this list is largely a summary of the thousands of transactions the hospital had during 19X1. Except in a few instances, individual transactions are not indicated. This also means that, other than where particular dates are specified, the itemization is not in the chronological order in which the events occurred. Items 4 through 10, for example, each describe a series of transactions that took place over the entire year at periodic intervals. The hospital rendered patient services daily, cash was received and disbursed every day, supplies were purchased periodically, salaries and wages were paid biweekly, and so forth.

You now are aware of all of the financial activities of Smalltown Hospital during 19X1. Knowing this, what is the hospital's net income for the year? How much cash does Smalltown Hospital have in the bank at the end of the year? At December 31, 19X1, what is the amount of accounts receivable due from patients? Inventory? Accounts payable to suppliers? What are the amounts of other hospital assets and liabilities?

Users of Accounting Information

Who cares about these balances? As you learned in Chapter 1, management, creditors, third-party payers, bankers, bondholders, and governmental agencies all care. The citizens of Smalltown have a rather personal interest in the hospital's finances as well. All of these and other groups care very much indeed about these questions and the answers to them! Without such information, none of these groups would be able to make intelligent economic decisions.

So, once we agree that financial information about Smalltown Hospital is important and useful, how do we deal with the problems of accumulating, communicating, and using it? How do we develop and maintain the necessary accounting records, and how do we report the recorded information to those who use it?

Chart of Accounts

As noted in Chapter 2, competent documentary evidence of completed transactions is the first and fundamental requirement of the accounting system. Documentary evidence is essential, because the reliability and accuracy of the information produced by the accounting process rests largely on the extent to which that information is based on verifiable, objectively determined facts. You realize, of course, that accounting never can become fully objective or completely scientific. Accounting is an art that requires the exercise of judgment and the use of estimates. Wherever possible, however, business transactions are evidenced by independent and objective documentation such as invoices, bank deposit slips, charge tickets, cash receipt slips, and other business papers.

Transaction Types Listed in the Chart of Accounts

Properly executed documentary evidences make the accountant aware that transactions have occurred. In order to record these transactions in an organized manner, an information classification system must be used. This system is set forth in a chart of accounts such as the one illustrated in Figure 3–1. This chart depicts the manner in which transaction data will be classified and recorded in the accounting records of Smalltown Hospital. It is designed primarily to meet the informational needs of the hospital management,

100 Assets
    101 Cash
    102 Accounts Receivable
    103 Inventory
        .
        .
        .
    110 Land
    111 Building
    112 Equipment
200 Liabilities
    201 Accounts Payable
    202 Bank Loan Payable
        .
        .
        .
    210 Bonds Payable
300 Equity
    301 Hospital Equity
    302 Revenue and Expense Summary
400 Revenues
    401 Routine Services Revenue
    402 Ancillary Services Revenue
    403 Other Revenues
500 Expenses
    501 Salaries and Wages Expense
    502 Supplies Expense
    503 Utilities Expense
    504 Insurance Expense
    505 Repairs Expense
    506 Interest Expense
    507 Other Expenses

Figure 3–1 Smalltown Hospital Chart of Accounts

but accounting standards as well as legal, tax, and regulatory agency requirements also influence the design of the chart of accounts.

The illustrative chart is divided into five major groups of accounts: assets, liabilities, equity, revenues, and expenses. Each account in the chart is assigned an identifying number. Any account in the 100 series is an asset account, any account in the 200 series is a liability account, and so on. This numerical coding of the accounts saves clerical time and effort in that it is easier to pronounce, write, or type *501,* for example, than it is to pronounce, write, or type

Coding Groups of Accounts

salaries and wages expense. The numerical coding also promotes accuracy and permits the accountant to identify the nature of any account readily. Data processing equipment requires the use of account numbers.

There are 21 accounts in Smalltown Hospital's chart. If the management of Smalltown Hospital required more detailed information about expenditures for, say, utilities, separate accounts could be provided for water, heat, and electricity, instead of combining all such expenditures into a single utilities account. Or, rather than a single revenue account for ancillary services, a number of separate accounts could be maintained for individual services such as operating room revenue, laboratory revenue, and pharmacy revenue.

This, of course, is done in actual practice, where charts of accounts generally consist of several hundred individual accounts. The Smalltown Hospital's chart of accounts, however, is limited to 21 accounts for the purposes of this introductory discussion. Notice also that we are not yet ready to introduce accounts for depreciation, prepaid and accrued expenses, bad debts, and various other financial statement items that you may recall from Chapter 1. These complications will be introduced at appropriate points in subsequent chapters.

Journal

Assuming that we have documentary evidence supporting the Smalltown Hospital's 19X1 transactions, and given the hospital's chart of accounts, we can proceed with the task of analyzing and recording the transactions for 19X1. Each of the 12 transactions previously listed will be analyzed in terms of its effects on the account classifications provided in the chart of accounts. Which account or accounts should be debited, and which should be credited, for each of these transactions? This debit and credit analysis will be recorded initially in an accounting record called a *journal*.

The General Journal

As you will see later, there are many types of journals: revenue journals, cash receipts journals, voucher registers, and so on. These special journals are illustrated in Chapters 11–14. We are concerned at this point, however, only with the *general journal*. This particular form of journal is illustrated in Figure 3–2.

The Journalizing Process

The process of recording transactions in the journal is called *journalizing*. It consists of a formal handwritten or typewritten analysis of the increase and decrease effects of transactions on the specific account classifications provided in the chart of accounts. You might think of journalizing as maintaining a business diary for the hospital. The journal is a chronological record of financial

Date			Accounts and Explanations	Acct. No.	Dr.	Cr.
Mo.	Day	Year	Account(s) Debited	No.	Amounts	
			Account(s) Credited	No.		Amounts
			Explanation of the transaction.			
			(Examples)			
1	1	X1	Cash	101	100,000	
			Hospital Equity	301		100,000
			Receipt of initial equity from			
			Civic Improvement Committee.			
1	2	X1	Cash	101	50,000	
			Bonds Payable	210		50,000
			Issue of 8%, 10-year bonds			
			at face value.			

Figure 3–2 General Journal Form

events in the economic life of the hospital. As each event, or transaction, occurs, it is recorded in the journal. This record, as you can see in Figure 3–2, consists of several elements, which are entered in the order listed:

1. The date of the transaction.
2. The titles of the accounts affected (increased and/or decreased) by the transaction, that is, the particular accounts to be debited and credited.
3. A brief explanation of the nature and salient facts of each transaction.
4. The account numbers of the accounts being debited and credited.
5. The dollar amounts of the debits and credits.

These are the essential elements of a journal entry. All five of these elements must be provided for each entry.

Several different kinds of journal entries are made in accounting. Later on in this book, you will learn how to make adjusting entries, correcting entries, reversing entries, and closing entries. At this point, however, we are concerned only with entries to record transactions, that is, transaction entries.

Entry No.	Accounts and Explanations	Acct. No.	Debit	Credit
1	Cash	101	100,000	
	Hospital Equity	301		100,000
	Receipt of equity funds from Smalltown Civic Improvement Committee.			
2	Cash	101	50,000	
	Bonds Payable	210		50,000
	Issue of 8%, 10-year bonds at face value.			
3	Land	110	25,000	
	Building	111	67,000	
	Equipment	112	45,000	
	Cash	101		137,000
	Purchase of plant assets.			
4	Inventory	103	28,200	
	Accounts Payable	201		28,200
	Purchase of supplies on account.			
5	Supplies Expense	502	21,500	
	Inventory	103		21,500
	Supplies used.			
6	Accounts Receivable	102	120,300	
	Routine Services Revenue	401		72,180
	Ancillary Services Revenue	402		48,120
	Charges to patients for services rendered.			
7	Cash	101	94,500	
	Accounts Receivable	102		94,500
	Collections on patients' accounts.			
8	Accounts Payable	201	22,600	
	Cash	101		22,600
	Payments on accounts payable to suppliers.			
9	Cash	101	13,800	
	Other Revenues	403		13,800
	Receipt of miscellaneous revenues.			

Figure 3-3 Smalltown Hospital 19X1 Journal

Entry No.	Accounts and Explanations	Acct. No.	Debit	Credit
10	Salaries and Wages Expense	501	76,400	
	Utilities Expense	503	12,700	
	Insurance Expense	504	3,600	
	Repairs Expense	505	2,900	
	Other Expenses	507	1,300	
	Cash	101		96,900
	Payments of operating expenses.			
11	Cash	101	12,000	
	Bank Loan Payable	202		12,000
	Receipt of short-term, 10% loan from local bank.			
12	Interest Expense	506	4,300	
	Cash	101		4,300
	Payment of interest as follows:			
	Interest on bonds $4,000			
	Interest on bank loan 300			
	Total $4,300			

Figure 3–3 Smalltown Hospital 19X1 Journal *(continued)*

All of the transaction entries for Smalltown Hospital for 19X1 are presented in Figure 3–3. Note the following points:

1. The date on which each transaction occurred ordinarily appears in the column on the far left. For purposes of this illustration, however, we give each transaction entry a number rather than a specific date. Transactions of the same type—purchases of supplies, for example—are summarized for the entire year in this illustration. They are recorded by a single journal entry to simplify and shorten the presentation. This is why the journal entries are not dated with a specific month and day indication.
2. The titles of the accounts debited and credited, along with a brief explanation of the transaction being recorded, are indicated in the next section of the journal.
   a. The titles of the accounts debited in each entry are written first and against the left-hand margin.
   b. The titles of the accounts credited are written underneath the accounts debited and are indented about an inch or so. This indentation distinguishes the credits from the debits at a glance.

     c. The explanation or description of the transaction follows the account titles and is indented about half an inch so that it will not be confused with account titles.

It is very important to use the precise account titles indicated by the chart of accounts and not to "invent" new accounts. Your analysis is limited to the accounts provided in the chart of accounts.

3. The account numbers of the accounts debited and credited in each journal entry are entered in the column provided for them. Do not "invent" new account numbers; use only the numerical coding provided by the chart of accounts.
4. The dollar amounts involved in the transaction are written in the debit and credit columns on the right-hand side of the journal. Dollar marks ($) are not necessary in these columns.
5. One line is skipped between journal entries so that each entry is set apart from the others on the journal page.

Although some accounting is still done manually in this type-written or handwritten form, most hospitals employ mechanized accounting equipment and computers. What you see in Figure 3–3 in manual form, however, is the same sort of record made by mechanized accounting equipment and computers.

Let us quickly examine each of the 12 transaction entries appearing in Smalltown Hospital's 19X1 journal:

Entry
No.

1. The transaction had the effect of increasing the hospital assets (cash) and increasing the hospital's equity. Assets are increased by debits, and equity is increased by credits; so, we record a debit to cash and a credit to hospital equity.

2. The transaction increased the hospital's assets (cash) and its liabilities (bonds payable). Assets are increased by debits, and liabilities are increased by credits; so, we debit cash and credit bonds payable. (This entry is very similar to entry 11.)

3. The transaction increased three asset categories (land, building, and equipment) and decreased another asset (cash). Assets are increased by debits and decreased by credits; so, we debit the accounts for land, building, and equipment, and credit the cash account.

4. The transaction was one in which the hospital acquired an asset (inventory) and incurred a liability (accounts payable); so, we record an addition to the hospital assets and an addition to hospital liabilities.

Later, you will see that purchased supplies sometimes may be debited directly to supplies expense rather than to inventory. For the present, however, we will debit inventory for purchases of supplies.

5. The transaction decreased an asset (inventory) and increased the hospital's expenses (supplies expense). Expenses are increased by debits; assets are decreased by credits; so, we record the cost of the supplies used as expense and reduce the inventory.

6. In this summary transaction, hospital services were rendered to patients who did not pay for the services at the time they were provided.

   Revenues earned by the hospital are recognized (recorded) when services are rendered. The transaction, then, increases the hospital's assets and its revenues. Because assets are increased by debits and revenues are increased by credits, we debit receivables and credit the appropriate revenue accounts.

7. Collections on patients' accounts increase cash and decrease accounts receivable. No revenue is recognized; the revenue to which these collections relate has already been recorded in entry 6.

8. When supplies were purchased on account (entry 4), accounts payable were established by a credit. Now, when a portion of these accounts is paid, accounts payable are debited (decreased) and cash is credited (decreased). This entry is a decrease in one account and a decrease in another; the transaction results in no increase in any account.

9. This transaction entry records the receipt of cash representing revenues collected from miscellaneous sources, such as sales by the hospital cafeteria. Some revenues may be recorded directly in this manner without using a receivables account.

10. This summary entry records the disbursements made during the year for various operating expenses. The appropriate expense accounts are debited, and cash is credited.

    In actual practice, however, all hospital disbursements usually are run through liability accounts. Salaries and wages, for example, generally require two entries:

Salaries and Wages Expense	$XXX,XXX	
Salaries and Wages Payable		$XXX,XXX
Salaries and Wages Payable	$XXX,XXX	
Cash		$XXX,XXX

    This procedure will be introduced later but, for now, we will record expenses directly by debits to expense and credits to cash. We also are disregarding, at this point, matters such as payroll taxes, prepaid and accrued expenses, and depreciation.

11. This entry records the receipt of a short-term (less than one year) loan from a bank. Cash is debited, and the liability to the bank is established by the credit. A similar transaction was recorded in entry 2.

    Note that neither this entry nor entry 2 gave recognition to interest, either as a liability or as an expense. The point is that at the time the bank loan was received and at the time the bonds were issued, the hospital owed no interest and therefore had no interest expense. The interest on these obligations is recorded in entry 12.

12. Recall that the hospital issued $50,000 of 10-year, 8 percent bonds at the beginning of the year. These bonds have been outstanding all year, so the bond interest expense is $4,000 (i.e., $50,000 × 8 percent). The bank loan, on the other hand, was obtained on October 1, 19X1. Because the hospital has had the use of the bank's money for only three months (October, November, and December), the hospital's interest expense is $300 (or $12,000 × 10 percent × 3 ÷ 12).

We are assuming that interest on the bonds and on the bank loan is paid on December 31, 19X1. So, the entry debits interest expense and credits cash for $4,300, or $4,000 + $300. If we assume, however, that the interest was payable on January 1, 19X2, the December 31 entry would be

Interest Expense	$ 4,300	
Accrued Interest Payable		$ 4,300

We are not yet ready to consider expense accruals, but this matter will be considered at a later point in this book.

What the Journal Reveals

Thus, Smalltown Hospital's 19X1 journal provides a chronological record of the effects of the year's transactions on the account classifications set forth in the hospital's chart of accounts. It presents an economic history of the hospital's financial activities for the year.

To assist you in studying the transaction entries in the 19X1 journal of Smalltown Hospital, a classification of routine transaction entries is provided in Figure 3–4. Note the following points:

1. Transactions completed by a hospital may be classified basically as either cash transactions or noncash transactions. If the transaction produces a cash receipt or requires a cash outlay, it is a cash transaction. All other transactions, of course, are noncash transactions.
2. If the transaction does not involve a cash inflow or outflow, it may be (for example) the purchase of supplies on account, a charge to patients for services rendered, or the use of supplies from the hospital's inventory.

   Although there are many other types of noncash transactions, these three are the ones with which you should be most concerned at this point in your study of accounting.
3. If the transaction is a cash transaction, it is either a cash disbursement or cash receipt transaction. This can be determined simply by reading the description of the transaction as given in the text or in end-of-chapter problems.
   a. If the transaction is a cash disbursement, you always make a credit to cash. Cash disbursements are decreases in cash, an asset. To decrease an asset, you credit the asset. Then you ask: "What do I debit?" Simply ask yourself: "For what

	Dr.	Cr.
Noncash Transaction Entries		
1. Purchases of supplies on account:		
Inventory	X	
Accounts Payable		X
2. Charges to patients for services rendered:		
Accounts Receivable	X	
Appropriate Revenue accounts		X
3. Usage of supplies from inventory:		
Supplies Expense	X	
Inventory		X
Cash Disbursement Transaction Entries		
1. Acquisition of an asset:		
Appropriate Asset account	X	
Cash		X
2. Elimination of a liability:		
Appropriate Liability account	X	
Cash		X
3. Payment of an expense:		
Appropriate Expense account	X	
Cash		X
Cash Receipt Transaction Entries		
1. Collections on patients' accounts:		
Cash	X	
Accounts Receivable		X
2. Incurrence of a liability:		
Cash	X	
Appropriate Liability account		X
3. Receipt of revenue:		
Cash	X	
Appropriate Revenue account		X

Figure 3–4 Classification of Routine Transaction Entries

was the money spent?'' Was it spent to acquire an asset? If so, debit the asset. Was it spent to eliminate or reduce a liability? If so, debit the appropriate liability account. Was it spent to pay an expense? If so, debit the appropriate expense account.

Cash disbursement transactions may require a debit to equity or to a revenue account, but such transactions are rather unusual. You need not be concerned with such transactions at this time.

b. If the transaction is identified as a cash receipt, you will always make a debit to cash. To determine the proper credit, you simply ask yourself: ''What was the source of the cash receipt?'' Did the cash arise from collections of patients' accounts? If so, credit accounts receivable. Was the cash obtained through the incurrence of a liability such as bank loans or bond issues? If so, credit the appropriate liability account. Does the cash receipt represent revenues provided on a cash basis, that is, cash received at the time the service is rendered? If so, credit the appropriate revenue account.

Cash receipt transactions rarely require a credit to expense, but a credit to equity sometimes is required (as you have seen in Smalltown Hospital's first journal entry). Also, hospitals occasionally sell plant assets that require a credit to land, buildings, or equipment. Later on, you will be introduced to some of these transactions.

Remember that Figure 3–4 is a classification of routine, regularly recurring transaction entries only. Such recurring transactions in practice are recorded in specialized journals that are illustrated in subsequent chapters. Until then, we will enter all transactions in a general journal. There also are other kinds of transactions not included in Figure 3–4. And, as mentioned earlier, entries other than transaction entries are made in journals, for example, adjusting entries and closing entries. You will be introduced to nontransaction entries shortly.

Ledger

At this point, we have a complete record of the transaction completed by Smalltown Hospital during 19X1. This record appears in chronological sequence in the hospital's journal. The journal, however, does not readily or directly provide the information needed for the development of financial statements. It does not provide individual account balances at the end of the year! Nowhere in the journal do we find, for example, the December 31, 19X1, cash balance. In actual practice, a general journal could consist of hundreds of pages and include perhaps thousands of transaction entries. Cash receipt and disbursement entries would appear in chronological order throughout the pages of the journal, and there would be no indication of the year-end cash balance. How, then, do we determine the December 31, 19X1, balance of cash or any other account in Smalltown Hospital's chart of accounts?

Posting Journal Data to the Ledger

To determine year-end account balances, we must transfer the information recorded in the journal to another accounting record: the *ledger*. The process of making this transfer is called *posting*. By posting to the ledger, the journalized information is summarized

Account Title: Cash						Account No.: 101			**Figure 3–5** Ledger Account
Date							Balance		
Mo.	Day	Year		Ref.	Dr.	Cr.	Dr.	Cr.	
				(Example)					
1	1	X1		GJ-1	100,000		100,000		
1	2	X1		GJ-1	50,000		150,000		
1	3	X1		GJ-1		137,000	13,000		

according to account classification so that all recorded increases and decreases in each account are brought together to permit the determination of individual account balances at the end of the year.

A ledger account, as it might appear in actual practice, is illustrated in Figure 3–5. A single page or card ordinarily is used for each account. The title and number of the account appears at the top of the form. Within the form, columns are provided to indicate the various elements of each posting to the account:

1. The date indicated generally is the date as of which the posting is being made. In other words, in posting the 19X1 journal entries, the postings to the ledger would be dated December 31, 19X1. Sometimes, however, the posting date may be the date the transaction occurred, as shown in Figure 3–5, but we will not do this in subsequent illustrations.
2. The next column may be used for memorandum entries or notations of supplemental information of value to the accountant. You may disregard this column for the time being.
3. The Ref. column (sometimes shown as LF, for *leaf folio*) is the posting reference. That means it contains the name of the journal and the page number of the journal from which the posting is made. This provides a cross-reference between the ledger and the journal.
4. The next two columns show the dollar amounts of debits and credits posted from the various journal entries affecting the account. In this way, all of the increases and decreases in each ledger account (as recorded in the journal) are brought together

on a single page so that the balance of each account can be determined.

5. The two columns on the far right are used to maintain a running balance (debit or credit, as the case may be) of the account. If debit postings exceed credit postings, the account will have a debit balance, and vice versa.

The example shown in the ledger account assumes that the account is the account for Cash, account number 101. What you see in this example are the postings to the cash account of the cash debits and credits from the first three entries of Smalltown Hospital's general journal.

The ledger account form used in the remainder of this book, however, will be the T-account form introduced in the preceding chapter. Figure 3–6 illustrates how we will make postings to these accounts. Notice that no posting dates will be indicated; we will assume that all postings are made on December 31. Instead of using a journal page number as the posting reference, we will simply use the journal entry number. And instead of maintaining a running balance in each account, we will not compute an account balance until all debit and credit postings are made.

You should recognize that Figure 3–5 illustrates only the postings of the cash debits and credits from the first three journal entries. All of the debits and credits in the journal, of course, must be posted to the appropriate ledger accounts. This will be seen in Figure 3–7.

Summary of Transaction-Recording Process

To summarize, then, the transactions for the period are initially recorded as transaction entries in the hospital's journal (Figure 3–3). Although this provides a necessary chronological record of the transactions, it does not provide the account balances resulting from those transactions. These end-of-period account balances are needed to prepare the financial statements. So, the information recorded in the journal must be rearranged and summarized in such a manner so that these balances can be determined. This is accomplished by posting (transferring) the journal entries to the ledger accounts.

The ledger contains a separate account for each account listed in the chart of accounts. Because Smalltown Hospital's chart provides for 21 accounts, the hospital's ledger consists of 21 accounts. This ledger is referred to as the *general ledger*. Just as there are several different kinds of journals, so are there several different kinds of ledgers. Ledgers other than the general ledger are called *subsidiary ledgers*. Such ledgers include the accounts receivable subsidiary ledger (or "patients' ledger"), the accounts payable ledger, the plant

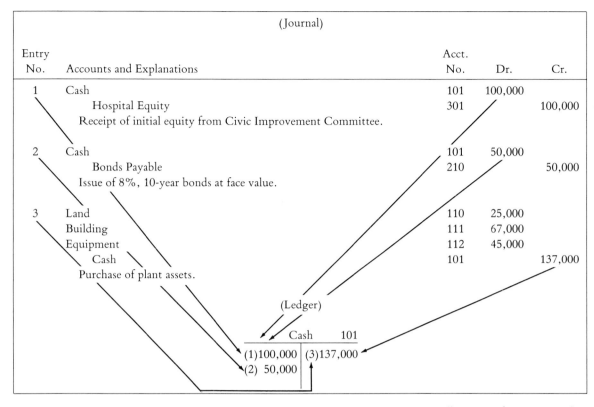

Figure 3-6 Illustration of Posting Procedure

assets subsidiary ledger, and others. Subsidiary ledgers are discussed later, but for now we are concerned only with the general ledger.

Although you may have some difficulty at first with the journalizing of transactions in journals, you should have little trouble with postings to the ledger accounts. Posting is simply a matter of copying the journal debits and credits into the ledger accounts. If the journal "says" debit cash, you debit the cash account in the ledger; if the journal indicates a credit to hospital equity, you post a credit to the ledger account for hospital equity. This procedure is easily learned. Be sure, however, that you post all debits and credits from the journal to the ledger; take care not to overlook any postings. And, unless you are attentive, you may find yourself posting debits as credits and credits as debits. If you do this, your ledger will not balance.

Figure 3-7 shows Smalltown Hospital's ledger after all postings of the 12 transaction entries have been made. It may be helpful for you to trace all of these postings from the hospital's journal (Figure 3-3) to the ledger accounts. Notice in Figure 3-7 that

Figure 3-7 Smalltown Hospital
19X1 Ledger

Cash	101	Accounts Receivable	102	Inventory	103
(1)100,000	(3)137,000	(6)120,300	(7) 94,500	(4) 28,200	(5) 21,500
(2) 50,000	(8) 22,600	(B) 25,800		(B) 6,700	
(7) 94,500	(10)96,900				
(9) 13,800	(12) 4,300				
(11)12,000					
(B) 9,500					

Land	110	Building	111	Equipment	112
(3) 25,000		(3) 67,000		(3) 45,000	

Accounts Payable	201	Bank Loan Payable	202	Bonds Payable	210
(8) 22,600	(4) 28,200		(11)12,000		(2) 50,000
	(B) 5,600				

Hospital Equity	301	Revenue and Expense Summary	302	Routine Services Revenue	401
	(1)100,000				(6) 72,180

Ancillary Services Revenue	402	Other Revenues	403	Salaries and Wages Expense	501
	(6) 48,120		(9) 13,800	(10)76,400	

Supplies Expense	502	Utilities Expense	503	Insurance Expense	504
(5) 21,500		(10)12,700		(10) 3,600	

Repairs Expense	505	Interest Expense	506	Other Expenses	507
(10) 2,900		(12) 4,300		(10) 1,300	

where an account has more than a single posting and the account
balance is not obvious, account balances at year end have been
determined. This was done by totaling the debits in the account,
totaling the credits in the account, and computing the difference
between the two totals. This difference, either a debit or a credit, is
shown as the account balance, labeled (B). If it is a debit balance, it

is shown on the left side of the account; credit balances are shown on the right side.

Only one posting appears in many of the ledger accounts because of the fact that the illustration is simplified. In actual practice, most ledger accounts have multiple postings. If, for example, the hospital pays salaries and wages to its employees on a monthly basis, the salaries and wages expense account contains 12 postings per year. We also have assumed annual postings to the ledger accounts, whereas general ledger postings are made monthly in actual practice. So do not be misled by the illustration; in an actual hospital, there typically is a considerable amount of activity in each ledger account.

One more point should be made with respect to Smalltown Hospital's ledger. You probably have noticed the revenue and expense summary account (number 302), wondering how and when it is used. The summary account is employed in the process of *closing the books,* a procedure that is discussed in Chapter 4. You need not be concerned about this account until then.

Trial Balance

At this point in Smalltown Hospital's accounting process, it would be interesting to determine whether the hospital's ledger is in balance. It should be in balance if we have made equal debits and credits in the journal, if we have posted these debits and credits correctly to the ledger accounts, and if we have made no mathematical errors in computing the balance of each account in the ledger. To ascertain whether the ledger is in balance, we can prepare a trial balance, as shown in Figure 3–8. It is a listing of all of the accounts in the ledger, with their debit or credit balances at the end of the year (or other period). The sequence in which the accounts are listed is the same as the sequence in which they appear in the ledger and in the chart of accounts.

Observe that the trial balance indicates that the Smalltown Hospital ledger is in balance. The debit balances total $301,700, as do the credit balances. A warning, however, is in order: The fact that the trial balance shows an equality of debit and credit balances is no guarantee that the dollar amounts are accurate. If the documentary evidence is incorrect or misinterpreted, the trial balance data will be incorrect. If debits and credits were made to the wrong accounts in the journal or ledger, the trial balance will include incorrect amounts. Thus, the trial balance is only a partial check on

Figure 3-8 Smalltown Hospital
Trial Balance,
December 31, 19X1

Acct. No.	Account Titles	Dr.	Cr.
101	Cash	$ 9,500	
102	Accounts Receivable	25,800	
103	Inventory	6,700	
110	Land	25,000	
111	Building	67,000	
112	Equipment	45,000	
201	Accounts Payable		$ 5,600
202	Bank Loan Payable		12,000
210	Bonds Payable		50,000
301	Hospital Equity		100,000
302	Revenue and Expense Summary		
401	Routine Services Revenue		72,180
402	Ancillary Services Revenue		48,120
403	Other Revenues		13,800
501	Salaries and Wages Expense	76,400	
502	Supplies Expense	21,500	
503	Utilities Expense	12,700	
504	Insurance Expense	3,600	
505	Repairs Expense	2,900	
506	Interest Expense	4,300	
507	Other Expenses	1,300	
	Totals	$301,700	$301,700

the accuracy of the accounting work of the period. Should the trial balance not balance, however, we know that an error has been made somewhere in the journal or ledger, or in the trial balance itself.

Smalltown Hospital's December 31, 19X1, trial balance is the starting point for the next chapter. In that chapter we will use the trial balance figures to prepare a set of annual financial statements. Chapter 4 also illustrates and discusses the use of worksheets, and describes and explains the process known as closing the books.

Questions

Q3–1. Why is documentary evidence essential to the accounting process? *evidence that a transaction has occur*

Q3–2. What is the purpose of a chart of accounts? What factors influence the design of a hospital's chart of accounts?

Q3–3. Distinguish between a chart of accounts and a ledger.

Q3–4. How does a chart of accounts differ from a trial balance?

Q3–5. Why are numerical codes assigned to the accounts in a chart of accounts? Are these codes identical in all hospitals?

Q3–6. Define each of the following terms: (a) journal, (b) journalizing, and (c) journal entry.

Q3–7. What are the five essential elements of a journal entry?

Q3–8. In recording cash receipt transactions in the journal, debits are made to cash. What types of accounts generally would be credited?

Q3–9. In recording cash disbursement transactions in the journal, credits are made to cash. What types of accounts generally would be debited?

Q3–10. What is the purpose of posting journal entries to ledger accounts?

Q3–11. What are the five essential elements of a posting to a ledger account?

Q3–12. Distinguish between general and subsidiary ledgers. Give two examples of a subsidiary ledger.

Q3–13. What is the purpose of a trial balance?

Q3–14. "If a trial balance indicates an equality of debit and credit balances, this indicates that the journal and ledger are free of errors." Do you agree? Explain.

Q3–15. "The ledger contains a separate account for each account in the hospital's chart of accounts. That is, if the chart of accounts contains 150 accounts, there will be 150 accounts in the ledger." Do you agree? Explain your opinion.

Q3–16. In what sequence are accounts listed in the ledger? In a trial balance? *Numerical*

Exercises

E3–1. Following are five multiple-choice questions:
1. The process of recording transactions in a journal is called
   a. Journalizing.
   b. Posting.
   c. Preparation of a trial balance.
   d. Closing the books.
2. The process of transferring recorded information in the journal to the ledger is called
   a. Journalizing.
   b. Posting.

    c. Accumulating.

    d. Reporting.

3. A chart of accounts is

    a. A listing of the accounts of a hospital with the account balances at the beginning of the fiscal year.

    b. A listing of the accounts of a hospital with the account balances at the end of the fiscal year.

    c. A listing of the accounts that will be used in recording and classifying the transactions of a hospital.

    d. A diagram indicating the organizational structure of the hospital.

4. A trial balance is

    a. A listing of the accounts of a hospital with the account balances at a specified date.

    b. An accounting form that presents only the revenues and expenses of the hospital for a given period.

    c. An accounting form that presents only the assets, liabilities, and equity of a hospital at a given point in time.

    d. The balance of a particular ledger account the first time you attempt to compute it.

5. An accounting record that presents the transactions of the hospital in chronological order is

    a. A journal.

    b. A ledger.

    c. A trial balance.

    d. An income statement and a balance sheet.

Required: Select the best answer for each of these multiple-choice questions.

E3–2. Compass Hospital provides you with the following information:

Accounts receivable, December 31, 19X1	$150,000
Accounts receivable, December 31, 19X2	175,000
Collections on patients' accounts during 19X2	825,000

Required: What was the amount of charges to patients for services rendered to them in 19X2?

E3–3. Catspaw Hospital provides you with the following information:

Accounts payable, December 31, 19X2	$ 45,000
Purchases of supplies on account during 19X2	316,000
Payments on accounts payable during 19X2	301,000

Required: What was the balance of accounts payable at December 31, 19X1?

E3–4. Contrail Hospital provides you with the following information:

Inventory, December 31, 19X1	$ 57,000
Inventory, December 31, 19X2	60,000
Cost of supplies purchased during 19X2	437,000

Required: What was the cost of supplies used during 19X2?

E3–5. Convex Hospital provides you with the following information:

Cost of supplies used during 19X2	$855,000
Accounts payable, December 31, 19X1	200,000
Accounts payable, December 31, 19X2	246,000
Inventory, December 31, 19X1	191,000
Inventory, December 31, 19X2	100,000

Required: What was the total amount paid on accounts payable during 19X2?

Problems

P3–1. Cupfull Hospital completed the following transactions during the month of October 19X1.
1. New equipment was purchased for $16,000 cash.
2. Supplies were purchased on account for $36,400.
3. Supplies that had cost $31,200 were issued from inventory for use in hospital activities.
4. Payments on accounts payable were $34,700.
5. Services rendered to patients during the month were billed as follows:

Routine services	$ 84,300
Ancillary services	47,900
Total	$132,200

6. Collections on patients' accounts totaled $105,750.
7. Other revenues collected in cash amounted to $13,600.
8. Operating expenses were paid as follows:

Salaries and wages	$ 82,400
Utilities	8,700
Insurance	2,900
Repairs	1,600
Other expense	7,300
Total	$102,900

9. A short-term, 9 percent loan of $15,000 was obtained from a local bank (disregard interest).

Required: Using the chart of accounts provided in Figure 3–1, prepare in good form general journal entries for each of the preceding transactions.

P3–2. Capstone Hospital began its corporate existence on January 1, 19X1. During the ensuing year, it completed the following transactions:

1. The hospital received initial capital of $250,000 from a fund-raising committee established by the citizens of Capstone. This money was deposited in a bank checking account opened in the name of Capstone Hospital.
2. The hospital issued $150,000 of 6 percent, 10-year bonds at face value. Interest on these bonds is payable annually on December 31.
3. Plant assets were purchased for cash, as follows:

Land	$ 35,000
Building	200,000
Equipment	125,000
Total	$360,000

4. Purchases of supplies on account totaled $37,500.
5. Supplies that had cost $32,000 were issued from inventory for use in hospital activities.
6. Services were billed to patients as follows:

Routine services	$ 91,000
Ancillary services	56,700
Total	$147,700

7. Cash collections on patients' accounts amounted to $121,600.
8. Payments on accounts payable totaled $24,900.
9. Other revenues received in cash amounted to $9,350.
10. Payments of operating expenses were as follows:

Salaries and wages	$ 79,250
Utilities	11,600
Insurance	4,200
Repairs	3,100
Other expenses	2,300
Total	$100,450

11. A short-term, 12 percent loan of $20,000 was obtained from a local bank.

12. On December 31 the following expense was paid:

Interest on bonds	$9,000
Interest on bank loan	600
Total	$9,600

Required: Using Figure 3–1's chart of accounts, (1) journalize the 19X1 transactions, (2) post the transaction entries to the general ledger, (3) prepare a trial balance at December 31, 19X1, (4) prepare an income statement for 19X1, and (5) prepare a balance sheet at December 31, 19X1.

P3–3. Cocktail Hospital's trial balance at January 1, 19X1, includes the following accounts:

Cash	$ 10,500	
Accounts Receivable	24,800	
Inventory	5,700	
Land	19,000	
Building	73,000	
Equipment	27,000	
Accounts Payable		$ 6,600
Bank Loan Payable		15,000
Bonds Payable		60,000
Hospital Equity		78,400
	$160,000	$160,000

The hospital completed the following transactions during the month ended January 31, 19X1:
1. Purchases of supplies on account were $4,900.
2. Supplies that had cost $5,200 were issued from inventory for use in hospital activities.
3. Services billed to patients were as follows:

Routine services	$40,800
Ancillary services	31,600
Total	$72,400

4. Cash collections on patients' accounts was $59,100.
5. Payments on accounts payable totaled $5,070.
6. Other revenues received in cash amounted to $7,300.
7. Operating expenses included these payments:

Salaries and wages	$53,200
Utilities	1,900
Insurance	1,200
Repairs	1,100

Other expenses	600
Total	$58,000

8. Payment of interest on bonds and bank loan, $870.

   Required: Using the chart of accounts provided in Figure 3–1, (1) enter the January 1, 19X1, balances in ledger accounts, (2) journalize the January 19X1 transactions, (3) post the transaction entries to the ledger accounts, (4) prepare a trial balance at January 31, 19X1, (5) prepare an income statement for January 19X1, and (6) prepare a balance sheet at January 31, 19X1.

P3–4. Copper Hospital's trial balance at November 30, 19X2, which includes data accumulated since December 31, 19X1, is the following:

101	Cash	$ 14,700	
102	Accounts Receivable	34,900	
103	Inventory	7,400	
110	Land	30,000	
111	Building	200,000	
112	Equipment	105,000	
201	Accounts Payable		$ 11,200
202	Bank Loan Payable		25,000
210	Bonds Payable		75,000
310	Hospital Equity		274,300
401	Routine Services Revenue		85,800
402	Ancillary Services Revenue		31,300
403	Other Revenues		9,400
501	Salaries and Wages Expense	95,000	
502	Supplies Expense	13,000	
503	Utilities Expense	3,600	
504	Insurance Expense	1,200	
505	Repairs Expense	1,700	
506	Interest Expense	4,500	
507	Other Expenses	1,000	
		$512,000	$512,000

The hospital completed the following transactions during the month of December 19X2:
1. Purchases of supplies on account amounted to $2,300.
2. Supplies that had cost $1,100 were issued from inventory for use in hospital activities.
3. Payments on accounts payable totaled $3,060.

4. Services billed to patients were

Routine services	$ 9,300
Ancillary services	6,070
Total	$15,370

5. Cash collections on patients' accounts totaled $16,140.
6. Other revenues received in cash totaled $980.
7. Payments of operating expenses included

Salaries and wages	$9,100
Utilities	300
Insurance	150
Repairs	240
Other expenses	80
Total	$9,870

8. Payment of interest on bonds and bank loan amounted to $850.

Required: Using the chart of accounts provided in Figure 3–1, (1) enter the November 30, 19X1, balances in ledger accounts, (2) journalize the December 19X1 transactions, (3) post the transaction entries to the ledger accounts, (4) prepare a trial balance at December 31, 19X1, (5) prepare an income statement for the year ended December 31, 19X1, and (6) prepare a balance sheet at December 31, 19X1.

Worksheets, Financial Statements, and Closing Entries

4

In the previous chapter, you had an opportunity to examine three of the initial steps in the accounting process: recording transaction entries in a general journal, posting these entries to a general ledger, and preparing a trial balance. The discussion centered around the business transactions completed by a hypothetical Smalltown Hospital during 19X1, the first year of that hospital's economic life. That illustration continues in this chapter as we explore worksheets, financial statements, and closing entries.

This chapter illustrates a simplified version of the *worksheets* (or, as they are sometimes called, *working papers*) widely used by accountants as a device to facilitate the preparation of financial statements. The worksheet you develop will lead to an illustration and discussion of Smalltown Hospital's 19X1 income statement and December 31, 19X1, balance sheet. The last section of this chapter describes and demonstrates the procedures performed to close the books for Smalltown Hospital.

General Worksheet

After transaction entries have been journalized and posted, a trial balance is prepared of the ledger account balances. Financial statements may be prepared directly from the trial balance listing of accounts. In most cases, where a large number of accounts is involved, the development of the financial statements can be facilitated by the preparation of a general worksheet. A major purpose of the worksheet is to classify and segregate the trial balance figures according to the financial statements in which they will be presented. Other purposes of the worksheet will be shown in subsequent chapters. In addition, later chapters will introduce you to special-purpose worksheets.

A worksheet to develop financial statements for 19X1 for Smalltown Hospital is illustrated in Figure 4–1. Note the following points:

1. The trial balance at December 31, 19X1, is entered on the left-hand side, with the dollar amounts being shown in the first two columns. This is the same trial balance that was developed in the preceding chapter and illustrated in Figure 3–8.
2. Next, the individual balances in the trial balance are extended to the appropriate financial statement columns. Debit balances are extended as debits, and credit balances are extended as credits, as follows:
    a. Asset and liability account balances are extended into the balance sheet section.
    b. The trial balance figure for hospital equity is extended into the equity statement section. This statement will be discussed in the next part of this chapter.
    c. The revenue and expense summary account has no balance and can be disregarded in the preparation of the worksheet. The summary account is used only in the process of closing the books.
    d. Revenue and expense account balances are extended into the income statement section of the worksheet.

Categorizing Trial Balance
Items on Worksheets

In this way, the individual trial balance items are categorized or assembled into groups according to the financial statements in which the items will be presented.
3. Totals now are taken of the debits and credits in the income statement section; debits total $122,700, and credits total $134,100. Because the debits are expenses and the credits are revenues, the difference ($11,400) is the 19X1 net income. The net income figure ($11,400) is shown in the income statement section as a *debit* simply to balance the columns at $134,100. In addition, the $11,400 net income is extended as a credit to the equity statement section of the worksheet.
4. Then, totals are taken of the debits (none) and credits in the equity statement section. In certain situations, there could be debits to the equity statement, but you need not be concerned with that possibility at this time. The credits to the equity statement include the $100,000 of hospital equity on January 1, 19X1, and the $11,400 net income for 19X1. This credit total of $111,400 is the amount of the hospital equity on December 31,

Acct. No.	Account Title	12/31/X1 Trial Balance		Income Statement		Equity Statement		Balance Sheet	
		Dr.	Cr.	Dr.	Cr.	Dr.	Cr.	Dr.	Cr.
101	Cash	9,500						9,500	
102	Accounts Receivable	25,800						25,800	
103	Inventory	6,700						6,700	
110	Land	25,000						25,000	
111	Building	67,000						67,000	
112	Equipment	45,000						45,000	
201	Accounts Payable		5,600						5,600
202	Bank Loan Payable		12,000						12,000
210	Bonds Payable		50,000						50,000
301	Hospital Equity		100,000				100,000		
302	Revenue and Expense Summary		- - -						
401	Routine Services Revenue		72,180		72,180				
402	Ancillary Services Revenue		48,120		48,120				
403	Other Revenues		13,800		13,800				
501	Salaries and Wages Expense	76,400		76,400					
502	Supplies Expense	21,500		21,500					
503	Utilities Expense	12,700		12,700					
504	Insurance Expense	3,600		3,600					
505	Repairs Expense	2,900		2,900					
506	Interest Expense	4,300		4,300					
507	Other Expenses	1,300		1,300					
	Totals	301,700	301,700	122,700	134,100				
	Net income for the year			11,400			11,400		
	Totals			134,100	134,100	-0-	111,400		
	Hospital equity, 12/31/X1					111,400			111,400
	Totals					111,400	111,400	179,000	179,000

Figure 4–1 Smalltown Hospital Worksheet to Develop Financial Statements, Year Ended December 31, 19X1

19X1. The $111,400 figure is entered in the equity statement section as a *debit* simply to balance the columns; the figure also is extended to the balance sheet section as a credit item.

5. A final step in completion of the worksheet is totaling the debits and credits in the balance sheet section. Notice that these columns balance with totals of $179,000.

Thus, a primary function of the worksheet is to assemble the account balances in financial statement groupings. This, of course, facilitates preparation of the formal financial statements.

Financial Statements

The assembled data provided by the worksheet can now be used in the preparation of 19X1 financial statements for Smalltown Hospital. These statements, in the order in which they usually are prepared, are as follows:

1. An income statement for the year ended December 31, 19X1, illustrated in Figure 4–2.
2. A statement of hospital equity for the year ended December 31, 19X1, illustrated in Figure 4–3.
3. A balance sheet at December 31, 19X1, illustrated in Figure 4–4.

As previously stated, financial statements are the final product of the accounting process. They are the means by which financial information is communicated to hospital management and interested external parties for use in making economic decisions.

Income Statement

The heading of the income statement (Figure 4–2) identifies the accounting entity as Smalltown Hospital, indicates that the state-

Figure 4–2 Smalltown Hospital Income Statement, Year Ended December 31, 19X1

Patient Service Revenues:		
Routine Services	$ 72,180	
Ancillary Services	48,120	
Total Patient Service Revenues	120,300	
Other Revenues	13,800	
Total Revenues		$134,100
Less Operating Expenses:		
Salaries and Wages	76,400	
Supplies	21,500	
Utilities	12,700	
Insurance	3,600	
Repairs	2,900	
Interest	4,300	
Other	1,300	
Total Operating Expenses		122,700
Net income for the year		$ 11,400

ment is an income statement, and specifies the time period covered by the statement as being the year ended December 31, 19X1. This statement presents the operating results of the hospital for 19X1 in terms of revenues earned and expenses incurred. The result of operations, measured as the difference between revenues earned and expenses incurred, is the *net income* (or net loss, in some cases).

Smalltown Hospital's income statement has been prepared in accordance with the *accrual basis* of accounting. Under this system of accounting, revenues are recognized and recorded in the time period in which they are earned by the hospital in rendering services and selling products to patients and others, regardless of when (if ever) the related inflow of cash occurs. Expenses are recognized and recorded in the time period in which they are incurred or consumed in revenue-producing activities of the hospital, regardless of when (if ever) the related outflow of cash occurs. The accrual basis is a generally accepted accounting principle that should be employed by all hospitals.

Accrual Versus Cash Basis Accounting

The alternative to the accrual system is the *cash basis* of accounting. In this system of accounting, revenues are recognized and recorded in the time period in which they are received in cash; expenses are recognized and recorded in the time period in which they are paid in cash. An income statement prepared on a cash basis, then, is little more than a statement of cash receipts and cash disbursements (and an incomplete statement at that, because not all cash receipts are revenues and not all disbursements are expenses). Thus, the cash basis of accounting is not appropriate for hospitals or, for that matter, most other enterprises for external reporting purposes.

Smalltown Hospital's income statement, then, is a statement of revenues earned and expenses incurred during 19X1. It is *not* a statement of cash received and disbursed. The term *revenue* does not mean cash receipts, nor is the term *expense* synonymous with cash disbursements. Notice, for example, that the income statement of Smalltown Hospital reports $120,300 of revenues earned from patient services. How much of this amount has been received in cash? Having seen the 19X1 transactions, you know that only $94,500 was collected during the year on patients' accounts. And where is the other $25,800? It is presented in the balance sheet as accounts receivable (see Figure 4–4)! Thus, $120,300 of patient services were rendered by Smalltown Hospital during 19X1, and this is the amount reported as revenues for the year, although $25,800 of that amount will not be collected until 19X2.

Or consider the $21,500 supplies expense item in the income statement of Smalltown Hospital. Is this the amount of supplies purchased and paid for during 19X1? No! Having worked with the 19X1 transactions, you know that $28,200 of supplies were purchased on account during the year and that cash payments of only $22,600 were made to the suppliers of these items. The income statement of the year is charged only for the cost of supplies consumed in activities of the period. As a result of this accrual basis accounting, the balance sheet reports a $6,700 inventory and $5,600 of accounts payable to suppliers. These items would not appear in the balance sheet if cash basis accounting were employed.

Net Income Not Directly Linked to Cash Balance in Short Run

All of this also means that there is no necessary short-run relationship between reported net income and the change in the cash balance during the year. Smalltown Hospital begins the year with $100,000 of cash but ends the year with a cash balance of only $9,500. Thus, in a year when a $11,400 net income is reported, the cash balance decreases by more than $90,000! Do not get the idea, therefore, that the income statement is a presentation of cash flows.

Cash flows, however, are vitally important in the management of a hospital. In addition to income statements and balance sheets, accountants also prepare statements of cash flows (cash receipts and disbursements) for internal management and external reporting purposes. A discussion of such statements will appear later in this book.

You should understand that the two-column format in which the income statement is presented in Figure 4–2 in no way implies a debit and credit relationship. The left-hand column is not necessarily a debit column, nor is the right-hand column necessarily a credit column. There are no debit or credit columns in financial statements. The number of columns employed is only a matter of presentation (display) style. The income statement, for example, could be formatted in a single column.

Equity Statement

A statement of hospital equity for the year ended December 31, 19X1, is illustrated for Smalltown Hospital in Figure 4–3. The statement begins with the equity figure at January 1. To this figure we add the 19X1 net income as indicated by the income statement. (If a net loss had been reported, the net loss would be subtracted from the January 1 equity balance.) The resulting amount is the amount of hospital equity at December 31. This dollar amount, of course, is the equity balance to be reported in the December 31, 19X1, balance sheet.

Hospital Equity, January 1[a]	$100,000
Add Net Income for the Year	11,400
Hospital Equity, December 31	$111,400

[a]This represents the contribution of initial equity funds received on January 1, 19X1, from the Smalltown Civic Improvement Committee, when the hospital began its operations.

Figure 4–3 Smalltown Hospital Statement of Hospital Equity, Year Ended December 31, 19X1

For the present purpose, assume that a hospital's equity is affected (changed) only by the net income or net loss of the period. Later on you will see, however, that the hospital equity balance is increased and decreased by other factors, particularly when a fund accounting system is used. When these factors are introduced, a more realistic equity statement will be illustrated.

The equity statement provides a connection between the income statement and the balance sheet. It also explains the change in the equity balance from one balance sheet to the next. It is an essential financial statement, one that all hospitals should prepare and include in their annual financial reports.

Equity Statement Links Income Statement and Balance Sheet

Balance Sheet

Smalltown Hospital's December 31, 19X1, balance sheet is illustrated in Figure 4–4. Notice that the heading provides the name of the accounting entity, the name of the statement, and the date of the statement. Unlike the dating of the income statement and equity statement, the dating of the balance sheet specifies a particular point in time. The information in the balance sheet applies only to the financial position of the hospital at the "close of business" on December 31, 19X1. Most of the balance sheet figures were different on the preceding day and will also be different on the next day. The balance sheet is somewhat like a photographic snapshot, whereas the income and equity statements are more like moving pictures covering a period of time.

The financial position of Smalltown Hospital is presented in terms of its assets, liabilities, and equity on December 31, 19X1. Assets are the economic resources of the hospital that are recognized and measured in conformity with generally accepted accounting principles. Liabilities are the economic obligations of the hospital that are recognized and measured in conformity with generally accepted accounting principles. Equity, sometimes called *fund balance, capital,* or *net worth,* is the excess of assets over liabilities. Because most of the assets are reported in the balance sheet at cost rather than at what they are "worth," however, the use of the term *net worth* can be misleading. So, this book uses the term *equity*.

Elements of Financial Position

Figure 4-4 Smalltown Hospital
Balance Sheet,
December 31, 19X1

Assets		
Cash	$ 9,500	
Accounts Receivable	25,800	
Inventory	6,700	
Total Current Assets		$ 42,000
Land	25,000	
Building	67,000	
Equipment	45,000	
Total Plant Assets		137,000
Total Assets		$179,000
Liabilities and Equity		
Accounts Payable	$ 5,600	
Bank Loan Payable	12,000	
Total Current Liabilities		$ 17,600
Long-Term Debt (8% Bonds Payable)		50,000
Total Liabilities		67,600
Hospital Equity		111,400
Total Liabilities and Equity		$179,000

Current and Noncurrent
Assets

Smalltown Hospital's assets are listed in the sequence usually seen in actual practice. The assets are classified into two main groups: current assets and noncurrent assets (which, in this situation, consist only of plant assets). The current assets consist of cash plus those other assets that are likely to be converted into cash within a short period (one year or less). Normally, the plant assets are reduced by depreciation, but for simplicity we are disregarding the matter of depreciation for the time being.

Current and Noncurrent
Liabilities

Smalltown Hospital's liabilities and equity also are listed in the usual sequence. Like the assets, the liabilities are classified into two major categories: current liabilities and noncurrent (or "long-term") liabilities. The *current liabilities* consist of debts that ordinarily are paid within a short time (one year or less). In this example, the *noncurrent liabilities* comprise a single item: the 8 percent bonds due in nine more years. A total of liabilities is obtained, and to it is added the hospital equity balance as reported in the equity statement. Then, of course, you see that total assets equal the total of liabilities and equity (the accounting equation).

As this book unfolds, you will develop more sophisticated financial statements. Many additional accounts will be introduced into the statements, and the impact of fund accounting and responsibility accounting on the statements will be described. We also must probe more deeply into problems of terminology, classification, valuation, and disclosure. The subject of financial analysis and interpretation also is covered in subsequent chapters.

Once the financial statements are prepared, the accountant can proceed to the last step in the accounting process. This procedure is known as *closing the books*. It consists of the closing of revenue and expense accounts in the hospital's ledger and the adjustment of the hospital equity to the balance at which it is stated in the year-end balance sheet. The balances of revenue and expense accounts in Smalltown Hospital's ledger relate only to the 19X1 year. These balances therefore must be eliminated to prepare the ledger for the next accounting period and to avoid the commingling of revenue and expense balances of one year with those of the next year.

Balance sheet accounts, referred to as *real (permanent) accounts*, are not closed. The balances of these accounts—assets, liabilities, and equity—are carried over into the next year as the opening balances for that year. The accounts to be closed are the income statement accounts, often called *nominal (temporary) accounts*. Thus, all revenue and expense account balances are closed; these accounts begin the next year with zero balances.

A closing of the books is accomplished by making what are called *closing entries* in the hospital's journal and by posting these entries to the ledger accounts. Figure 4–5 presents the closing entries for Smalltown Hospital for 19X1.

The first closing entry is one to eliminate the revenue account balances. Recall that all revenue accounts have credit balances. The closing entry, therefore, debits each revenue account for its credit balance as shown in the hospital's ledger. A credit is made in this entry to the revenue and expense summary account for the total revenues of the period. This credit balances the entry (entry number 13).

A second closing entry is made to remove the expense account balances from the ledger. Because the expense accounts have debit balances, this entry credits each of the expense accounts for its debit balance. The total of these credits (total expenses for the period) is debited to the revenue and expense summary. This is entry 14.

The third and last closing entry (number 15) is one to close the revenue and expense summary account and to add the net income for 19X1 to the hospital equity account. Because the revenue and expense summary account has been debited (entry 14) for total expenses and credited (entry 13) for total revenues, that account

Closing the Books

Real and Nominal Accounts

Closing Entries

Entry No.	Accounts and Explanations	Acct. No.	Dr.	Cr.
13	Routine Services Revenue	401	72,180	
	Ancillary Services Revenue	402	48,120	
	Other Revenues	403	13,800	
	Revenue and Expense Summary	302		134,100
	To close revenue accounts.			
14	Revenue and Expense Summary	302	122,700	
	Salaries and Wages Expense	501		76,400
	Supplies Expense	502		21,500
	Utilities Expense	503		12,700
	Insurance Expense	504		3,600
	Repairs Expense	505		2,900
	Interest Expense	506		4,300
	Other Expense	507		1,300
	To close expense accounts.			
15	Revenue and Expense Summary	302	11,400	
	Hospital Equity	301		11,400
	To close revenue and expense summary, and to add net income for 19X1 to the hospital equity.			

Figure 4–5 Smalltown Hospital 19X1 Journal Closing Entries

now has a credit balance in the amount of the net income for the period. The debit to the summary account in entry 15 for the net income therefore will close that account. If the hospital had a net loss for the period, of course, the debit and credit in this entry would be reversed.

The posting of these three closing entries from Smalltown Hospital's journal to its ledger accounts is shown in Figure 4–6. It is suggested that you trace the individual postings into the ledger. They are referenced as numbers 13, 14, and 15. Notice also that the closing of the revenue accounts, expense accounts, and the revenue and expense summary account is indicated in the ledger by the "double-ruling" of the individual accounts.

Starting the Next Year's Books

Smalltown Hospital's ledger now contains balance sheet accounts only; all other accounts have been closed. These remaining ledger balances are left open to become the beginning ledger balances of the ensuing year. None of the revenue or expense accounts have balances, so these accounts are ready to receive postings of the next year's revenues and expenses. In this way, the revenues and

Cash 101		Accounts Receivable 102		Inventory 103	
(1)100,000	(3)137,000	(6)120,300	(7) 94,500	(4) 28,200	(5) 21,500
(2) 50,000	(8) 22,600				
(7) 94,500	(10)96,900	(B) 25,800		(B) 6,700	
(9) 13,800	(12) 4,300				
(11)12,000					
(B) 9,500					

Land 110		Building 111		Equipment 112	
(3) 25,000		(3) 67,000		(3) 45,000	

Accounts Payable 201		Bank Loan Payable 202		Bonds Payable 210	
(8) 22,600	(4) 28,200		(11)12,000		(2) 50,000
	(B) 5,600				

Hospital Equity 301		Revenue and Expense Summary 302		Routine Services Revenue 401	
	(1)100,000	(14)122,700	(13)134,100	(13)72,180	(6) 72,180
	(15)11,400	(15) 11,400			
	(B)111,400				

Ancillary Services Revenue 402		Other Revenues 403		Salaries and Wages Expense 501	
(13) 48,120	(6) 48,120	(13)13,800	(9) 13,800	(10)76,400	(14)76,400

Supplies Expense 502		Utilities Expense 503		Insurance Expense 504	
(5) 21,500	(14)21,500	(10)12,700	(14)12,700	(10) 3,600	(14) 3,600

Repairs Expense 505		Interest Expense 506		Other Expense 507	
(10) 2,900	(14) 2,900	(12) 4,300	(14) 4,300	(10) 1,300	(14) 1,300

Figure 4–6 Smalltown Hospital 19X1 Ledger (With Closing Entries)

Figure 4-7 Smalltown Hospital
Postclosing Trial Balance,
December 31, 19X1

Acct. No.	Account Titles	Dr.	Cr.
101	Cash	$ 9,500	
102	Accounts Receivable	25,800	
103	Inventory	6,700	
110	Land	25,000	
111	Building	67,000	
112	Equipment	45,000	
201	Accounts Payable		$ 5,600
202	Bank Loan Payable		12,000
210	Bonds Payable		50,000
301	Hospital Equity		111,400
302	Revenue and Expense Summary		
401	Routine Services Revenue		
402	Ancillary Services Revenue		
403	Other Revenues		
501	Salaries and Wages Expense		
502	Supplies Expense		
503	Utilities Expense		
504	Insurance Expense		
505	Repairs Expense		
506	Interest Expense		
507	Other Expenses		
	Totals	$179,000	$179,000

expenses of one year are not commingled with the revenues and expenses of the next year. This aids the measurement of net income for each year.

Checking Whether the
Accounts Balance

At this point, another trial balance may be taken of the ledger to determine whether the accounts are in balance after the books are closed. This trial balance is called a *postclosing trial balance*; the trial balance illustrated in Chapter 3 as Figure 3-8 is referred to as a *preclosing trial balance*. A postclosing trial balance for Smalltown Hospital is presented in Figure 4-7. Notice that it contains balance sheet account balances only. These are the account balances with which Smalltown Hospital will begin 19X2.

Summary of Accounting Procedure

It should be useful at this time to present a summary of the operations we have covered so far. All of the procedures or operations performed during the annual accounting period are together called the accounting cycle. The steps in this cycle discussed and illustrated up to this point are summarized in the diagram in Figure 4-8.

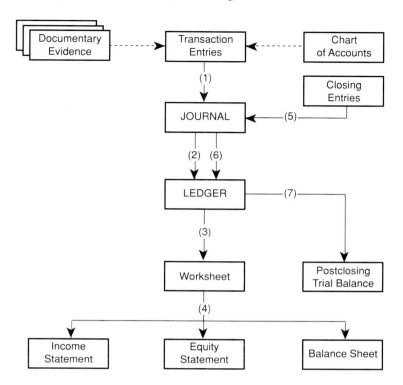

Figure 4–8 Summary of Accounting Procedure

Assuming the existence of documentary evidences of transactions and a well-designed chart of accounts, the steps in the accounting cycle are as follows:

1. Journalize transaction entries in the journal.
2. Post transaction entries from the journal to the ledger and determine individual account balances.
3. Enter the preclosing trial balance on a worksheet and complete the worksheet.
4. Prepare financial statements from the information provided on the worksheet.
5. Journalize closing entries in the journal.
6. Post closing entries from the journal to the ledger.
7. Prepare a postclosing trial balance of the account balances now remaining in the ledger.

There are, however, additional steps involved in a complete accounting cycle. One of these additional steps is the journalizing and posting of another kind of journal entry called the *adjusting entry.* This procedure, often a matter of considerable difficulty for introductory accounting students, is treated in detail in the next three chapters.

Questions

Q4-1. What is the major purpose of a general worksheet?

Q4-2. Distinguish between the cash basis and the accrual basis of accounting.

Q4-3. Distinguish between revenues and cash receipts.

Q4-4. Distinguish between expenses and cash disbursements.

Q4-5. Why should cash basis accounting not be used by hospitals?

Q4-6. What is the purpose of the statement of hospital equity?

Q4-7. Define briefly each of the following terms: (a) assets, (b) liabilities, and (c) equity.

Q4-8. Describe briefly the procedure known as closing the books.

Q4-9. Distinguish between "real" and "nominal" accounts.

Q4-10. Distinguish between a preclosing trial balance and a post-closing trial balance.

Q4-11. List, in the sequence normally completed, the steps involved in an accounting cycle.

Q4-12. What is the significance of "double rulings" in ledger accounts?

Exercises

E4-1. Dowdy Hospital provides you with the following information:

Revenues for 19X2	$500,000
Expenses for 19X2	450,000
Hospital equity, December 31, 19X1	860,000
Revenue and expense summary	-0-

Required: (1) Prepare closing entries for 19X2 in general journal form. (2) What is the hospital's equity balance on December 31, 19X2?

E4-2. Doit Hospital provides you with the following information:

Assets	$350,000
Liabilities	150,000
Hospital equity	180,000

Revenues $420,000

Expenses 400,000

Required: (1) Prepare a preclosing trial balance. (2) Prepare a postclosing trial balance.

E4–3. Devon Hospital provides you with the following information:

Revenue and Expense
Summary   302

787,000	800,000
13,000	

Required: Answer the following questions:

1. What were total revenues for the year?
2. What were total expenses for the year?
3. What was the net income (loss) for the year?
4. If hospital equity was $400,000 at the beginning of the year, what was hospital equity at the end of the year?

E4–4. Following are five multiple-choice questions:

1. Posting is an accounting procedure in which
   a. Information is transferred from the ledger to the journal.
   b. Information is transferred from the journal to the ledger.
   c. Information is transferred from the ledger to the hospital financial statements.
   d. Information is transferred from the trial balance to the ledger.
2. A trial balance can be prepared
   a. Only before the books are closed.
   b. Only after the books are closed.
   c. Either before or after the books are closed.
   d. Only at the end of the fiscal year.
3. In closing entries
   a. Expense accounts are always debited.
   b. Expense accounts are always credited.
   c. Expense accounts may be debited in some cases, and credited in other cases.
   d. Expense accounts are not debited or credited.

4. Under the accrual basis of accounting, revenues are recorded
   a. In the period in which they are collected in cash.
   b. In the period in which they are earned through the provision of services or the sale of products.
   c. In the period in which management decides they should be recognized.
   d. In the period in which the income tax laws indicate that they are taxable.

5. Dawson Hospital provides you with the following information:

Value of services rendered to patients	$600,000
Cash collections on patients' accounts	540,000
Cash disbursements for expenses	530,000
Expenses incurred during the period	550,000

   Under the accrual basis of accounting, the net income (loss) of the period should be
   a. $(10,000).
   b. $10,000.
   c. $50,000.
   d. $70,000.

Required: Select the best answer to each of the above questions.

Problems

P4-1. The following balances, among others, appeared in the general ledger of Dent Hospital at the end of its fiscal year:

Acct. No.

301	Hospital equity	$143,674
302	Revenue and expense summary	-0-
401	Routine services revenue	85,375
402	Ancillary services revenue	52,939
403	Other revenues	21,655
501	Salaries and wages expense	101,488
502	Supplies expense	22,475
503	Utilities expense	13,880
504	Insurance expense	4,203
505	Repairs expense	1,922
506	Interest expense	3,077
507	Other expenses	1,249

Required: Prepare, in good form, general journal entries to close the books of Dent Hospital for the year.

P4–2. Following is the preclosing trial balance of Dunston Hospital on December 31, 19X2:

Acct. No.		Dr.	Cr.
101	Cash	$ 11,200	
102	Accounts Receivable	27,400	
103	Inventory	7,300	
110	Land	15,000	
111	Building	80,000	
112	Equipment	35,000	
201	Accounts Payable		$ 6,900
202	Bank Loan Payable		14,000
210	Bonds Payable		60,000
301	Hospital Equity		96,900
302	Revenue and Expense Summary		-0-
401	Routine Services Revenue		86,400
402	Ancillary Services Revenue		41,700
403	Other Revenues		19,200
501	Salaries and Wages Expense	94,600	
502	Supplies Expense	28,700	
503	Utilities Expense	13,400	
504	Insurance Expense	3,100	
505	Repairs Expense	2,700	
506	Interest Expense	4,400	
507	Other Expenses	2,300	
	Totals	$325,100	$325,100

Required: (1) Prepare a general worksheet to develop financial statements for the year ended December 31, 19X2. (2) Prepare, in good form, financial statements for 19X2. (3) Prepare, in general journal form, closing entries for 19X2.

P4–3. The following balances, among others, appeared in the general ledger of Dixon Hospital at the end of its fiscal year:

Acct. No.		
301	Hospital Equity	$294,600
302	Revenue and Expense Summary	-0-
401	Routine Services Revenue	121,800
402	Ancillary Services Revenue	87,500
403	Other Revenues	26,300
501	Salaries and Wages Expense	155,400
502	Supplies Expense	31,400

503	Utilities Expense	$ 18,700
504	Insurance Expense	6,400
505	Repairs Expense	3,900
506	Interest Expense	7,500
507	Other Expenses	3,300

Required: (1) Enter the balances in ledger accounts. (2) Journalize the necessary closing entries for the year. (3) Post the closing entries to the ledger accounts.

P4–4. The following balances appeared in the general ledger of Deerly Hospital at December 31, 19X2:

Acct. No.

101	Cash	$ 31,100
102	Accounts Receivable	89,700
103	Inventory	11,200
110	Land	25,000
111	Building	240,000
112	Equipment	114,000
201	Accounts Payable	22,800
202	Bank Loan Payable	28,000
210	Bonds Payable	75,000
301	Hospital Equity	372,300
302	Revenue and Expense Summary	-0-
401	Routine Services Revenue	140,700
402	Ancillary Services Revenue	79,900
403	Other Revenues	21,300
501	Salaries and Wages Expense	150,800
502	Supplies Expense	38,500
503	Utilities Expense	22,100
504	Insurance Expense	4,700
505	Repairs Expense	3,200
506	Interest Expense	7,900
507	Other Expenses	1,800

Required: (1) Prepare a general worksheet to develop financial statements for the year ended December 31, 19X2. (2) Prepare, in good form, financial statements for 19X2. (3) Prepare, in general journal form, closing entries for 19X2.

Prepaid and Accrued Expenses

5

In the two preceding chapters, Smalltown Hospital's 19X1 transactions were entered in the journal and posted to the ledger. A trial balance of the ledger accounts was then prepared. We assumed that the trial balance dollar amounts were the correct account balances at the end of the year, and these figures were used in the development of financial statements for 19X1. In actual practice, however, many of the account balances included in the trial balance are likely to be incorrect! This means that financial statements should not be prepared until the incorrect balances in the trial balance are adjusted to reflect the correct amounts. The necessary corrections are accomplished by journalizing and posting *adjusting entries*. All of the required adjustments must be made before financial statements are prepared.

Incorrect account balances will appear in the trial balance regardless of the amount of care exercised in recording the transactions of the period. Some of the reasons for this are as follows:

1. *Prepaid and Accrued Expenses.* The trial balance may include expense accounts whose balances are overstated or understated because of
   a. The prepayment of expenses during the period
   b. The failure to recognize expenses that were incurred during the current period but that will not be paid until the next period

Adjustments for prepaid and accrued expenses are illustrated and discussed in this chapter.

2. *Deferred and Accrued Revenues.* The trial balance may include revenue accounts whose balances are overstated or understated because of

    a. The receipt of revenues in advance

    b. The failure to recognize revenues that were earned during the current period but that will not be received until the next period

Adjustments for deferred and accrued revenues are illustrated and discussed in Chapter 6.

3. *Revenue Deductions.* The trial balance may include incorrect balances in accounts representing revenue deductions, such as charity service and bad debts. Chapter 7 deals with adjustments of this type.

4. *Depreciation.* The trial balance may not reflect the correct amount of depreciation expense relating to hospital buildings and equipment. Adjustments for depreciation are discussed in Chapter 7.

These are the types of adjusting entries we will examine in this chapter and in Chapters 6 and 7. After we explore the types of adjusting entries, all of the various adjustments will be brought together in a comprehensive illustration in Chapter 8.

Matching Principle

Chapter 4 made a very important distinction between cash basis accounting and accrual basis accounting. You have seen that the business life of the hospital entity is divided into time segments called accounting periods. So far we have assumed that these accounting periods are calendar years—that is, the 12 months from January 1 through December 31. This is the fiscal year employed by Smalltown Hospital. Many hospitals have adopted a fiscal year or accounting period, however, that ends June 30 or September 30. Such a fiscal period generally is referred to as the *natural business year.* No matter what the annual period may be, it is broken down into monthly reporting periods. In actual practice, the hospital will prepare monthly as well as annual financial statements.

Cash Versus Accrual Basis of Accounting

    Regardless of the period involved, a major accounting objective is the measurement of the net income for the period. How is this determination made? Under the pure cash basis method of accounting, the revenues of the period are only those received in cash during the period; the expenses recognized are only those paid in cash during the period. However, the cash basis procedure is not a generally accepted method of accounting for hospitals.

    Under the accrual basis method of accounting, the revenues of the period are considered to be those that were earned during the period, regardless of whether the related cash was received during the same period. The expenses of the period primarily are those incurred in the production of the revenue of the period, regardless of whether the related cash was expended during the same period. In addition, certain other expenses may be recognized during the period by a process of systematic and rational allocation, even though those expenses cannot be directly associated with the revenues of that period. The accrual basis is a generally accepted accounting principle on which the financial statements of hospitals must be based.

This brings us to the *matching principle*. The revenues of the hospital are "matched" with the accounting period during which they are earned. To put it another way, revenues must be recognized and recorded in the time period during which they are earned by the hospital through the provision of services and the sale of goods to patients and others. Revenues are earned when a hospital renders services to patients, when assets are sold, and when the hospital rents its assets to others. The hospital may receive cash prior to the earning of the revenue, at the time the revenue is earned, or after the earning of the revenue. Unfortunately, hospitals also may earn revenues for which they are never paid. Revenue deductions related to the matching principle are treated in Chapter 6.

The matching principle also has important implications for recognition of hospital expenses. The expenses of the hospital are "matched" to the extent practicable with the revenues to which they are related. In other words, expenses are incurred in the production of revenues. Once the revenues of a given time period are measured and recorded, the expenses incurred in the production of those revenues should be recognized and recorded in the same period. There is, then, a "matching" of expenses with revenues in each accounting period to permit a meaningful and useful measurement of periodic net income.

Not all hospital costs can be directly and easily associated with specific revenues. Yet, such costs must be charged as expenses to one or more accounting periods at one time or another. When no direct association of expenses with revenues can be made, the costs are "matched" with the accounting period or periods that they benefit. If more than one accounting period benefits from a cost expenditure, the cost is allocated to expense on some systematic and rational basis. If a cost expenditure is made during the current period and no future benefit is expected, that cost is charged in its entirety to expense of the current period (the immediate recognition con-

Matching Revenues with Period in Which They Are Earned

cept). Expense adjustments related to the matching principle are treated later in this chapter and in Chapter 7.

Prepaid Expenses

Prepaid expenses, sometimes called *deferred expenses* or *deferred charges,* are expenditures made by the hospital for goods and services not yet consumed or used in hospital operations. They are therefore recognized as expense in a future accounting period (or periods). Because these cost expenditures benefit one or more future accounting periods, they should be appropriately classified in the balance sheet as assets. Prepaid expenses, then, may be referred to as unexpired or "unexpensed" costs. Some examples of prepaid expenses are prepaid insurance, prepaid interest, and prepaid rent.

Adjusting the Trial Balance for Prepayments

At the end of each accounting period, the trial balance must be scanned to determine the need for adjustments arising because of prepayments of expenses by the hospital. An analysis often must be made of the debits and credits in each of the accounts to develop the necessary adjusting entries. As a basis for illustration, we will assume a hypothetical Hoosier Hospital at the end of its first year of operations. This hospital's December 31, 19X1, trial balance is shown in Figure 5–1. From this point on, the trial balance taken after all transaction entries have been journalized and posted will be called a *preadjusted trial balance* (to distinguish it from an adjusted trial balance and from a postclosing trial balance). Certain of the accounts included in Figure 5–1 have not been specifically discussed before, but the nature and use of each of these accounts will soon become apparent to you.

Prepaid Insurance

Observe that Hoosier Hospital's preadjusted trial balance includes a prepaid insurance account (number 107) with a debit balance of $3,600. Normally, we would expect Hoosier Hospital also to have some amount of insurance expense for the 19X1 year, but the insurance expense account (number 604) has no balance whatever! It would seem obvious that an adjustment is needed here.

To determine the necessary adjustment, we need to examine copies of the hospital's insurance policies. Let us assume that we discover a single comprehensive insurance policy for which the hospital paid a three-year premium in advance on January 1, 19X1. The amount of the premium was $3,600, meaning that the hospital's insurance expense is $1,200 per year; that is, a third of the insurance premium expired in 19X1. The transaction entry made by Hoosier Hospital on January 1, 19X1, when the premium was paid, must have been as follows:

Acct. No.	Account Titles	Dr.	Cr.
101	Cash	$ 38,300	
102	Temporary Investments	12,000	
103	Accrued Interest Receivable	-0-	
104	Accounts Receivable	96,600	
105	Allowance for Uncollectible Accounts		$ -0-
106	Inventory	10,500	
107	Prepaid Insurance	3,600	
108	Prepaid Rent	1,080	
109	Prepaid Interest	720	
150	Land	25,000	
160	Building	180,000	
161	Accumulated Depreciation—Building		-0-
170	Equipment	60,000	
171	Accumulated Depreciation—Equipment		-0-
201	Accounts Payable		29,840
202	Notes Payable		18,000
203	Accrued Interest Payable		-0-
204	Accrued Salaries and Wages Payable		-0-
205	Deferred Rental Income		4,200
206	Deferred Tuition Income		2,160
250	Bonds Payable		80,000
301	Hospital Equity		225,000
302	Revenue and Expense Summary		-0-
401	Routine Services Revenue		151,300
402	Ancillary Services Revenue		137,400
403	Interest Income		-0-
404	Rental Income		-0-
405	Tuition Income		-0-
406	Other Revenues		27,100
501	Charity Service	29,200	
502	Contractual Adjustments	19,400	
503	Bad Debts	-0-	
601	Salaries and Wages Expense	139,600	
602	Supplies Expense	28,600	
603	Utilities Expense	14,400	
604	Insurance Expense	-0-	
605	Repairs Expense	8,300	
606	Rent Expense	-0-	
607	Depreciation Expense	-0-	
608	Interest Expense	-0-	
609	Other Expenses	7,700	
	Totals	$675,000	$675,000

Figure 5-1 Hoosier Hospital Preadjusted Trial Balance, December 31, 19X1

Prepaid Insurance	107	$3,600	
Cash	101		$3,600
Payment of 3-year premium in advance on a comprehensive insurance policy.			

At the end of the year, however, $1,200 of this prepayment has expired and should be included in the hospital's 19X1 expenses. Also at year's end, the amount of prepaid insurance to be reported as an asset is only $2,400 ($3,600 − $1,200).

An adjusting entry therefore must be made in the hospital's journal at December 31, 19X1. The required entry is the following:

Insurance Expense	604	$1,200	
Prepaid Insurance	107		$1,200
Adjustment for portion of prepaid premium that expired during 19X1.			

When this entry is posted, it corrects the two account balances in the ledger of the hospital. The $1,200 of insurance expense will appear among the expenses in Hoosier Hospital's 19X1 income statement. The $2,400 adjusted balance of prepaid insurance will be presented as an asset in the hospital's December 31, 19X1, balance sheet. It is an asset because the insurance company "owes" Hoosier Hospital insurance protection for the next two years (19X2 and 19X3), and this asset is valued at the unexpired cost of the insurance. Prepaid insurance represents a future economic benefit (insurance protection).

The same adjusting entry will be required at the end of 19X2 and at the end of 19X3. Then, of course, it will be time to renew the insurance and make another premium payment. In this way, a $3,600 expenditure on January 1, 19X1, is charged or allocated to expense over the three-year period benefiting from the expenditure at the rate of $1,200 per year. (Had the entire $3,600 been charged to 19X1 expense, this would result in an overstatement of 19X1 expense and an understatement of expense in 19X2 and 19X3.) Because this hospital uses accrual basis accounting, expenses are recognized in the period in which they are incurred, regardless of when they are paid.

Assume, however, that the entire $3,600 premium was charged to insurance expense at the time it was paid. The transaction entry for January 1, 19X1, would have been:

Insurance Expense	604	$3,600	
Cash	101		$3,600
Payment of insurance premium.			

Had this been done, the required adjusting entry at December 31, 19X1, would be as follows:

Prepaid Insurance	107	$2,400	
Insurance Expense	604		$2,400
Adjustment for prepaid insurance premium.			

The result is the same as before: $1,200 of 19X1 insurance expense and $2,400 of prepaid insurance at December 31, 19X1.

It is important that you clearly understand that this discussion of adjusting entries is presented in terms of an annual time frame. Well-managed hospitals, of course, prepare monthly income statements and balance sheets. For these monthly statements to be accurate and useful, all significant adjustments must be made at the end of each month. If we assume the preparation of monthly financial statements for Hoosier Hospital, an adjusting entry would be made at the end of each month to recognize $100 ($1,200 ÷ 12) of insurance expense and to reduce prepaid insurance by the same amount:

Insurance Expense	604	$ 100	
Prepaid Insurance	107		$ 100
Adjustment for monthly expiration of prepaid insurance premiums.			

Adjusting for Insurance
Expense

The illustration presented in Chapter 9 assumes monthly adjusting entries, but we will discuss adjustments in annual terms until then.

Hospitals carry substantial amounts of many different types of insurance and have a large number of policies. Thus, the determination of the monthly and annual insurance expense figures can be somewhat difficult. It may be necessary to maintain an insurance register and perhaps an insurance expiration schedule or worksheet. Not only do these specialized records provide the necessary information for accounting adjustments, they also aid in the management of the hospital's insurance requirements to ensure that adequate coverage is maintained, that claims for insured losses are promptly reported and recovered, and so on.

Prepaid Rent

Let us assume now that Hoosier Hospital rented certain equipment for use in its business offices on May 1, 19X1. Following is the transaction entry:

Prepaid Rent	108	$1,080	
Cash	101		$1,080
Payment of a year's rent in advance for office equipment ($90 per month).			

The December 31, 19X1, preadjusted trial balance therefore includes $1,080 of prepaid rent (account 108) but no balance in Rent Expense (account 606).

Because the rent is $90 per month, Hoosier Hospital's 19X1 expenses therefore should include rent expense of $720 ($90 × 8 months). Prepaid rent at December 31, 19X1, should be $360 ($90 × 4 months), the rent that is prepaid for January through April of 19X2. The required December 31, 19X1, adjusting entry is as follows:

Rent Expense	606	$ 720	
Prepaid Rent	108		$ 720
Adjustment to record rent expense for May through December 19X1, at $90 per month.			

In 19X2, the remaining $360 of prepaid rent will be charged to expense. In this way, the equipment rental cost is charged to expense during the periods in which the equipment is being used by the hospital. Had the entire $1,080 payment been charged to expense in the year of payment, Hoosier Hospital's 19X1 expenses would have been overstated and its 19X2 expenses understated.

Suppose, however, that the prepayment of the rent on May 1, 19X1, had been recorded as a debit to rent expense, as follows:

Rent Expense	606	$1,080	
Cash	101		$1,080
Payment of one year's rent in advance for office equipment ($90 per month).			

Had this been the transaction entry, the December 31, 19X1, adjusting entry would be somewhat different. The following would be the necessary adjusting entry:

Prepaid Rent	108	$ 360	
Rent Expense	606		$ 360
Adjustment to record prepaid rent for January through April 19X2, at $90 per month.			

However the transaction entry is handled, the net result at year's end is to have $720 in Rent Expense and $360 in the Prepaid Rent account.

Prepaid Interest

Assume that Hoosier Hospital obtained a six-month loan of $18,000 from a bank on November 1, 19X1. The hospital issued to the bank a promissory note, paying 8 percent interest in advance for the six-month term of the note. The hospital's transaction entry on November 1 was as follows:

Cash	101	$17,280	
Prepaid Interest	109	720	
Notes Payable	202		$18,000

Proceeds of 6-month note
issued to bank, with 8%
interest deducted in
advance:

Face amount of		
note	$18,000	
Less interest—		
$18,000 ×		
8% × 1/2	720	
Proceeds of note	$17,280	

Interest on the note for a full year would be $1,440 (8% × $18,000). The loan, however, is for a six-month period, and only a half year's interest is prepaid. Interest expense is $120 per month ($720 ÷ 6 months).

At December 31, 19X1, interest expense for November and December has been incurred by the hospital. The necessary adjusting entry at year-end is the following:

Interest Expense	608	$ 240	
Prepaid Interest	109		$ 240

Adjustment for interest expense on
bank loan for November and
December 19X1: $18,000 × 8%
× 2/12 = $240.

The remaining $480 ($720 − $240) of prepaid interest is an asset at the end of 19X1. The bank "owes" to the hospital the use of the borrowed money for another four months. This $480 will be charged to interest expense in 19X2.

If the interest involved in the November 1, 19X1, transaction entry had been debited to interest expense (instead of prepaid interest), the required adjusting entry at December 31 would be as follows:

| Prepaid Interest | 109 | $480 | |
| Interest Expense | 608 | | $480 |

Adjustment for 4 months' prepaid
interest on bank loan at December 31:
$18,000 \times 8\% \times 4/12 = \$480$.

Again, no matter what debit is made for the $720 of interest in the
November 1, 19X1, transaction entry, we must end up with $240
in interest expense and $480 in prepaid interest at the end of the
year.

A hospital will likely have other types of prepaid expenses.
Whatever the particular expense item, adjustments are made in the
manner shown in the preceding illustrations. The procedure is
summarized in the following:

Summary of Process for
Handling Prepaid Expenses

1. Assuming the prepayment is debited to a prepaid expense
   account in the transaction entry:

Prepaid Expense		Expense	
Transaction Entry	Adjusting Entry	Adjusting Entry	

The amount of the adjusting entry is that portion of the prepayment that has expired and should be recorded as expense of the
current period.

2. Assuming the prepayment is debited to an expense account in
   the transaction entry:

Prepaid Expense		Expense	
Adjusting Entry		Transaction Entry	Adjusting Entry

The amount of the adjusting entry is that portion of the prepayment that has not expired and is to be recorded as expense in a future period.

Prepaid expenses are assets because they represent unexpired costs—costs that benefit a future accounting period. They represent benefits, such as insurance protection, use of equipment, or use of money, to be received in the future and consequently should not be charged to expense in the current period.

Accrued Expenses

Accrued expenses are expenses that have been incurred but for which the hospital has not yet paid. Accrued expenses represent the costs of goods and services consumed or used in hospital operations of the current period, but for which the hospital will not make expenditures until some future accounting period. The liability for these future disbursements is called an *accrued liability,* or an *accrued expense payable.* In most cases, the liability is presented among the current liabilities in the balance sheet of the hospital. Examples include accrued interest payable and accrued salaries and wages payable (sometimes called *accrued payroll*).

At the end of each accounting period, the trial balance accounts must be scanned and analyzed to determine the need for adjustments for accrued expenses. Once the necessary adjustments are determined, they are journalized and posted to the hospital's ledger.

Accrued Interest

Let us assume that Hoosier Hospital issued $80,000 of 9 percent, 15-year bonds on July 1, 19X1, at face value. The transaction entry was as follows:

Cash	101	$80,000	
Bonds Payable	250		$80,000
Proceeds from issuance of			
$80,000 of 9%, 15-year bonds			
at face value.			

Assume also that interest on these bonds is payable semiannually on January 1 and July 1 of each year, commencing January 1, 19X2. These semiannual interest payments therefore will be $3,600 ($80,000 × 9% × 1/2). At the trial balance date, December 31,

19X1, no interest has yet been paid on these bonds; the first interest payment is due January 1, 19X2.

So, in this situation an expense has been incurred but is unrecorded and unpaid. The required December 31, 19X1, adjusting entry is the following:

Interest Expense	608	$3,600	
Accrued Interest Payable	203		$3,600
Adjustment for 6 months'			
interest accrued on bonds since			
July 1, 19X1.			

The money borrowed by the hospital through the issuance of the bonds costs the hospital 9 percent per year. Because the hospital had the use of this money for six months (July through December 19X1), the cost of using the money for this half-year period should be recorded as an expense in 19X1. The fact that this expense has not been paid by the hospital has nothing at all to do with the recognition of the expense in the 19X1 accounting period. Because the interest has not been paid, however, the adjusting entry must establish the liability as accrued interest payable.

On January 1, 19X2, the first semiannual interest payment date, the bond interest is paid. The transaction entry is as follows:

Accrued Interest Payable	203	$3,600	
Cash	101		$3,600
Payment of semiannual interest			
on bonds for the 6 months ended			
December 31, 19X1.			

In this way, the bond interest applicable to 19X1 is charged to 19X1 expense, although it was not actually paid until 19X2. Had the December 31, 19X1, adjusting entry not been made, 19X1 interest expense would have been understated.

In Hoosier Hospital's preadjusted trial balance (Figure 5–1), the Salaries and Wages Expense account (number 601) has a debit

Accrued Salaries and Wages

balance of $139,600. This is the amount of 19X1 salaries and wages paid to hospital employees in 19X1. But is this the correct amount of salaries and wages expense for 19X1?

For the purpose of illustration, assume that Hoosier Hospital pays all of its employees on the first day of each month for salaries and wages they earned in the preceding month. The $139,600 appearing in the trial balance is, therefore, salaries and wages only for the first 11 months of 19X1! Employees' salaries and wages for December 19X1 have not yet been paid and, consequently, are not included in the salaries and wages expense account balance. These December salaries and wages will be paid January 1, 19X2, but should be recorded as 19X1 expense. On December 31, 19X1, the hospital employees have earned their December pay. The hospital has received the benefit of their time and efforts during the month. The December payroll is a cost that has been incurred by the hospital, but that cost is unrecorded and unpaid. It is an expired cost that must be recognized as a 19X1 expense, and as of December 31, 19X1, a liability of the hospital to its employees.

Assume that the December 19X1 payroll is determined to be $13,000. (In actual practice, the accrued payroll figure sometimes must be estimated. More will be said about this in a later chapter.) The necessary adjusting entry at December 31, 19X1, is as follows:

Salaries and Wages Expense	601	$13,000	
Accrued Salaries and Wages			
Payable	204		$13,000
Adjustment for accrued payroll			
for the month of December			
19X1.			

This entry puts salaries and wages into the expense of the period during which they were incurred as hospital expenses. It also establishes a liability for unpaid salaries and wages for inclusion in the hospital's December 31, 19X1, balance sheet.

On January 1, 19X2, the December 19X1 payroll is paid. Assuming that the amount actually disbursed on that date is the same as the amount that was accrued in the preceding adjusting entry, the transaction entry is the following:

Accrued Salaries and Wages
    Payable   204 $13,000
        Cash   101 $13,000
Payment of December 19X1
accrued salaries and wages.

Thus, the salaries and wages are recorded as expenses of the period in which they are incurred as expenses rather than in the period in which they are paid.

    Now, a complication should be introduced. Disregard the previous situation and assume instead that Hoosier Hospital pays its employees every two weeks—that is, every 14 days. Let us say that the last payroll period in 19X1 was the 14-day period ending December 27, 19X1. On the following day, December 28, employees received their paychecks for that 14-day pay period. What this means is that the trial balance figure for salaries and wages expense of $139,600 represents 361 days of payroll expense (not 365 days). Employees have presumably worked another four days in 19X1 (December 28–31) for which they have not yet been, and will not be, paid until after the end of the next 14-day payroll period (January 10, 19X2). These four days of payroll cost, however, must be recorded as 19X1 expense!

    Let us assume that these four days of payroll are computed (perhaps estimated in some way) to be $3,700. The necessary December 31, 19X1, adjusting entry is as follows:

Adjusting Entry for Salaries and Wages

Salaries and Wages Expense   601 $ 3,700
    Accrued Salaries and Wages
        Payable   204 $ 3,700
Adjustment for accrued payroll
for the last 4 days of December
19X1.

Now assume that the actual payroll for the 14-day period ending January 10, 19X2, turns out to be $13,000. When this is paid on January 11, 19X2, the transaction entry is:

Accrued Salaries and Wages Payable	204	$3,700	
Salaries and Wages Expense	601	9,300	
Cash	101		$13,000
Payment of payroll for the 14-day period ending January 10, 19X2.			

This entry records the payment of two things: (1) the 4 days of payroll for 19X1 that were recorded previously as a liability and as 19X1 expense and (2) the 10 days of payroll for 19X2 that are debited to 19X2 expense. In this way, employees' salaries and wages are recorded as expenses of the period in which they are incurred by the hospital, and not necessarily in the period in which they are paid.

Hospitals, of course, have many types of expense accruals other than those illustrated here. Whatever expense items they might be, they are handled in the manner described for accrued interest and accrued payroll. The required adjusting entry will always be a debit to an expense account and a credit to a liability account. Then, when that liability is paid, the liability account is debited and the cash account credited.

Reversing Entries

In some accounting systems, *reversing entries* are prepared on the first day of each new accounting period. They are called reversing entries because they "reverse" certain previously recorded adjusting entries. The reversing entries are made to avoid certain complications in the accounting routine. This book, however, employs reversing entries only in a small number of cases. One of these relates to adjustments for accrued payroll. Let us examine the "reversing" procedure in that area.

Reversing Entries for Accrued Payroll

Assume the facts of the preceding illustration. Hoosier Hospital had paid $139,600 of salaries and wages during 19X1, $3,700 of salaries and wages were accrued at year end, and $13,000 of salaries and wages were paid on January 11, 19X2. The (1) 19X1 summary transaction entry, (2) 19X1 year-end adjusting entry, (3) December 31, 19X1, closing entry, (4) January 1, 19X2, reversing entry, and (5) January 11, 19X2, transaction entry are shown in the following list:

(1)	Salaries and Wages Expense	601	$139,600	
	Cash	101		$139,600
	Payments of salaries and wages during 19X1.			
(2)	Salaries and Wages Expense	601	3,700	
	Accrued Salaries and Wages Payable	204		3,700
	Adjustment for accrued salaries and wages at December 31, 19X1.			
(3)	Revenue and Expense Summary	302	143,300	
	Salaries and Wages Expense	601		143,300
	To close the expense account.			
(4)	Accrued Salaries and Wages Payable	204	3,700	
	Salaries and Wages Expense	601		3,700
	Reversal of December 31, 19X1, adjusting entry.			
(5)	Salaries and Wages Expense	601	13,000	
	Cash	101		13,000
	Payment of salaries and wages on January 11, 19X2.			

Notice that the reversing entry (number 4) is the "reverse" of the December 31, 19X1, adjusting entry (number 2). The reversing entry eliminates the Accrued Salaries and Wages Payable account and places a credit balance of $3,700 in the 19X2 Salaries and Wages Expense account. Entry number 5 debits the Salaries and Wages Expense account for $13,000. As a result, the 19X2 Salaries and Wages Expense account winds up with a debit balance of $9,300, the correct amount for the first 10 days of 19X2.

Thus, because of the reversing entry, the total amount of salaries and wages paid on January 11, 19X2, can be debited to the expense account. In other words, there is no need to "break" the debit amount between the expense account and the Accrued Liability account. This is one of the complications that is avoided by using reversing entries.

You should not conclude, however, that all adjusting entries are to be reversed. Some are reversed; some are not. In this book, the use of reversing entries will be limited to a few illustrations concerning accrued expenses (such as salaries and wages) and accrued revenues (seen in the following chapter).

Questions

Q5–1. What is the purpose of adjusting entries? Distinguish between transaction and adjusting entries.

Q5–2. Describe briefly the *matching principle*.

Q5–3. Define *prepaid expense*. Give three examples of hospital expense items that may be prepaid.

Q5–4. Define *accrued expense*. Give three examples of hospital expense items that often must be accrued at the end of an accounting period.

Q5–5. Distinguish between prepaid and accrued expenses.

Q5–6. Distinguish among (a) preadjusted trial balance, (b) adjusted trial balance, (c) preclosing trial balance, and (d) postclosing trial balance.

Q5–7. Why are prepaid expenses reported in a balance sheet as assets?

Q5–8. Why are accrued expenses reported in a balance sheet as liabilities?

Q5–9. What is the purpose of reversing entries? Distinguish between adjusting entries and reversing entries.

Exercises

E5–1. Eston Hospital paid a three-year insurance premium of $1,350 in advance on January 1, 19X1.

Required: What amount should Eston Hospital report as prepaid insurance in its December 31, 19X2, balance sheet?

E5–2. Eastland Hospital paid a three-year insurance premium in advance on January 1, 19X1. The hospital's adjusted trial balance at December 31, 19X2, included a prepaid insurance account with a balance of $1,480.

Required: What was the amount of the insurance premium paid on January 1, 19X2?

E5–3. Early Hospital rented certain equipment for use in its business offices on October 1, 19X1, paying one year's rent of $1,800 in advance.

1800 - 450 = 1350

Required: What amount should appear as prepaid rent in Early Hospital's postclosing trial balance at December 31, 19X1?

E5–4. Edson Hospital obtained a six-month loan of $24,000 from a bank on August 1, 19X1, paying 10 percent interest in advance. The interest was debited to interest expense.

24,000 × 10% × 1/12 = 200

Required: Assuming that adjustments are made annually on December 31 only, prepare the necessary adjusting entry for December 31, 19X1.

E5–5. Using the data of Exercise 5–4, assume that the August 1, 19X1, transaction entry debited the interest to prepaid expense.

24,000 × 10% × 5/12 = 1000

Required: If adjustments are made annually on December 31 only, what is the necessary adjusting entry at December 31, 19X1?

E5–6. Esterbrook Hospital issued $100,000 of 6 percent, 20-year bonds on July 1, 19X1, at face value. Interest is payable semiannually on January 1 and July 1 of each year, beginning January 1, 19X2.

6 mos

100,000 × 6% × 6/12 = 3,000

Required: Assuming that adjustments are made annually on December 31 only, prepare the necessary adjusting entry on December 31, 19X1.

E5–7. Easy Hospital's preadjusted trial balance at December 31, 19X1, includes a Salaries and Wages Expense account with a debit balance of $805,200. It is determined, however, that employees have earned an additional $38,900 of salaries and wages in 19X1 that have not yet been paid.

38,900 Dr Salaries Ex
38,900 Cr - Acc Sal Ex

Required: Prepare the necessary adjusting entry for December 31, 19X1.

E5–8. Ernst Hospital's 19X2 income statement reports salaries and wages expense of $699,400. The hospital's balance sheets include the following accounts:
12/31/X1 Accrued salaries and wages payable	$41,600
12/31/X2 Accrued salaries and wages payable	38,400

Required: What was the amount of salaries and wages actually paid in cash during 19X2?

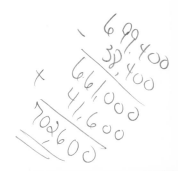

699,400
38,400
661,000
41,600
702,600

E5–9. Extant Hospital paid $355,100 of salaries and wages during 19X2. Its balance sheets reported accrued salaries and wages payable as follows:

12/31/X2	$28,300
12/31/X1	25,700

Required: What amount should be reported as salaries and wages expense in Extant Hospital's 19X2 income statement?

E5–10. Eucher Hospital's 19X2 income statement reported insurance expense of $8,000. Its balance sheets reported prepaid insurance as follows:

12/31/X1	$1,400
12/31/X2	1,100

Required: What was the amount actually paid in cash for insurance premiums during 19X2?

E5–11. Easter Hospital paid $4,600 of rent expense during 19X2. Its balance sheets reported prepaid rent expense as follows:

12/31/X1	$1,200
12/31/X2	900

Required: What amount should be reported as rent expense in Easter Hospital's 19X2 income statement?

Problems

P5–1. Exerto Hospital's preadjusted trial balance on December 31, 19X1, included the following accounts, among others:

Acct. No.		
107	Prepaid Insurance	$5,040
108	Prepaid Rent	2,100
109	Prepaid Interest	1,200
604	Insurance Expense	-0-
606	Rent Expense	-0-
608	Interest Expense	-0-

The hospital paid a three-year insurance premium in advance on January 1, 19X1. On August 1, 19X1, a year's rent was paid in advance. A $20,000, 12 percent loan for six months was obtained from a bank on November 1, 19X1, and the interest was paid in advance by the hospital.

Required: Prepare, in general journal form, the necessary adjusting entries at December 31, 19X1.

P5–2. Eversure Hospital's preadjusted trial balance at December 31, 19X1, included the following accounts, among others:

Acct.
No.

203	Accrued Interest Payable	$ -0-
204	Accrued Salaries and Wages Payable	-0-
601	Salaries and Wages Expense	245,600
608	Interest Expense	-0-
202	Notes Payable	120,000

On September 1, 19X1, the hospital issued its $120,000, 8 percent, six-month note to a local bank in connection with a short-term loan. An analysis indicated that employees had earned $33,600 of salaries and wages during 19X1 that had not been paid to them.

Required: Prepare, in general journal form, the necessary adjusting entries at December 31, 19X1.

P5–3. Exacto Hospital's preadjusted trial balance at December 31, 19X1, included the following accounts, among others:

Acct.
No.

107	Prepaid Insurance	$ 5,760
108	Prepaid Rent	2,700
109	Prepaid Interest	3,600
202	Note Payable	80,000
203	Accrued Interest Payable	-0-
204	Accrued Salaries and Wages Payable	-0-
250	Bonds Payable	400,000
601	Salaries and Wages Expense	755,200
604	Insurance Expense	-0-
606	Rent Expense	-0-
608	Interest Expense	-0-

The following additional information is available:
1. A three-year insurance premium was prepaid on January 1, 19X1.
2. One year's rent was paid in advance on June 1, 19X1.
3. On December 1, 19X1, an $80,000, 9 percent, six-month loan was obtained from a local bank. Interest was prepaid.
4. Unpaid salaries and wages at December 31, 19X1, totaled $68,700.

5. On October 1, 19X1, $400,000 of 6 percent, 10-year bonds were issued at face value. Interest on these bonds is payable annually on October 1, beginning October 1, 19X2.

Required: Prepare, in general journal form, the necessary adjusting entries for December 31, 19X1.

P5–4. The following accounts appeared in the adjusted trial balance of Evansville Hospital at December 31, 19X1:

Cash	$ 26,300
Accounts Receivable	105,900
Inventory	14,700
Prepaid Insurance	1,800
Prepaid Rent	900
Prepaid Interest	500
Plant and Equipment	575,000
Accounts Payable	29,700
Notes Payable	125,000
Accrued Interest Payable	2,300
Accrued Salaries and Wages Payable	9,800
Bonds Payable	350,000
Hospital Equity	193,600
Routine Services Revenue	135,000
Ancillary Services Revenue	75,800
Other Revenues	30,900
Salaries and Wages Expense	140,000
Supplies Expense	31,000
Utilities Expense	29,000
Insurance Expense	8,200
Repairs Expense	5,400
Rent Expense	7,100
Interest Expense	4,900
Other Expenses	1,400

Required: Prepare, in good form, a balance sheet at December 31, 19X1, and an income statement for the year then ended.

P5–5. Eunice Hospital's preadjusted trial balance at December 31, 19X1, included the following accounts, among others:

Acct. No.		
107	Prepaid Insurance	$ -0-
108	Prepaid Rent	-0-
109	Prepaid Interest	-0-
202	Notes Payable	80,000
203	Accrued Interest Payable	-0-
204	Accrued Salaries and Wages Payable	-0-
250	Bonds Payable	100,000
601	Salaries and Wages Expense	399,500
604	Insurance Expense	5,760
606	Rent Expense	2,700
608	Interest Expense	4,800

The following additional information is available:

1. A three-year insurance premium was prepaid on January 1, 19X1.
2. One year's rent was paid in advance on June 1, 19X1.
3. On December 1, 19X1, an $80,000, 12 percent, six-month loan was obtained from a local bank; interest was prepaid.
4. Unpaid salaries and wages at December 31, 19X1, amounted to $27,400.
5. On April 1, 19X1, $100,000 of 6 percent, 15-year bonds were issued at face value. Interest on these bonds is payable annually on April 1, beginning April 1, 19X2.

Required: Prepare, in general journal form, the necessary adjusting entries at December 31, 19X1.

Deferred and Accrued Revenues

6

This chapter introduces some additional adjustments of the Hoosier Hospital's December 31, 19X1, trial balance (see Figure 5–1). These adjustments are of two major types:

- *Deferred Revenues.* Certain revenues have been received in cash but as yet have not been earned by the hospital.

- *Accrued Revenues.* Certain revenues have been earned but as yet have not been received in cash by the hospital.

The adjustments required for these items are similar to those illustrated in the preceding chapter for prepaid and accrued expenses. This chapter, however, concerns revenues, not expenses. The accrual basis objective of the adjustments described here is to give accounting recognition to revenues in the accounting period in which they are earned, regardless of when the related cash receipts occur, if ever. Although hospital revenues are for the most part received in cash in the period earned, a substantial amount of revenues is earned prior to the receipt of cash. Less frequently, certain other revenues may be earned in an accounting period subsequent to the period in which the related cash receipts occur.

Deferred Revenues

Deferred revenues, sometimes called *deferred income, prepaid income,* or *revenues received in advance,* consist of revenue items for which cash has been received but that the hospital has not yet earned. Because of the cash receipt, the hospital must provide certain corresponding goods and services in some future accounting period (or periods). Examples of deferred revenues include rentals received in advance and advance receipts of tuition for educational programs conducted by the hospital. More complicated deferred revenue situations are discussed at later points in this book.

Deferred Rent   Let us assume that Hoosier Hospital rents office space in its building
to certain physicians on its medical staff. This practice began on
August 1, 19X1, when a year's rent of $4,200 ($350 per month)
was received in advance. At that time, Hoosier Hospital made the
following transaction entry:

Cash	101	$4,200	
Deferred Rental Income	205		$4,200
Receipt of one year's rent in advance for office space provided for staff physicians ($350 per month).			

On August 1, 19X1, then, the hospital has a liability to the physicians to provide office space for their use during the next 12 months. The deferred rental income account reflects that liability.

On December 31, 19X1, the hospital has provided the office space for five months (August through December). The hospital therefore has earned $1,750 of rental income ($350 × 5 months). Because this income has not been recorded by the hospital, an adjusting entry is required:

Deferred Rental Income	205	$1,750	
Rental Income	404		$1,750
Adjustment for 5 months of rental income earned from provision of office space for physicians.			

This entry recognizes the rental income earned in 19X1 and reduces the Deferred Rental Income account to the correct December 31, 19X1, balance of $2,450. In other words, on December 31, 19X1, the hospital has a remaining liability to furnish office space for seven months in 19X2. This liability is measured at $350 per month ($350 × 7 months = $2,450).

Thus, $2,450 of rental income received in 19X1 is deferred to 19X2, the year in which it will be earned by the hospital. Were this not done, the income of 19X1 would be overstated, and the 19X2 income understated. The accrual basis of accounting prevents such misstatements.

Suppose, however, that the August 1, 19X1, transaction entry credited the $4,200 to rental income rather than to deferred rental income. The following would have been the transaction entry:

Cash	101	$4,200	
Rental Income	404		$4,200
Receipt of a year's rent for office space to be provided to physicians.			

Accountant's Review of Rental Agreements

In scanning the trial balance at the end of the year, the accountant must be alert in order to recognize the need for an adjustment of the Rental Income account. This might come to the accountant's attention through an examination of rental agreements, leases, and other documents. In any event, the following adjustment is required at December 31, 19X1:

Rental Income	404	$2,450	
Deferred Rental Income	205		$2,450
Adjustment for 7 months' rental income to be deferred to 19X2.			

So, regardless of the credit made in the transaction entry, we must wind up 19X1 with $1,750 in Rental Income and $2,450 in Deferred Rental Income.

There is another possibility that might be mentioned here, although it is not likely to be seen in actual practice. The transaction entry could be as follows:

Cash	101	$4,200	
Rental Income	404		$1,750
Deferred Rental Income	205		2,450
Receipt of a year's rentals of which 5 months is income of the current year; the remainder is deferred to 19X2.			

If this transaction entry is made on August 1, 19X1, no adjusting entry will be necessary at the year's end. For various reasons, however, this procedure may be undesirable or unworkable in actual practice. It is mentioned here only to assist you in understanding adjustment procedures.

Adjusting Entries for Rental Space

Income also may arise from the rental of space in the hospital as sleeping quarters for interns and residents, or the hospital may own separate buildings that are used as residences for nurses and other personnel. Space in the hospital's lobby and public areas may be rented to private concerns for gift shops and newsstands. A hospital-operated television service also may produce rental income. In any of these cases, adjusting entries may be appropriate at the end of each accounting period.

Deferred Tuition

Assume that Hoosier Hospital operates an educational program, such as a school of nursing or a school for laboratory technologists. Further assume that, on September 1, 19X1, the hospital received $2,160 of fees and tuition for the nine-month school year that ends May 31, 19X2. For this transaction, Hoosier Hospital made the following entry:

Cash	101	$2,160	
Deferred Tuition Income	206		$2,160
Receipt of tuition ($240 per month) for the 9-month school year ending May 31, 19X2.			

Here again, the hospital has received revenue in advance. The hospital has an obligation to the students in the program to provide educational services during the next nine months. This liability is represented by the credit to the Deferred Tuition Income account. When the tuition is received, the hospital has earned no income.

By the end of 19X1, however, the school presumably has been operating for four months (September through December), and the hospital therefore has earned $960 of tuition income ($240 × 4 months, or 4/9 × $2,160). The following adjusting entry is required at December 31, 19X1:

Deferred Tuition Income	206	$ 960	
Tuition Income	405		$ 960
Adjustment for tuition income earned in 19X1 (4 months @ $240 per month).			

This entry gives accounting recognition to the tuition income earned during the current year and defers recognition of the remaining tuition revenue to 19X2. Hoosier Hospital will report $960 of tuition income in its 19X1 income statement and $1,200 of deferred tuition income (a current liability) in its December 31, 19X1, balance sheet.

Now assume that the September 1, 19X1, transaction entry credited all of the tuition received to income as follows:

Cash	101	$2,160	
Tuition Income	405		$2,160
Receipt of tuition ($240 per month) for the 9-month school year ending May 31, 19X2.			

Had this been done, the December 31, 19X1, trial balance would have $2,160 in the Tuition Income account (rather than in the Deferred Tuition Income account). In this event, the following adjusting entry would be required for December 31, 19X1:

Tuition Income	405	$1,200	
Deferred Tuition Income	206		$1,200
Adjustment for tuition to be deferred to 19X2 (5 months @ $240 per month).			

Thus, we again produce the necessary account balances on December 31, 19X1: $960 of tuition income and $1,200 of deferred tuition income.

The accounting procedures for deferred revenues are summarized in the following T-accounts:

1. Assuming the transaction entry credited the cash received to a deferred revenue account:

	Revenue		Deferred Revenue
	Adjusting Entry	Adjusting Entry	Transaction Entry

The adjusting entry transfers the amount of revenue earned during the current period from the liability account (deferred revenue) to the revenue account.

2. Assuming the transaction entry credited the cash received to a revenue account:

Revenue		Deferred Revenue	
Adjusting Entry	Transaction Entry		Adjusting Entry

The adjusting entry transfers the amount of unearned revenue from the revenue account to the deferred revenue account.

Thus, the nature and amount of the required adjusting entry depend on the account initially credited in the transaction entry.

Accrued Revenues

Accrued revenues consist of revenue items that the hospital has earned but for which the hospital has not recorded a receivable or collected cash. The hospital, of course, routinely provides goods and services to patients and has a claim against them (or third-party payers) for the value of those goods and services. These claims are recorded as receivables (assets), as previously indicated. In addition, the hospital provides other types of services that produce revenues and require the recognition of related receivables. Examples of these accrued revenue items are accrued interest receivable, accrued rent receivable, and accrued tuition receivable. This discussion illustrates the accrual of interest revenues and receivables.

Let us say that Hoosier Hospital invested $12,000 in 8 percent government bonds on October 1, 19X1. These bonds, purchased at face value, pay interest annually on October 1, commencing October 1, 19X2. The following was the transaction entry:

Temporary Investments	102	$12,000	
Cash	101		$12,000
Purchase of $12,000 (face value) of 8% government bonds for temporary investment.			

Perhaps at this time Hoosier Hospital had a cash balance in excess of its then-current needs. In accordance with good business practice, it was decided to invest those funds for a short period of time to obtain interest income. Although the bonds may be 10-year bonds, the hospital intends to hold them only as a temporary or short-term investment. As a result, the investment will be classified as a current asset in Hoosier Hospital's balance sheet.

At December 31, 19X1, Hoosier Hospital has held this investment for three months (October through December). The hospital has earned interest income of $240 ($12,000 $\times$ 8 percent $\times$ 3/12), and the following year-end adjusting entry must be recorded:

Accrued Interest Receivable	103	$ 240	
Interest Income	403		$ 240
Adjustment for 3 months' interest earned on temporary investments in government bonds.			

This entry gives accounting recognition to interest income earned (but not yet received) during 19X1. The interest, however, will be received on the next annual interest payment date, October 1, 19X2. So, the entry makes a debit to the appropriate asset account, Accrued Interest Receivable. In Hoosier Hospital's December 31,

19X1, balance sheet, the accrued interest receivable will be reported as a current asset.

On October 1, 19X2, the hospital will receive in cash a full year's interest, or $960 ($12,000 × 8 percent), on the bond investment. The following might be the transaction entry at that time:

Cash	101	$960	
Accrued Interest Receivable	103		$240
Interest Income	403		720
Receipt of a year's interest on tempo-			
rary investment in 8% government			
bonds, $240 of which was recognized			
as income in 19X1.			

Recording Income in Year in Which It Is Earned

Notice that all of the interest income was received in cash in 19X2, but $240 of it was recorded as 19X1 income and $720 was recognized as 19X2 income. Thus, income is recorded in the year in which it is earned and not necessarily in the year in which it is received in cash.

Hoosier Hospital might have chosen to make a reversing entry on January 1, 19X2. In addition, if Hoosier Hospital prepared monthly financial statements, adjusting entries would have been made monthly. Chapter 9 covers monthly adjustment procedures in detail. So, assuming annual adjustments only, Hoosier Hospital could have made the following reversing entry on January 1, 19X2:

Interest Income	403	$240	
Accrued Interest Receivable	103		$240
Reversal of December 31, 19X1,			
entry for accrued interest on tempo-			
rary investment in government			
bonds.			

This entry eliminates the balance in the Accrued Interest Receivable account and places a debit balance in the 19X2 Interest Income account. Then, when the annual interest is received on the investment on October 1, 19X2, the following transaction entry is made:

Cash	101	$ 960	
Interest Income	403		$ 960
Receipt of a year's interest on			
temporary investment in 8% gov-			
ernment bonds.			

When this $960 credit is posted to the interest income account, the account then has the proper $720 balance: the $960 credit posting minus the $240 debit posting from the reversing entry. Compare this transaction entry (assuming a reversing entry was made) with the previously illustrated transaction entry (assuming no reversing entry was made) for October 1, 19X2. Thus, the use of reversing entries tends to simplify subsequent transaction entries.

Summary of Adjustments for Prepayments and Accruals

Explanation of Adjusting Entries

This chapter has illustrated adjusting entries for deferred and accrued revenues; the preceding chapter illustrated adjustments for prepaid and accrued expenses. Now, let us bring these adjustments together as they would appear in Hoosier Hospital's general journal for 19X1. In Figure 6–1, the adjusting journal entries (AJEs) numbered 1 through 5 were discussed in the preceding chapter; those numbered 6 through 8 were described earlier in this chapter.

Entries 1, 2, and 3 are the adjustments arising from the prepayment of expenses during 19X1. In each case, an expense account is debited, and an asset account is credited. This is because we have assumed that the hospital has an accounting policy of debiting prepaid expense accounts in the initial transaction entry. For example, when insurance premiums are paid, a debit is made to prepaid insurance, not to insurance expense.

Adjusting entries 4 and 5 are those necessary to give accounting recognition to accrued expenses (expenses incurred during 19X1 but not yet paid). In each case, the entry debits an expense account and credits a liability account. This is always true for adjustments for accrued expenses.

Entries 6 and 7 are adjusting entries for deferred (prepaid) revenues. Each of these entries debits a liability account and credits a revenue account. This is because we have assumed that it is Hoosier Hospital's accounting policy to credit a deferred revenue account whenever revenue items are received in advance. For example, when rental prepayments are received, a credit is made to the

Entry No.	Accounts and Explanations	Acct. No.	Dr.	Cr.
1	Insurance Expense	604	$ 1,200	
	Prepaid Insurance	107		$ 1,200
	Adjustment for part of prepaid premium that expired during 19X1 (Chapter 5).			
2	Rent Expense	606	720	
	Prepaid Rent	108		720
	Adjustment to record rent expense for May through December 19X1, at $90 per month (Chapter 5).			
3	Interest Expense	608	240	
	Prepaid Interest	109		240
	Adjustment for interest on bank loan for November and December 19X1 (Chapter 5).			
4	Interest Expense	608	3,600	
	Accrued Interest Payable	203		3,600
	Adjustment for 6 months' interest accrued on bonds since July 1, 19X1 (Chapter 5).			
5	Salaries and Wages Expense	601	13,000	
	Accrued Salaries and Wages Payable	204		13,000
	Adjustment for accrued payroll for the month of December 19X1 (Chapter 5).			
6	Deferred Rental Income	205	1,750	
	Rental Income	404		1,750
	Adjustment for 5 months of rental income earned from provision of office space for physicians (Chapter 6).			
7	Deferred Tuition Income	206	960	
	Tuition Income	405		960
	Adjustment for tuition income earned in 19X1 (Chapter 6).			
8	Accrued Interest Receivable	103	240	
	Interest Income	403		240
	Adjustment for 3 months' interest on temporary investment in government bonds (Chapter 6).			

Figure 6–1 Hoosier Hospital 19X1 Journal (Adjusting Entries)

Deferred Rental Income account, not to the Rental Income account.

Entry 8 relates to the accrual of income that was earned during 19X1 but that had not been received in cash by the end of the year. The entry debits an asset account and credits an income account. This is always true of adjustments for accrued revenues.

All of these adjusting entries, of course, are posted in due course to Hoosier Hospital's ledger. When this is accomplished, most of the ledger accounts will have correct balances reflecting accrual basis accounting. These eight entries, however, are not all of the adjusting entries normally required at the end of a fiscal year. In the next chapter, two additional types of adjustments are considered. These adjustments relate to revenue deductions and to depreciation.

Questions

Q6–1. Define *deferred revenue*. Give two examples of deferred revenue.

Q6–2. Define *accrued revenue*. Give two examples of accrued revenue.

Q6–3. Why is deferred revenue reported in a balance sheet as a liability?

Q6–4. Why is accrued revenue reported in a balance sheet as an asset?

Q6–5. Fodder Hospital received a year's rent in advance on May 1, 19X1. The hospital's December 31, 19X1, balance sheet reported deferred rental income of $580. What was the amount of rent received on May 1, 19X1?

Q6–6. Ferntown Hospital received $1,800, representing a year's rent in advance, on November 1, 19X1. In the transaction entry, $1,800 was credited to the Deferred Rental Income account. Assuming that adjustments are made annually on December 31 only, what adjusting entry should be made on December 31, 19X1?

Q6–7. Refer to the data of Question 6–6 but assume that the Rental Income account was credited for $1,800 in the transaction entry. Assuming that adjustments are made annually on December 31 only, what adjusting entry should be made on December 31, 19X1?

Exercises

E6–1. Foster Hospital's 19X2 income statement reported rental income of $8,200. The hospital's balance sheets reported deferred rental income as follows:

| 12/31/X1 | $1,700 |
| 12/31/X2 | 1,300 |

Required: What was the amount of rent actually received in cash during 19X1?

E6-2. Fat Hospital received in cash rental payments of $10,700 during 19X2. Its balance sheets reported deferred rental income as follows:

12/31/X2 $2,600
12/31/X1   1,800

Required: What amount should be reported as rental income in Fat Hospital's 19X2 income statement?

E6-3. On September 1, 19X1, Fasby Hospital received $10,620 of fees and tuition for one of its educational programs that has a nine-month school year ending May 31, 19X2.

Required: What amount should be reported as deferred tuition income in the hospital's December 31, 19X1, balance sheet?

E6-4. Favor Hospital invested $60,000 in 8 percent government bonds on August 1, 19X1. These bonds, which were purchased at face value, pay interest annually on August 1, commencing August 1, 19X2.

Required: Assuming that adjustments are made annually on December 31 only, prepare the necessary adjusting entry for accrued interest as of December 31, 19X1.

E6-5. Flabby Hospital received interest payments of $8,600 during 19X2. Its balance sheets reported accrued interest receivable as follows:

12/31/X1 $1,100
12/31/X2   1,400

Required: What amount should be reported as interest income in the hospital's 19X2 income statement?

Problems

P6-1. Frangipani Hospital's December 31, 19X1, preadjusted trial balance includes the following accounts, among others:

Acct. No.		
102	Temporary Investments	$24,000
103	Accrued Interest Receivable	-0-
205	Deferred Rental Income	5,400
206	Deferred Tuition Income	4,320
403	Interest Income	-0-
404	Rental Income	-0-
405	Tuition Income	-0-

The following additional information is available:

1. On September 1, 19X1, the hospital invested $24,000 (face value) in 8 percent government bonds that pay interest annually on September 1, commencing September 1, 19X2.
2. On June 1, 19X1, the hospital received a year's rent in advance.
3. On September 1, 19X1, the hospital received nine months' tuition in advance for one of its educational programs.

Required: Prepare, in general journal form, the necessary adjusting entries at December 31, 19X1.

P6–2. Frosty Hospital's December 31, 19X1, preadjusted trial balance includes the following accounts, among others:

Acct. No.

102	Temporary Investments	$ 30,000
103	Accrued Interest Receivable	-0-
205	Deferred Rental Income	-0-
206	Deferred Tuition Income	-0-
403	Interest Income	-0-
404	Rental Income	5,400
405	Tuition Income	4,320

The following additional information is available:

1. On April 1, 19X1, the hospital invested $30,000 (face value) in 8 percent government bonds that pay interest annually on April 1, commencing April 1, 19X2.
2. On June 1, 19X1, the hospital received a year's rent in advance.
3. On September 1, 19X1, the hospital received nine months' tuition in advance for one of its educational programs.

Required: Prepare, in general journal form, the necessary adjusting entries at December 31, 19X1.

P6–3. The following is Flapper Hospital's preadjusted trial balance as of December 31, 19X1:

Acct. No.

101	Cash	$ 34,900
102	Temporary Investments	60,000
103	Accrued Interest Receivable	-0-
104	Accounts Receivable	172,000
106	Inventory	15,000
107	Prepaid Insurance	6,480

108	Prepaid Rent	$ 4,500	
109	Prepaid Interest	2,400	
150	Plant and Equipment	350,020	
201	Accounts Payable		$ 28,200
202	Notes Payable		48,000
203	Accrued Interest Payable		-0-
204	Accrued Salaries and Wages Payable		-0-
205	Deferred Rental Income		3,600
206	Deferred Tuition Income		4,900
250	Bonds Payable		200,000
301	Hospital Equity		335,300
302	Revenue and Expense Summary		-0-
401	Routine Services Revenue		97,500
402	Ancillary Services Revenue		58,200
403	Interest Income		-0-
404	Rental Income		-0-
405	Tuition Income		-0-
406	Other Revenues		19,300
601	Salaries and Wages Expense	100,000	
602	Supplies Expense	25,000	
603	Utilities Expense	12,000	
604	Insurance Expense	-0-	
605	Repairs Expense	9,000	
606	Rent Expense	-0-	
608	Interest Expense	-0-	
609	Other Expenses	3,700	
		$795,000	$795,000

The following additional information is available:

1. On August 1, 19X1, the hospital invested $60,000 (face value) in 8 percent government bonds that pay interest annually on August 1, commencing August 1, 19X2.
2. On January 1, 19X1, a three-year insurance premium was paid in advance.
3. One year's rent was received in advance on March 1, 19X1.
4. One year's rent was paid in advance by the hospital on May 1, 19X1.
5. On November 1, 19X1, the hospital issued its six-month, 10 percent note for $48,000 to a local bank in

connection with a short-term loan. The interest was prepaid by the hospital.

6. On October 1, 19X1, the hospital issued $200,000 of 6 percent, 10-year bonds at face value. These bonds pay interest semiannually on October 1 and April 1, commencing April 1, 19X2.

7. Unpaid salaries and wages at December 31, 19X1, amounted to $16,800.

8. On September 1, 19X1, the hospital received nine months' tuition in advance for one of its educational programs.

Required: (1) Enter the preadjusted December 31, 19X1, balances in general ledger accounts. (2) Prepare, in general journal form, the necessary adjusting entries at December 31, 19X1. (3) Post the adjusting entries to the ledger accounts and prepare an adjusted trial balance at December 31, 19X1. (4) Prepare an income statement for 19X1 and a balance sheet at December 31, 19X1. (5) Prepare, in general journal form, the necessary closing entries at December 31, 19X1. (6) Post the closing entries to the ledger accounts. (7) Prepare a postclosing trial balance at December 31, 19X1.

Depreciation and Revenue Deductions

7

Adjustment procedures for prepaid expenses, accrued expenses, deferred revenues, and accrued revenues were discussed in the two preceding chapters. This chapter describes and illustrates two additional types of adjustments required at the end of the accounting period. The first concerns depreciation of the hospital's plant assets. The second relates to the problem of revenue deductions: charity service, contractual adjustments, and bad debts. When this chapter is concluded, you will have been introduced to most of the adjusting entries related to hospital accounting.

Depreciation

Hoosier Hospital's December 31, 19X1, trial balance (refer again to Figure 5–1) includes the following account balances to which your attention should now be directed:

Acct. No.	Account Titles	Dr.	Cr.
150	Land	$ 25,000	
160	Building	180,000	
161	Accumulated Depreciation—Building		$ -0-
170	Equipment	60,000	
171	Accumulated Depreciation—Equipment		-0-
507	Depreciation Expense	-0-	

Accounts 150, 160, and 170 are asset accounts whose debit balances reflect the original historical costs of the hospital's plant

Depreciation Recorded Through Adjusting Entries

assets: land, buildings, and equipment used in hospital operations (and not held for investment purposes or for sale in the ordinary course of business). Accounts 161 and 171 are called *contraasset accounts,* that is, *negative asset accounts.* As you learned in Chapter 1, these accounts reflect the amount of plant asset cost that has been charged to expense (depreciation) in the hospital's income statements of the current and prior accounting periods. Account 507 reports the amount of depreciation expense for the current period. Depreciation therefore enters the accounting records through adjusting entries that debit depreciation expense and credit the appropriate accumulated depreciation accounts.

Assume, for purposes of illustration, that Hoosier Hospital acquired all of its plant assets in a cash transaction on January 1, 19X1:

Land	150	$ 25,000	
Building	160	180,000	
Equipment	170	60,000	
Cash	101		$265,000
Purchase of plant assets for cash.			

These plant assets were used throughout 19X1. Because the activities of the year were made possible by, and benefited from, the use of these assets, is it not logical to expect that some part of the cost of the assets should be charged as expense against the revenues of the period?

Nature of Depreciation Depreciation is an accounting procedure by which the cost (less salvage value, if any) of certain plant assets is allocated to expense over the estimated useful lives of such assets in a systematic and rational manner. The amount of plant asset cost allocated to a particular accounting period is called *depreciation expense.* A fundamental point to remember is that depreciation is a process of cost allocation, not of valuation. You should understand that depreciation, in the accounting sense, is not a measurement of the loss in the market value of an asset during a given period.

Consider, for example, an item of equipment used in the radiology department of the hospital. This equipment cost, say, $4,000 when acquired on January 1, 19X1. Obviously, the equipment will not last forever; it eventually will wear out and/or become obsolete with time, use, and changes in technology. When the equipment reaches the point at which it is no longer useful to the hospital, it will be discarded (either sold or scrapped) and probably replaced by new equipment. The amount, if any, for which the old equipment can be sold at the end of its useful life is called *salvage value, residual value,* or *scrap value.*

To compute depreciation on this radiology equipment, we must estimate its useful life (usually in years) and its salvage value (if any). These estimates must be made when the equipment is acquired. Hence, they must be based on informed judgment and experienced opinion. (We will probe more deeply into this matter in a subsequent chapter.)

So, let us assume that we estimate a useful life of six years and a salvage value of $400 for the equipment. This means that we expect the equipment to be used over a six-year period from the beginning of 19X1 to the end of 19X6, at which time it may sell for $400. Then, subtracting the salvage value from the cost of the equipment, we obtain $3,600 ($4,000 − $400), the depreciation base, or depreciable cost. This is the net cost (acquisition cost minus salvage value) to the hospital for the use of the equipment over its six-year life. We can depreciate no more than $3,600.

If we divide the $3,600 depreciable cost by the estimated useful life of six years to determine annual depreciation expense ($3,600 ÷ 6), we find that depreciation expense is $600 per year. This method of computing the annual amount of depreciation expense is referred to as *straight-line depreciation.* It is perhaps the most widely used depreciation method. We will examine other depreciation methods in a subsequent chapter.

At the end of 19X1, then, $600 of the cost of the radiology equipment must be recognized as depreciation expense. This is accomplished by the following adjusting entry:

Depreciation Expense	507	$600	
Accumulated Depreciation—			
Equipment	171		$600
Adjustment for depreciation of			
radiology equipment for 19X1.			

The 19X1 income statement will report $600 of depreciation expense. In the balance sheet at December 31, 19X1, the presentation is the following:

Equipment, at cost	$4,000	
Less accumulated depreciation	600	
Equipment, net		$3,400

Note that accumulated depreciation, the contraasset account, is shown in the balance sheet as a deduction from the asset account. The resulting $3,400 figure is the undepreciated cost of the equipment; it also is referred to as the "book value" of the equipment. It is not necessarily, however, the "market value" of the equipment; that is, it is not the price for which the equipment could be sold by the hospital on December 31, 19X1.

Each year for the next five years, $600 will be recorded as annual depreciation expense. That is, depreciation will accumulate at the rate of $600 per year. In the December 31, 19X3, balance sheet, for example, the presentation will be as follows:

Equipment, at cost	$4,000	
Less accumulated depreciation	1,800	
Equipment, net		$2,200

Here, depreciation has accumulated for three years: 19X1–19X3, to a total of $1,800 ($600 × 3 years). This will continue until the end of 19X6, at which time the equipment will be fully depreciated and, presumably, retired from service by the hospital.

Incorrect Useful Life and Salvage Value Estimates

What if the equipment is not retired at the end of 19X6? Suppose the useful life and salvage value estimates turn out to be incorrect. What happens if the equipment is sold prior to 19X6? These are very interesting questions, but we must defer a consideration of the answers to subsequent chapters.

One additional point, however, should be made here. Assume that the equipment mentioned above was acquired on, say, July 1, 19X1. In that case, how much depreciation should be taken on the equipment for 19X1? The answer is a half-year's depreciation, or $300 ($600 ÷ 2), because the hospital had the use of the equipment for only six months. (The hospital may adopt a different policy with respect to this matter, but we will not discuss it at this time.)

Had the equipment been acquired on December 31, 19X1, no depreciation expense would be recorded in 19X1 for this equipment.

Returning now to Hoosier Hospital, let us develop the December 31, 19X1, adjusting entries for depreciation. Land is nondepreciable, but depreciation must be computed and recorded for the hospital's building and equipment. Buildings and equipment are depreciable assets.

Adjusting Entries

Depreciation of Building.   The useful life of Hoosier Hospital's building is estimated to be 50 years. Salvage value is estimated to be 20 percent of the cost of the building, or $36,000 (20 percent of $180,000). The depreciable cost, then, is $144,000 ($180,000 − $36,000), and annual depreciation is $2,880 ($144,000 ÷ 50). At December 31, 19X1, the following adjusting entry is required:

Depreciation Expense	507	$2,880	
Accumulated Depreciation— Building	161		$2,880
Adjustment for 19X1 depreciation of hospital building:			
Cost		$180,000	
Less salvage value (20%)		36,000	
Depreciable cost		$144,000	
$144,000 ÷ 50 = $2,880			

If monthly adjustments were made by Hoosier Hospital during 19X1, this entry would be made for $240 ($2,880 ÷ 12 months) at the end of each month.

The $2,880 of depreciation on the building will appear among the expenses in Hoosier Hospital's 19X1 income statement. In the process of closing the books at the end of the year, the Depreciation Expense account will be closed. The Accumulated Depreciation account, however, is not closed; it is presented in the hospital's

December 31, 19X1, balance sheet in the manner described earlier. It also is carried forward into 19X2 as one of the opening balances for that year.

Depreciation of Equipment.   Assume that the estimated useful life of Hoosier Hospital's equipment is 10 years and that the salvage value is 10 percent, or $6,000 (10 percent of $60,000). The required adjusting entry at December 31, 19X1, is as follows:

Depreciation Expense		507 $5,400	
Accumulated Depreciation— Equipment		171	$5,400

Adjustment for 19X1 depreciation of hospital equipment:

Cost	$60,000
Less salvage value (10%)	6,000
Depreciable cost	$54,000

$54,000 ÷ 10 = $5,400

In actual practice, the computation of depreciation is complicated by the fact that hospitals own many different types of equipment that have been acquired on different dates and that have different useful lives and salvage values. And, of course, different depreciation methods may be applied to different classes of equipment.

Several depreciation expense accounts usually are employed in an actual situation. In order to reduce the amount of detail, however, we are using a single Depreciation Expense account for depreciation of both buildings and equipment.

Revenue Deductions

Turn your attention now to several other accounts in Hoosier Hospital's December 31, 19X1, trial balance (Figure 5–1). The relevant accounts are as follows:

Acct. No.	Account Titles	Dr.	Cr.
104	Accounts Receivable	$96,600	
105	Allowance for Uncollectible Accounts		$ -0-
501	Charity Service	29,200	
502	Contractual Adjustments	19,400	
503	Bad Debts	-0-	

You know, of course, that account 104 reflects the uncollected billings made to patients (or to third-party payers) for hospital services rendered. On December 31, 19X1, then, $96,600 of Hoosier Hospital's 19X1 patient service revenues remain uncollected and in Accounts Receivable. Account 104 is always debited (and revenues credited) for all services provided at full, established rates for those services, regardless of the financial status or medical classification of the patients served by the hospital. This provides an accounting measurement of the monetary value of the hospital services rendered during the period.

In fact, hospitals do not always collect their full, established rates for services rendered. There are several reasons for this situation.

The first reason why hospitals fail to collect their revenues is that most hospitals provide services to all who are in need of those services, regardless of the recipients' ability to pay. Hospitals render a considerable volume of services to the financially indigent, either at nominal service rates or at no charge whatever. The difference between the hospital's established rates for such services and the amount collected (if any) is called *charity service.* The amount of charity service provided by the hospital is accumulated and reported as a *revenue deduction* in the Revenue Deductions—Charity Service account (number 501). Because this account reflects "lost revenues," it has a debit balance.

Charity Service

To illustrate, assume that Hoosier Hospital provides certain ancillary services to a group of charity patients. Established rates for these services total $174, but the hospital receives nothing. Two entries are necessary:

Accounts Receivable	104	$174	
Ancillary Services Revenue	402		$174
Services rendered to charity patients.			
Revenue Deductions—Charity			
Service	501	174	
Accounts Receivable	104		174
Writeoff of patients' accounts to			
charity service.			

In subsequent discussion, the "revenue deductions" prefix to the Charity Service account will be omitted for ease of presentation. It is, however, an account that usually is reported in the income statement as a deduction from patient service revenues.

In its Statement Number 7, "The Presentation of Patient Service Revenue and Related Issues," however, the HFMA's Principles and Practices Board concluded that charity service should be reported as an expense in general purpose financial statements issued to external users.[1] The statement does not apply to internal accounting reports in which charity service may be reported as a revenue deduction or as an expense, whichever is more managerially useful. Over the next several years, it will be interesting to see whether the classification of charity service as an expense becomes the general practice among healthcare entities. This book treats charity service as a revenue deduction.

Third-Party Contract Terms

A second reason why hospitals often do not collect their full rates concerns certain third-party contracts. Under these contracts, the hospital has agreed to provide certain services to a particular group of patients at contract rates that are less than the hospital's full rates. The difference generally is not collectible by the hospital from those patients. This uncollectible difference usually is accumulated in another revenue deduction account called Contractual Adjustments (account 502).

To illustrate, assume that Hoosier Hospital provides $10,000 of services to certain third-party patients under a contract that

[1]HFMA Principles and Practices Board, *A Compilation of Statements 1–9* (HFMA: Chicago, 1987), p. 61.

provides for 90 percent reimbursement to the hospital. The entries are as follows:

Accounts Receivable	104	$10,000	
Routine Services Revenue	401		$ 6,000
Ancillary Services Revenue	402		4,000
Services rendered to patients.			
Cash	101	9,000	
Contractual Adjustments	502	1,000	
Accounts Receivable	104		10,000
Collection of third-party			
patients' accounts.			

The $1,000 of lost revenue (10 percent of $10,000) is debited to the Contractual Adjustments account that, like charity service, will be included in the income statement as a deduction from gross patient service revenues.

Statement 7 of the HFMA Principles and Practices Board, however, concludes that revenues be reported net of contractual adjustments in general-purpose financial statements.[2] In other words, revenues should be reported at the amount that the third-party payer has an obligation to pay. Over time, this may become the general practice of healthcare entities. In this book, we will treat contractual adjustments as revenue deductions.

A third reason why hospitals fail to collect their revenues is that some patients simply do not pay their hospital bills, just as they may not pay their other bills. If these patients' accounts remain uncollected after the hospital's best collection efforts, they are written off as bad debts. These uncollectibles are accumulated in another revenue deduction account: Bad Debts (account 503).

Bad Debts

It is very important not to confuse bad debts with charity service. Bad debts arise from services rendered to patients who are *able but unwilling* to pay; charity services are services provided to patients who are *unable to pay.*

Statement 2 of the Principles and Practices Board sets forth the differentiation between bad debts and charity service, and the time when the differentiation should be made.[3] At the time of admission, or as soon thereafter as possible, the financial status of patients

[2]Ibid, pp. 60–61.
[3]Ibid, pp. 7–11.

should be clearly established so as to permit accurate accounting classifications of all patient service transactions.

Making Adjustments for Revenue Deductions

In addition to accounting recognition of charity service, contractual adjustments, and bad debts during an accounting period, adjusting entries for these revenue deductions also are necessary at the end of the period. These entries consist of estimates of charity service, contractual adjustments, and bad debts related to services rendered during the period and included in the end-of-period accounts receivable.

This estimated portion of accounts receivable likely to prove uncollectible in the next accounting period is debited to the revenue deduction accounts and credited to the Allowance for Uncollectible Accounts (account number 105). This is done to "match" gross revenues with related revenue deductions in the same accounting period. It is the same principle described in Chapter 5 as the matching of revenue and expense.

The Allowance for Uncollectible Accounts is a contraasset account. It is presented in the hospital's balance sheet as a deduction from accounts receivable in much the same manner that accumulated depreciation is deducted from the hospital's plant assets. Journal entries relating to the allowance account are illustrated later in this chapter.

Charity Service

Recall that Hoosier Hospital's December 31, 19X1, trial balance includes account 501, Charity Service, with a debit balance of $29,200. This indicates that the hospital, in a series of journal entries, gave accounting recognition to $29,200 of charity service rendered during 19X1. In a single summary entry, this is what was recorded:

Charity Service	501	$29,200	
Accounts Receivable	104		$29,200
Writeoff of patients' accounts			
to charity service.			

Prior to this, when the services were provided to charity patients, entries were made to record the revenues and establish the accounts receivable.

At year's end, however, there are $96,600 of accounts receivable. How much of this $96,600 will not be collected because of charity service? If it is possible and practicable to identify specific accounts (or portions of specific accounts) as charity, such accounts (or portions of them) should be written off immediately and directly to the Charity Service account. This procedure is frequently feasible. If not, an estimate generally is made of the percentage of accounts receivable likely not to be collected because of being charity service. Assuming this percentage to be 5 percent, the necessary adjusting entry at December 31, 19X1, is

Charity Service	501	$4,830
Allowance for Uncollectible		
Accounts	105	$4,830
Adjustment for estimated portion		
of accounts receivable likely to		
prove uncollectible because of		
charity service (5% of $96,600 =		
$4,830).		

This entry matches the charity service revenue deduction with the related revenues recorded during 19X1. The entry also establishes the allowance account so that the accounts receivable will be reported in the December 31, 19X1, balance sheet at net realizable value, or collectible value.

In 19X2, when it is determined that a 19X1 patient account of, say, $700 is deemed uncollectible by reason of financial indigence, the following entry is made:

Allowance for Uncollectible		
Accounts	105	$ 700
Accounts Receivable	104	$ 700
Writeoff of 19X1 charity		
accounts to the allowance for		
uncollectibles.		

Had the adjusting entry not been made at the end of 19X1 to establish the allowance account for estimated charity service, the 19X2 writeoff would have been debited to the 19X2 charity service (Revenue Deductions) account. And this would have put the debit to charity service in the wrong year! The charity service was provided in 19X1, not in 19X2.

Contractual Adjustments

Hoosier Hospital's December 31, 19X1, trial balance includes account 502, Contractual Adjustments, which has a debit balance of $19,400. All of these revenue deductions were recorded by the hospital in a series of entries, but the following entry summarizes them:

Contractual Adjustments	502	$19,400	
Accounts Receivable	104		$19,400
Writeoff of patients' accounts			
to contractual adjustments.			

This entry records the contractual adjustments given accounting recognition during 19X1. At December 31, however, how much of the $96,600 of accounts receivable will prove to be uncollectible by reason of contractual adjustments?

Estimating Contractual Adjustments

If it is possible to identify the contractual adjustment portion of individual accounts, such amounts should be written off immediately and directly to the Contractual Adjustments account. This procedure generally is not feasible. Instead, an estimate is made of the percentage of accounts receivable likely to prove uncollectible because of contractual adjustments. Let us assume that only $20,000 of year-end accounts receivable are subject to contractual adjustment and that an estimated 12 percent of these balances probably will be uncollected because of such adjustments. The following is the required December 31, 19X1, adjusting entry:

Contractual Adjustments	502	$ 2,400	
Allowance for Uncollectible			
Accounts	105		$ 2,400
Adjustment for estimated			
portion of accounts receivable			
likely to prove uncollectible by			
reason of contractual			
adjustments (12% of $20,000).			

This entry matches the revenue deduction for contractual adjustments with the related revenues recorded during 19X1.

In 19X2, when $1,900 of 19X1 accounts receivable are found to be uncollectible by reason of contractual adjustments, the following entry is made:

Allowance for Uncollectible			
Accounts	105	$1,900	
Accounts Receivable	104		$1,900
Writeoff of a portion of 19X1 accounts receivable against the allowance for uncollectibles.			

Had the allowance account not been established by the December 31, 19X1, adjusting entry, the 19X2 writeoff above would have been made to revenue deductions (Contractual Adjustments) of 19X2. This would have produced a mismatching of revenues and revenue deductions.

Bad Debts

A third revenue deduction account, Bad Debts (account 503), appears in the December 31, 19X1, trial balance of Hoosier Hospital. Because this account has no balance, it can be correctly assumed that the hospital has not recognized any bad debts during 19X1. As of December 31, however, the hospital has $96,600 of accounts receivable. How much of these receivables will prove to be uncollectible by reason of bad debts?

Determining Bad Debts

If it can be determined that specific accounts are bad debts on December 31, those particular accounts should be written off immediately and directly to the Bad Debts account—in other words, debit Bad Debts and credit accounts receivable. This procedure, however, often is not feasible, particularly with those accounts that have been on the books only a short time and for which additional collection efforts will be made in the future. Thus, an estimate must be made as to the amount of bad debts likely to arise out of the December 31 accounts receivable.

This estimate may be developed as a percentage of accounts receivable or as a percentage of patient service revenues for the period. It also may be determined through the preparation of a so-called aging schedule for the year-end accounts receivable. These methods of estimating bad debts are described fully in a later chapter. Until we consider them in detail, we will estimate bad debts simply as a percentage of year-end accounts receivable, recognizing that this procedure is not always appropriate.

Let us assume, then, that Hoosier Hospital estimates its bad debts at 10 percent of December 31, 19X1, accounts receivable. The required adjusting entry is the following:

Bad Debts	503	$9,660	
Allowance for Uncollectible			
Accounts	105		$9,660
Adjustment for estimated portion			
of accounts receivable likely to			
prove uncollectible by reason of			
bad debts (10% of $96,600 =			
$9,660).			

This entry puts the revenue deduction (Bad Debts) in the same year in which the related revenues and accounts receivable arose.

In 19X2, when an individual patient's account of (say) $950 is deemed to be a bad debt and therefore uncollectible, the entry is:

Allowance for Uncollectible			
Accounts	105	$ 950	
Accounts Receivable	104		$ 950
Writeoff of a patient's account			
deemed to be a bad debt.			

Had the allowance account not been established at the end of 19X1, the writeoff in 19X2 necessarily would have been charged to Bad Debts of 19X2 (the wrong year, in that the related revenues were recognized in 19X1).

Bad Debts as Expenses Versus Revenue Deductions

It should be noted that Statement 7 of the Principles and Practices Board concludes that bad debts should be reported as expenses in general-purpose financial statements.[4] In effect, Statement 7 would eliminate the reporting of all revenue deductions (except perhaps through disclosures in footnotes). This book, however, treats bad debts as revenue deductions.

[4]Ibid, p. 61.

The assumed December 31, 19X1, adjusting entries for charity service, contractual adjustments, and bad debts are repeated (summarized) as follows:

Allowance for Uncollectible Accounts

Charity Service	501	$ 4,830	
Allowance for Uncollectible			
Accounts	105		$ 4,830
Adjustment for estimated charity service in year-end accounts receivable.			
Contractual Adjustments	502	2,400	
Allowance for Uncollectible			
Accounts	105		2,400
Adjustment for estimated amount of contractual adjustments in year-end receivables.			
Bad Debts	503	9,660	
Allowance for Uncollectible			
Accounts	105		9,660
Adjustment for estimated bad debts in year-end accounts receivable.			

Although a separate allowance account generally is maintained for each type of revenue deduction, a single allowance account is used here to reduce the amount of detail.

Taken together, these entries establish a total credit balance of $16,890 ($4,830 + $2,400 + $9,660) in the allowance account. The balance sheet of Hoosier Hospital at December 31, 19X1, therefore, will report:

Accounts Receivable	$96,600	
Less Allowance for Uncollectible Accounts	16,890	
Accounts Receivable, net		$79,710

Entry No.	Accounts and Explanations	Acct. No.	Dr.	Cr.
9	Depreciation Expense	507	$2,880	
	Accumulated Depreciation—Building	161		$ 2,880
	Adjustment for 19X1 depreciation of hospital building.			
10	Depreciation Expense	507	5,400	
	Accumulated Depreciation—Equipment	171		5,400
	Adjustment for 19X1 depreciation of hospital equipment.			
11	Charity Service	501	4,830	
	Allowance for Uncollectible Accounts	105		4,830
	Adjustment for estimated charity service in year-end receivables.			
12	Contractual Adjustments	502	2,400	
	Allowance for Uncollectible Accounts	105		2,400
	Adjustment for estimated contractual adjustments in year-end receivables.			
13	Bad Debts	503	9,660	
	Allowance for Uncollectible Accounts	105		9,660
	Adjustment for estimated bad debts in year-end receivables.			

Figure 7–1 Hoosier Hospital 19X1 Journal (Adjusting Entries)

The $79,710 figure is the net realizable value of the hospital's accounts receivable at December 31. It is the amount of the accounts receivable estimated to be collectible in cash in the future (early in 19X2, we hope). This balance sheet valuation of accounts receivable is a generally accepted accounting principle.

Summary of Adjustments for Depreciation and Revenue Deductions

In the previous chapter (Figure 6–1), adjusting journal entries for prepayments and accruals were illustrated. Those adjustments were numbered as entries 1 through 8. Figure 7–1 presents the adjusting entries discussed in this chapter as entries 9 through 13. Entries 9 and 10 are for depreciation expense; entries 11 through 13 are for revenue deductions. The next chapter pulls together all 13 adjusting entries and prepares the 19X1 financial statements for Hoosier Hospital.

Q7–1. What is a contraasset account? Give two examples of such an account.

Q7–2. Define *depreciation* as the term is used in accounting.

Q7–3. For plant assets, what is salvage value? How is the amount of salvage value determined for a particular asset?

Q7–4. How is the estimated useful life of a plant asset determined?

Q7–5. Gordon Hospital purchased a new item of equipment for $15,000 on January 1, 19X1. This equipment has an estimated useful life of 10 years and an expected salvage value of 20 percent. Compute the amount of straight-line depreciation for 19X1.

Q7–6. For depreciable plant assets, what is meant by the term *book value*?

Q7–7. Is land a depreciable asset? Explain.

Q7–8. Gravity Hospital purchased a new item of equipment on January 1, 19X1.The equipment has an estimated useful life of 10 years and an expected salvage value of 20 percent. Gravity Hospital's December 31, 19X5, balance sheet reports $10,000 of accumulated depreciation on this equipment. What was the cost of the equipment when acquired on January 1, 19X1?

Q7–9. Gamma Hospital purchased a new item of equipment for $40,000 on May 1, 19X1. The equipment has an estimated useful life of 10 years and an expected salvage value of $4,000. What amount should be reported as accumulated depreciation on this equipment in Gamma Hospital's December 31, 19X2, balance sheet?

Q7–10. Hospitals do not always collect their full, established rates for services rendered. Explain why this situation exists.

Q7–11. Distinguish among (a) charity service, (b) contractual adjustments, and (c) bad debts.

Q7–12. At what amount should patients' accounts receivable be valued in a hospital's balance sheet?

E7–1. Garry Hospital provides $1,600 of routine services and $1,400 of ancillary services to a patient under a third-party contract that provides for 85 percent reimbursement to the hospital. The remaining 15 percent is not billable to the patient.

Required: Make general journal entries to record (1) the services rendered to the patient and (2) the collection of the patient's account.

E7–2. Great Hospital has $100,000 of accounts receivable at December 31, 19X1. It is estimated that 9 percent of these accounts will eventually prove to be bad debts and, therefore, uncollectible. During 19X2, $8,300 of the 19X1 accounts receivable are written off as bad debts.

Required: Make general journal entries to record (1) the estimated bad debts at December 31, 19X1, and (2) the writeoff of bad accounts during 19X2.

E7–3. Goodcare Hospital has $100,000 of accounts receivable at December 31, 19X1. It is estimated that 7 percent of these accounts will be uncollectible by reason of charity service, 10 percent will not be collectible because of contractual adjustments, and 4 percent will prove to be bad debts.

Required: Make the necessary adjusting entries at December 31, 19X1, and indicate how the receivables should be reported in the hospital's balance sheet for December 31, 19X1.

E7–4. Gracious Hospital purchased the following plant assets on January 1, 19X1:

	Cost	Salvage Value	Estimated Useful Life (Years)
Land	$ 100,000		
Building	8,000,000	$1,600,000	40
Equipment	4,500,000	500,000	20

Required: Assuming straight-line depreciation, what is the depreciation expense for 19X4? At what amount, net of accumulated depreciation, would these assets be presented in the balance sheet of the hospital at December 31, 19X6?

E7–5. Golly Hospital purchased equipment with the following costs:

Purchase Date	Cost	Estimated Useful Life (Years)
1/1/X1	$100,000	8
4/1/X1	200,000	10
7/1/X1	300,000	6

Required: All equipment has a 20 percent salvage value. What is depreciation expense for 19X1?

P7–1. Goodness Hospital's general ledger contains the following unadjusted account balances, among others, at December 31, 19X1:

Acct.
No.

104	Accounts Receivable	$ 850,000
105	Allowance for Uncollectible Accounts	-0-
150	Land	25,000
160	Building	3,000,000
161	Accumulated Depreciation—Building	-0-
170	Equipment	1,800,000
171	Accumulated Depreciation—Equipment	-0-
501	Revenue Deductions—Charity Service	-0-
502	Revenue Deductions—Contractual Adjustments	-0-
503	Revenue Deductions—Bad Debts	-0-
607	Depreciation Expense	-0-

The following additional information is available:
1. Of the December 31, 19X1, accounts receivable, it is estimated that 15 percent will prove to be uncollectible due to these factors:
Charity service, 4%
Contractual adjustments, 6%
Bad debts, 5%
2. The hospital building, which was acquired on January 1, 19X1, has an estimated useful life of 40 years and an expected salvage value of $200,000.
3. Equipment, which cost $1,500,000, was acquired on January 1, 19X1. Additional equipment was acquired on July 1, 19X1, for $300,000. All equipment has a 20 percent salvage value and an estimated useful life of 10 years.

Required: Prepare, in general journal form, all necessary adjusting entries at December 31, 19X1.

P7–2. Certain of the accounts in Gateway Hospital's preadjusted trial balance at December 31, 19X6, are as follows:

Acct. No.		
102	Temporary Investments	$ 60,000
103	Accrued Interest Receivable	-0-
104	Accounts Receivable	940,000
105	Allowance for Uncollectible Accounts	3,000
107	Prepaid Insurance	1,800
150	Land	50,000
160	Building	4,000,000
161	Accumulated Depreciation—Building	450,000
170	Equipment	1,900,000
171	Accumulated Depreciation—Equipment	750,000
202	Notes Payable	100,000
203	Accrued Interest Payable	-0-
205	Deferred Rental Income	3,000
403	Interest Income	2,875
404	Rental Income	1,780
501	Charity Service	56,290
502	Contractual Adjustments	71,300
503	Bad Debts	-0-
604	Insurance Expense	11,450
607	Depreciation Expense	-0-
608	Interest Expense	9,230

The following additional information is available:

1. The hospital's temporary investments consist of $60,000 (face value) of 8 percent bonds that were acquired on October 1, 19X7. These bonds pay interest annually on October 1, commencing October 1, 19X7.

2. Account 105 is used only for estimated bad debts; charity service and contractual adjustments are charged directly to accounts 501 and 502, respectively. The $3,000 credit balance in account 105 here represents the excess of estimated bad debts at December 31, 19X5, over the actual bad debts written off during 19X6. It is estimated that all of the December 31, 19X6, accounts receivable are collectible except for 5 percent that probably will prove to be bad debts.

3. Account 107 includes a three-year insurance premium paid in advance on June 1, 19X6.

4. The hospital building, which was acquired on January 1, 19X1, has an estimated useful life of 40 years and an expected 10 percent salvage value.

5. All the equipment was acquired on January 1, 19X1. It has an estimated useful life of 12 years and a $100,000 salvage value.

6. Account 202 represents the face amount of a 12 percent, 6-month bank loan obtained by the hospital on November 1, 19X6. Interest on the note was not prepaid.

7. Account 205 represents a year's rent received in advance on March 1, 19X6.

Required: Prepare, in general journal form, the necessary adjusting entries for December 31, 19X6.

P7–3. Gaterburg Hospital's general ledger contains the following unadjusted account balances, among others, for December 31, 19X5:

Acct. No.		
104	Accounts Receivable	$120,000
105	Allowance for Uncollectible Accounts	-0-
150	Land	15,000
160	Building	900,000
161	Accumulated Depreciation—Building	80,000
170	Equipment	450,000
171	Accumulated Depreciation—Equipment	120,000
501	Revenue Deductions—Charity Service	-0-
502	Revenue Deductions—Contractual Adjustments	-0-
503	Revenue Deductions—Bad Debts	-0-
607	Depreciation Expense	-0-

The following additional information is available:

1. Of the December 31, 19X5, accounts receivable, it is estimated that 17 percent will prove to be uncollectible due to the following:
   Charity service, 6%
   Contractual adjustments, 7%
   Bad debts, 4%

2. The hospital building was acquired on January 1, 19X1. It has an estimated useful life of 40 years and an estimated salvage value of $100,000.

3. On January 1, 19X1, the hospital acquired $400,000 of equipment having an estimated useful life of 12 years and an estimated salvage value of 10 percent. Additional equipment, costing $50,000 and acquired on May 1,

19X5, has an estimated useful life of eight years and an estimated salvage value of $2,000.

Required: (1) Prepare, in general journal form, the necessary adjusting entries at December 31, 19X5. (2) Indicate the manner in which receivables should be presented in the hospital's December 31, 19X5, balance sheet. (3) Indicate the presentation of plant assets in the hospital's December 31, 19X5, balance sheet.

Accounting Cycle Summary

8

Chapter 5 began an illustration explaining the 19X1 financial activities of a hypothetical Hoosier Hospital. That illustration was continued in Chapters 6 and 7. Now we want to summarize quickly the discussion in those chapters and proceed to complete the accounting cycle for Hoosier Hospital. A summary of all of the procedures involved in the cycle is presented in Figure 8–1. This

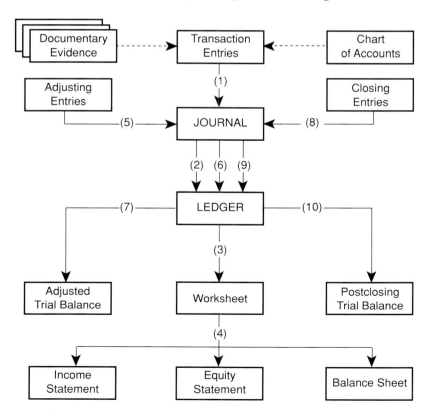

Figure 8–1 Summary of Accounting Procedure

diagram is quite similar to the one presented for the annual accounting cycle in Chapter 4 as Figure 4–8. Here, however, we have included the adjustment process.

Recall that Hoosier Hospital opened on January 1, 19X1. Over the course of the year, thousands of business transactions were completed with patients, third-party payers, suppliers, employees, and others. As these transactions occurred, documentary evidence was used as a basis for the development of transaction entries. These entries were journalized in the hospital's 19X1 journal (step 1 in Figure 8–1) to provide a chronological record of the increase and decrease effects of the transactions on the accounting classifications set forth in the hospital's chart of accounts. At the end of the year, the transaction entries were posted from the journal to the ledger (step 2 in Figure 8–1), and the year-end balance of each account was determined. These balances then were arranged in a preadjusted trial balance and entered on a worksheet (step 3 in Figure 8–1). The previously illustrated trial balance is repeated here as Figure 8–2.

Expansion of the Worksheet

Instead of preparing a separate preadjusted trial balance, we could enter the trial balance directly on the worksheet, as shown in Figure 8–3. This worksheet is used to develop the necessary adjusting entries. Each of the trial balance accounts is carefully scrutinized to determine the need for an adjustment of its balance. As these adjustments are determined, they are entered in the adjustments column of the worksheet (but not in the journal at this time). When all of the adjustments have been made, the adjusted balances of the accounts are extended into the columns for adjusted balances on the worksheet.

The worksheet then is completed by the extension of the adjusted balances into the appropriate statement columns. In footing the statement columns, the net income for the year and the hospital's year-end equity balance are determined. Naturally, the various columns of the worksheet must balance.

Financial Statements

The next procedure in the accounting cycle (step 4 in Figure 8–1) is the preparation of financial statements (income statement, equity statement, and balance sheet) for 19X1 for Hoosier Hospital. These statements are prepared directly from the information contained in the worksheet.

Acct. No.	Account Titles	105Dr.	Cr.
101	Cash	$ 38,300	
102	Temporary Investments	12,000	
103	Accrued Interest Receivable	-0-	
104	Accounts Receivable	96,600	
105	Allowance for Uncollectible Accounts		$ -0-
106	Inventory	10,500	
107	Prepaid Insurance	3,600	
108	Prepaid Rent	1,080	
109	Prepaid Interest	720	
150	Land	25,000	
160	Building	180,000	
161	Accumulated Depreciation—Building		-0-
170	Equipment	60,000	
171	Accumulated Depreciation—Equipment		-0-
201	Accounts Payable		29,840
202	Notes Payable		18,000
203	Accrued Interest Payable		-0-
204	Accrued Salaries and Wages Payable		-0-
205	Deferred Rental Income		4,200
206	Deferred Tuition Income		2,160
250	Bonds Payable		80,000
301	Hospital Equity		225,000
302	Revenue and Expense Summary		-0-
401	Routine Services Revenue		151,300
402	Ancillary Services Revenue		137,400
403	Interest Income		-0-
404	Rental Income		-0-
405	Tuition Income		-0-
406	Other Revenues		27,100
501	Charity Service	29,200	
502	Contractual Adjustments	19,400	
503	Bad Debts	-0-	
601	Salaries and Wages Expense	139,600	
602	Supplies Expense	28,600	
603	Utilities Expense	14,400	
604	Insurance Expense	-0-	
605	Repairs Expense	8,300	
606	Rent Expense	-0-	
607	Depreciation Expense	-0-	
608	Interest Expense	-0-	
609	Other Expenses	7,700	
	Totals	$675,000	$675,000

Figure 8–2 Hoosier Hospital Preadjusted Trial Balance, December 31, 19X1

Acct. No.	Account Titles	Preadjusted Trial Balance 12/31/X1 Dr.	Cr.	Adjustments 12/31/X1 Dr.	Cr.	Adjusted Trial Balance Dr.	Cr.	Income Statement 19X1 Dr.	Cr.	Equity Statement 19X1 Dr.	Cr.	Balance Sheet 12/31/X1 Dr.	Cr.
101	Cash	38,300				38,300						38,300	
102	Temporary Investments	12,000				12,000						12,000	
103	Accrued Interest Receivable			(8) 240		240						240	
104	Accounts Receivable	96,600				96,600						96,600	
105	Allowance for Uncollectible Accounts				(11)4,830 (12)2,400 (13)9,660		16,890						16,890
106	Inventory	10,500				10,500						10,500	
107	Prepaid Insurance	3,600			(1) 1,200	2,400						2,400	
108	Prepaid Rent	1,080			(2) 720	360						360	
109	Prepaid Interest	720			(3) 240	480						480	
150	Land	25,000				25,000						25,000	
160	Building	180,000				130,000						180,000	
161	Accumulated Depreciation— Building				(9) 2,880		2,880						2,880
170	Equipment	60,000				60,000						60,000	
171	Accumulated Depreciation— Equipment				(10)5,400		5,400						5,400
201	Accounts Payable		29,840				29,840						29,840
202	Notes Payable		18,000				18,000						18,000
203	Accrued Interest Payable				(4) 3,600		3,600						3,600
204	Accrued Salaries and Wages Payable				(5)13,000		13,000						13,000
205	Deferred Rental Income		4,200	(6) 1,750			2,450						2,450
206	Deferred Tuition Income		2,160	(7) 960			1,200						1,200
250	Bonds Payable		80,000				80,000						80,000
301	Hospital Equity		225,000				225,000				225,000		
302	Revenue and Expense Summary												
401	Routine Services Revenue		151,300				151,300		151,300				
402	Ancillary Services Revenue		137,400				137,400		137,400				
403	Interest Income				(8) 240		240		240				
404	Rental Income				(6) 1,750		1,750		1,750				
405	Tuition Income				(7) 960		960		960				
406	Other Revenues		27,100				27,100		27,100				
501	Charity Service	29,200		(11)4,830		34,030		34,030					
502	Contractual Adjustments	19,400		(12)2,400		21,800		21,800					
503	Bad Debts			(13)9,660		9,660		9,660					
601	Salaries and Wages Expense	139,600		(5)13,000		152,600		152,600					
	Totals Carried forward	616,000	675,000	32,840	46,880	633,970	717,010	218,090	318,750	-0-	225,000	425,880	173,260

Figure 8-3 Hoosier Hospital Worksheet to Develop Financial Statements, Year Ended December 31, 19X1

Acct. No.	Account Titles	Preadjusted Trial Balance 12/31/X1 Dr.	Cr.	12/31/X1 Adjustments Dr.	Cr.	Adjusted Trial Balance Dr.	Cr.	19X1 Income Statement Dr.	Cr.	19X1 Equity Statement Dr.	Cr.	12/31/X1 Balance Sheet Dr.	Cr.
	Totals Brought Forward	616,000	675,000	32,840	46,880	633,970	717,010	218,090	318,750	-0-	225,000	425,880	173,260
602	Supplies Expense	28,600				38,600		28,600					
603	Utilities Expense	14,400				14,400		14,400					
604	Insurance Expense			(1) 1,200		1,200		1,200					
605	Repairs Expense	8,300				8,300		8,300					
606	Rent Expense			(2) 720		720		720					
607	Depreciation Expense			(9) 2,880 (10) 5,400		8,280		8,280					
608	Interest Expense			(3) 240 (4) 3,600		3,840		3,840					
609	Other Expenses	7,700				7,700		7,700					
	Totals	675,000	675,000	46,880	46,880	717,010	717,010	291,130	318,750				
	Net Income for the Year							27,620			27,620		
	Totals							318,750	318,750		252,620		
	Hospital Equity, December 31, 19X1									-0-			252,620
	Totals									252,620	252,620	425,880	425,880

Figure 8-3 Hoosier Hospital Worksheet to Develop Financial Statements, Year Ended December 31, 19X1 (*continued*)

Figure 8–4 Hoosier Hospital Income Statement, Year Ended December 31, 19X1

Gross Patient Service Revenues:		
Routine Services	$151,300	
Ancillary Services	137,400	
Gross Patient Service Revenues		$288,700
Less Revenue Deductions:		
Charity Service	34,030	
Contractual Adjustments	21,800	
Bad Debts	9,660	
Total Revenue Deductions		65,490
Net Patient Service Revenues		223,210
Other Operating Revenues:		
Rent	1,750	
Tuition	960	
Other	27,100	
Total Other Operating Revenues		29,810
Total Operating Revenues		253,020
Less Operating Expenses:		
Salaries and Wages	152,600	
Supplies	28,600	
Utilities	14,400	
Insurance	1,200	
Repairs	8,300	
Rent	720	
Depreciation	8,280	
Interest	3,840	
Other	7,700	
Total Operating Expenses		225,640
Operating Income		27,380
Add Nonoperating Income (Interest)		240
Net Income for the Year		$ 27,620

Figure 8–5 Hoosier Hospital Statement of Hospital Equity, Year Ended December 31, 19X1

Hospital Equity, January 1	$225,000
Add Net Income for 19X1	27,620
Hospital Equity, December 31	$252,620

Preparing the Financial Statements

Figure 8–4 illustrates Hoosier Hospital's 19X1 income statement; Figure 8–5, the statement of hospital equity; and Figure 8–6, the balance sheet. Because these statements are somewhat more sophisticated than the ones previously illustrated, you should give them careful study.

Assets		
Cash		$ 38,300
Temporary Investments		12,000
Accrued Interest Receivable		240
Accounts Receivable	$ 96,600	
Less Allowance for Uncollectible		
Accounts	16,890	79,710
Inventory		10,500
Prepaid Insurance		2,400
Prepaid Rent		360
Prepaid Interest		480
Total Current Assets		143,990
Land	25,000	
Building	$180,000	
Less Accumulated Depreciation	2,880	177,120
Equipment	60,000	
Less Accumulated Depreciation	5,400	54,600	256,720
Total Assets		$400,710
Liabilities and Equity		
Accounts Payable	$ 29,840	
Notes Payable	18,000	
Accrued Interest Payable	3,600	
Accrued Salaries and Wages Payable	13,000	
Deferred Rental Income	2,450	
Deferred Tuition Income	1,200	
Total Current Liabilities		$ 68,090
Long-Term Debt		
(9% Bonds Payable, Due 1991)		80,000
Total Liabilities		148,090
Hospital Equity		252,620
Total Liabilities and Equity		$400,710

Figure 8-6 Hoosier Hospital Balance Sheet, December 31, 19X1

After the financial statements are distributed to Hoosier Hospital's management, governing board, and other interested parties, the accountant returns to the journal to journalize the adjusting entries for the year (step 5 in Figure 8–1). This is illustrated in Figure 8–7.

Once they are journalized, the adjusting entries are posted to the ledger (step 6 in Figure 8–1). The postings of these entries to Hoosier Hospital's ledger accounts are shown in Figure 8–8. There the unadjusted balances in the ledger accounts are unlabeled, and the adjusted balances are encircled. Keep in mind as you examine Figure

Journalizing and Posting Adjusting Entries

Entry No.	Accounts and Explanations	Acct. No.	Dr.	Cr.
1	Insurance Expense	604	$ 1,200	
	Prepaid Insurance	107		$ 1,200
	Adjustment for portion of prepaid premium that expired during 19X1 (see Chapter 5).			
2	Rent Expense	606	720	
	Prepaid Rent	108		720
	Adjustment to record rent expense for May through December 19X1, at $90 per month (see Chapter 5).			
3	Interest Expense	608	240	
	Prepaid Interest	109		240
	Adjustment for interest on bank loan for November and December 19X1 (see Chapter 5).			
4	Interest Expense	608	3,600	
	Accrued Interest Payable	203		3,600
	Adjustment for 6 months' interest accrued on bonds since July 1, 19X1 (see Chapter 5).			
5	Salaries and Wages Expense	601	13,000	
	Accrued Salaries and Wages Payable	204		13,000
	Adjustment for accrued payroll for the month of December 19X1 (see Chapter 5).			
6	Deferred Rental Income	205	1,750	
	Rental Income	404		1,750
	Adjustment for 5 months of rental income earned from provision of office space for physicians (see Chapter 6).			
7	Deferred Tuition Income	206	960	
	Tuition Income	405		960
	Adjustment for tuition income earned in 19X1 (see Chapter 6).			
8	Accrued Interest Receivable	103	240	
	Interest Income	403		240
	Adjustment for 3 months' interest on temporary investment in government bonds (see Chapter 6).			

Figure 8–7 Hoosier Hospital 19X1 Journal (Adjusting Entries)

Entry No.	Accounts and Explanations	Acct. No.	Dr.	Cr.
9	Depreciation Expense	507	$ 2,880	
	Accumulated Depreciation—Building	161		$ 2,880
	Adjustment for 19X1 depreciation of hospital building (see Chapter 7).			
10	Depreciation Expense	507	5,400	
	Accumulated Depreciation—Equipment	171		5,400
	Adjustment for 19X1 depreciation of hospital equipment (see Chapter 7).			
11	Charity Service	501	4,830	
	Allowance for Uncollectible Accounts	105		4,830
	Adjustment for estimated charity service in year-end receivables (see Chapter 7).			
12	Contractual Adjustments	502	2,400	
	Allowance for Uncollectible Accounts	105		2,400
	Adjustment for estimated contractual adjustments in year-end receivables (see Chapter 7).			
13	Bad Debts	503	9,660	
	Allowance for Uncollectible Accounts	105		9,660
	Adjustment for estimated bad debts in year-end receivables (see Chapter 7).			

Figure 8–7 Hoosier Hospital 19X1 Journal (Adjusting Entries) *(continued)*

8–8 that the postings of adjusting entries are numbered 1 through 13. You may wish to trace each of these postings from the journal (Figure 8–7).

After the adjusting entries are posted and adjusted balances are obtained in the ledger accounts, the adjusted balances may be arranged in an adjusted trial balance (step 7 in Figure 8–1). Hoosier Hospital's adjusted trial balance is not illustrated here because an adjusted trial balance appears on the worksheet in Figure 8–2.

Preparing an Adjusted Trial Balance

The next procedure in the accounting cycle is the preparation of closing entries. The entries are recorded in the journal (step 8 in Figure 8–1) as shown in Figure 8–9. Notice that the closing entries are numbered 14 through 17. In addition to the closing of revenue and expense accounts, the revenue deduction accounts also must be closed, as indicated in entry 15.

Journalizing and Posting Closing Entries

Figure 8-8 Hoosier Hospital
19X1 Ledger (With Adjusting
Entries)

Cash	101
38,300	
(38,300)	

Temporary Investments	102
12,000	
(12,000)	

Accrued Interest Receivable	103
(8) 240	
(240)	

Accounts Receivable	104
96,600	
(96,600)	

Allowance for Uncollectible Accounts	105
	(11) 4,830
	(12) 2,400
	(13) 9,660
	(16,890)

Inventory	106
10,500	
(10,500)	

Prepaid Insurance	107
3,600	(1) 1,200
(2,400)	

Prepaid Rent	108
1,080	(2) 720
(360)	

Prepaid Interest	109
720	(3) 240
(480)	

Land	150
25,000	
(25,000)	

Building	160
180,000	
(180,000)	

Accum. Depreciation— Building	161
	(9) 2,880
	(2,880)

Equipment	170
25,000	
(25,000)	

Accum. Depreciation— Equipment	171
	(10) 5,400
	(5,400)

Accounts Payable	201
	29,840
	(29,840)

Notes Payable	202
	18,000
	(18,000)

Accrued Interest Payable	203
	(4) 3,600
	(3,600)

Accrued Salaries and Wages Payable	204
	(5) 13,000
	(13,000)

Deferred Rental Income	205
(6) 1,750	4,200
	(2,450)

Deferred Tuition Income	206
(7) 960	2,160
	(1,200)

Bonds Payable	250
	80,000
	(80,000)

Figure 8-8 Hoosier Hospital 19X1 Ledger (With Adjusting Entries) *(continued)*

Hospital Equity 301	Revenue and Expense Summary 302	Routine Services Revenue 401
225,000		151,300
(225,000)		(151,300)

Ancillary Services Revenue 402	Interest Income 403	Rental Income 404
137,400	(8) 240	(6) 1,750
(137,400)	(240)	(1,750)

Tuition Income 405	Other Revenues 406	Charity Service 501
(7) 960	27,100	29,200
		(11)4,830
(960)	(27,100)	(34,030)

Contractual Adjustments 502	Bad Debts 503	Salaries and Wages Expense 601
19,400	(13) 9,660	139,600
(12) 2,400		(5) 13,000
(21,800)	(9,660)	(152,600)

Supplies Expense 602	Utilities Expense 603	Insurance Expense 604
28,600	14,400	(1) 1,200
(28,600)	(14,400)	(1,200)

Repairs Expense 605	Rent Expense 606	Depreciation Expense 607
8,300	(2) 720	(9) 2,880
		(10) 5,400
(8,300)	(720)	(8,280)

Interest Expense 608	Other Expense 609	
(3) 240	7,700	
(4) 3,600		
(3,840)	(7,700)	

Entry No.	Accounts and Explanations	Acct. No.	Dr.	Cr.
14	Routine Services Revenue	401	$151,300	
	Ancillary Services Revenue	402	137,400	
	Interest Income	403	240	
	Rental Income	404	1,750	
	Tuition Income	405	960	
	Other Revenues	406	27,100	
	Revenue and Expense Summary	302		$318,750
	To close revenue accounts.			
15	Revenue and Expense Summary	302	65,490	
	Charity Service	501		34,030
	Contractual Adjustments	502		21,800
	Bad Debts	503		9,660
	To close revenue deduction accounts.			
16	Revenue and Expense Summary	302	225,640	
	Salaries and Wages Expense	601		152,600
	Supplies Expense	602		28,600
	Utilities Expense	603		14,400
	Insurance Expense	604		1,200
	Repairs Expense	605		8,300
	Rent Expense	606		720
	Depreciation Expense	607		8,280
	Interest Expense	608		3,840
	Other Expenses	609		7,700
	To close expense accounts.			
17	Revenue and Expense Summary	302	27,620	
	Hospital Equity	301		27,620
	To close Revenue and Expense Summary account and add net income to equity.			

Figure 8–9 Hoosier Hospital 19X1 Journal (Closing Entries)

Posting Closing Entries to the Ledger

The closing entries are now posted to the ledger (step 9 in Figure 8–1), as illustrated in Figure 8–10. When this is completed, the revenue, revenue deduction, and expense accounts are double-ruled to indicate that those accounts are closed.

Preparing a Postclosing Trial Balance

The last step in the accounting cycle is the preparation of a postclosing trial balance (step 10 in Figure 8–1). The December 31, 19X1, postclosing trial balance for Hoosier Hospital is illustrated in

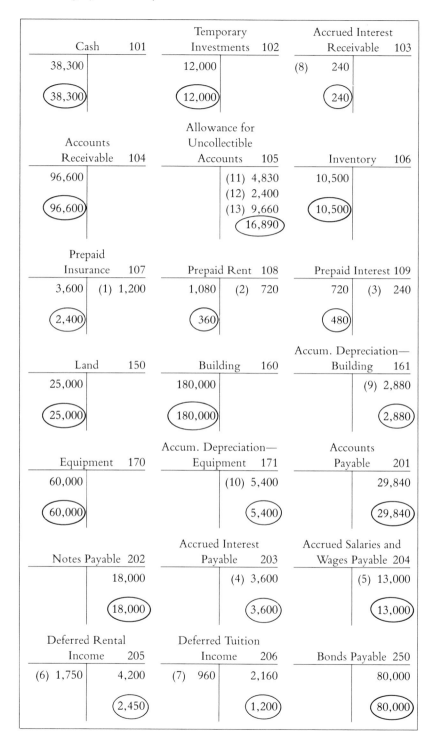

Figure 8-10 Hoosier Hospital 19X1 Ledger (With Closing Entries)

Figure 8-10 Hoosier Hospital
19X1 Ledger (With Closing
Entries) *(continued)*

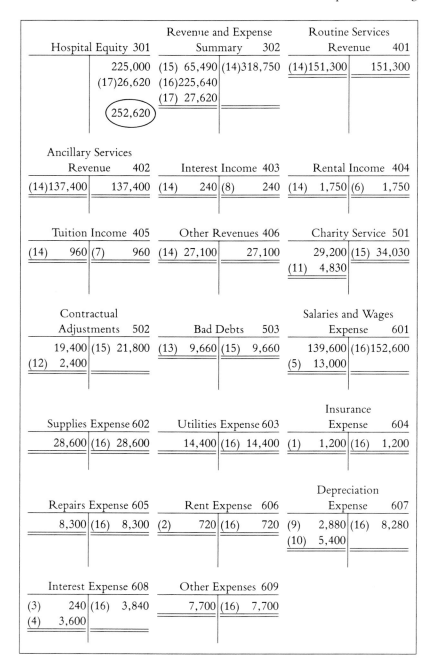

Hospital Equity 301	Revenue and Expense Summary 302	Routine Services Revenue 401
225,000	(15) 65,490 | (14)318,750	(14)151,300 | 151,300
(17)26,620	(16)225,640	
(252,620)	(17) 27,620	

Ancillary Services Revenue 402	Interest Income 403	Rental Income 404
(14)137,400 | 137,400	(14) 240 | (8) 240	(14) 1,750 | (6) 1,750

Tuition Income 405	Other Revenues 406	Charity Service 501
(14) 960 | (7) 960	(14) 27,100 | 27,100	29,200 | (15) 34,030
		(11) 4,830

Contractual Adjustments 502	Bad Debts 503	Salaries and Wages Expense 601
19,400 | (15) 21,800	(13) 9,660 | (15) 9,660	139,600 | (16)152,600
(12) 2,400		(5) 13,000

Supplies Expense 602	Utilities Expense 603	Insurance Expense 604
28,600 | (16) 28,600	14,400 | (16) 14,400	(1) 1,200 | (16) 1,200

Repairs Expense 605	Rent Expense 606	Depreciation Expense 607
8,300 | (16) 8,300	(2) 720 | (16) 720	(9) 2,880 | (16) 8,280
		(10) 5,400

Interest Expense 608	Other Expenses 609	
(3) 240 | (16) 3,840	7,700 | (16) 7,700	
(4) 3,600		

Figure 8-11. Note that the remaining balances are those for asset, liability, and equity accounts only. It is with these balances that Hoosier Hospital will begin the new year, 19X2. On January 1, 19X2, a new accounting cycle commences.

Acct. No.	Accounts and Titles	Dr.	Cr.
101	Cash	$ 38,300	
102	Temporary Investments	12,000	
103	Accrued Interest Receivable	240	
104	Accounts Receivable	96,600	
105	Allowance for Uncollectible Accounts		$ 16,890
106	Inventory	10,500	
107	Prepaid Insurance	2,400	
108	Prepaid Rent	360	
109	Prepaid Interest	480	
150	Land	25,000	
160	Building	180,000	
161	Accumulated Depreciation—Building		2,880
170	Equipment	60,000	
171	Accumulated Depreciation— Equipment		5,400
201	Accounts Payable		29,840
202	Note Payable		18,000
203	Accrued Interest Payable		3,600
204	Accrued Salaries and Wages Payable		13,000
205	Deferred Rental Income		2,450
206	Deferred Tuition Income		1,200
250	Bonds Payable		80,000
301	Hospital Equity		252,620
	Totals	$425,880	$425,880

Figure 8–11 Hoosier Hospital Postclosing Trial Balance, December 31, 19X1

Questions

Q8–1. List and describe briefly each of the 10 major steps in a complete accounting cycle.

Q8–2. "Annual financial statements cannot be prepared until the books are closed for the year." Do you agree? Explain. *10*

Q8–3. Following is a random listing of accounting procedures. Indicate the normal sequence in which these procedures are performed.

4 a. Prepare financial statements.

1 b. Journalize closing entries.

6 c. Post adjusting entries to the ledger.

8 d. Prepare general worksheet.

2 e. Journalize transaction entries.

9 f. Post closing entries to the ledger.

5 g. Prepare adjusted trial balance.

3 h. Post transaction entries to the ledger.

i. Prepare postclosing trial balance.

j. Journalize adjusting entries.

Q8–4. Garden Hospital paid a three-year insurance premium of $3,600 in advance on January 1, 19X1, debiting the $3,600 to the prepaid account. At the end of the year, the necessary adjusting entry was not made. The omission was not discovered. What effect would this error have on (a) total assets, (b) total liabilities, and (c) hospital equity, as reported in the hospital's balance sheet for December 31, 19X1?

Q8–5. Goshen Hospital paid an account payable of $4,500 during December 19X1. In the transaction entry, however, the debit was made to supplies expense. The error was not discovered until after the financial statements for 19X1 were prepared. What effect would this error have on (a) total assets, (b) total liabilities, and (c) hospital equity, as reported in the hospital's December 31, 19X1, balance sheet?

Q8–6. Gibson Hospital received $2,300 in payment of a patient's account receivable on December 27, 19X1. In the transaction entry, however, the credit was made erroneously to routine service revenues. The error was not discovered until after the financial statements for 19X1 were prepared. What effect would this error have on (a) the total assets, (b) the total liabilities, and (c) the hospital equity, as reported in the hospital's December 31, 19X1, balance sheet?

Exercises

E8–1. Getwell Hospital provides you with the following information:

	12/31/X2	12/31/X1
Accrued interest receivable	$4,100	$3,900
Prepaid interest	6,400	5,700
Accrued interest payable	3,200	3,600
Deferred interest income	4,800	5,300

In 19X2, the hospital received $38,000 of interest in cash and paid $54,000 of interest.

Required: What should be reported in the hospital's 19X2 income statement as (1) interest expense and (2) interest income?

E8–2. Goodwill Hospital provides you with the following information from its 19X2 general ledger:

Revenue and Expense
Summary   302

899,204	964,382
65,178	

Required: Assuming the hospital equity at December 31, 19X1, was $516,894, what was the hospital equity at December 31, 19X2?

E8–3. Goodhope Hospital provides you with the following information:

	12/31/X2	12/31/X1
Deferred rental income	$8,000	$7,500
Prepaid rental expense	7,400	8,200
Accrued rent receivable	6,300	6,200
Accrued rent payable	5,100	5,900

The hospital's 19X2 income statement reports rental income of $40,000 and rental expense of $60,000.

Required: (1) What was the amount of rent received in cash during 19X2? (2) What was the amount of rent paid in cash during 19X2?

E8–4. Goodcare Hospital follows an accounting policy under which all income received in cash is credited to income and all expense paid in cash is debited to expense. At the end of each month, adjusting entries are made for prepayments and accruals. The prepayments and accruals at the end of January 19X2 were as follows:

Prepaid expenses	$4,000
Prepaid income	3,000
Accrued expenses	6,000
Accrued income	5,000

Required: If the necessary adjusting entries are not made on January 31, 19X2, by what amount would the January net income be overstated (or understated)?

P8–1. Given here is the preadjusted trial balance of Greatville Hospital at December 31, 1977, the end of the hospital's current fiscal year:

Problems

Acct. No.		Dr.	Cr.
101	Cash	$31,600	
102	Temporary Investments	15,000	
103	Accrued Interest Receivable	-0-	
104	Accounts Receivable	102,400	
105	Allowance for Uncollectible Accounts		$ -0-
106	Inventory	11,600	
107	Prepaid Insurance	1,980	
108	Prepaid Rent	2,100	
109	Prepaid Interest	1,200	
150	Land	22,000	
160	Building	175,000	
161	Accumulated Depreciation— Building		-0-
170	Equipment	80,000	
171	Accumulated Depreciation— Equipment		-0-
201	Accounts Payable		31,300
202	Notes Payable		20,000
203	Accrued Interest Payable		-0-
204	Accrued Salaries and Wages Payable		-0-
205	Deferred Rental Income		1,680
206	Deferred Tuition Income		1,215
250	Bonds Payable		100,000
301	Hospital Equity		207,085
302	Revenue and Expense Summary		-0-
401	Routine Services Revenue		169,300
402	Ancillary Services Revenue		128,700
403	Interest Income		-0-
404	Rental Income		-0-
405	Tuition Income		-0-
406	Other Revenues		29,800
501	Charity Service	28,200	
502	Contractual Adjustments	20,300	
503	Bad Debts	-0-	
601	Salaries and Wages Expense	141,200	
602	Supplies Expense	27,300	
603	Utilities Expense	15,100	
604	Insurance Expense	-0-	

605	Repairs Expense	$ 7,600	
606	Rent Expense	-0-	
607	Depreciation Expense	-0-	
608	Interest Expense	-0-	
609	Other Expenses	6,500	
	Totals	$689,080	$689,080

The following additional information is available:

1. The temporary investment consists of $15,000 (face value) of 8 percent bonds acquired by the hospital on October 1, 19X1. These bonds pay interest annually on October 1, commencing October 1, 19X2.

2. Of the December 31, 19X1, accounts receivable, it is estimated that 12 percent will eventually prove uncollectible by reason of (a) charity service, 4 percent; (b) contractual adjustments, 5 percent; and (c) bad debts, 3 percent.

3. A three-year insurance premium of $1,980 was paid in advance by the hospital on January 1, 19X1.

4. The hospital prepaid a year's rent of $2,100 on June 1, 19X1.

5. On November 1, 19X1, the hospital borrowed $20,000 from a bank by issuing its six-month, 12 percent note. Interest on the note was prepaid.

6. The hospital building, which was acquired on January 1, 19X1, has an estimated useful life of 40 years and a salvage value of $15,000.

7. The equipment, which was acquired on January 1, 19X1, has an estimated useful life of 8 years and a 10 percent salvage value.

8. On April 1, 19X1, the hospital issued $100,000 of 15–year, 6 percent bonds at face value. These bonds pay interest annually on April 1, commencing April 1, 19X2.

9. Unpaid salaries and wages at December 31, 19X1, totaled $15,600.

10. The hospital received one year's rent of $1,680 in advance on March 1, 19X1.

11. On September 1, 19X1, the hospital received nine months' tuition in advance in connection with one of its educational programs.

Required: (1) Prepare a worksheet to develop financial statements in the manner illustrated in Figure 8–3. (2) Prepare, in good form, a complete set of financial statements for 19X1.

P8–2. Certain of the adjusted balances in the ledger of Gatorberg Hospital at December 31, 19X1, the end of the hospital's current fiscal year, are provided here:

Acct. No.		
301	Hospital Equity	$275,000
302	Revenue and Expense Summary	-0-
401	Routine Services Revenue	159,700
402	Ancillary Services Revenue	101,800
403	Interest Income	2,600
404	Rental Income	1,900
405	Tuition Income	1,500
406	Other Revenues	29,800
501	Charity Service	31,700
502	Contractual Adjustments	42,300
503	Bad Debts	11,600
601	Salaries and Wages Expense	145,900
602	Supplies Expense	21,500
603	Utilities Expense	12,300
604	Insurance Expense	2,300
605	Repairs Expense	4,100
606	Rent Expense	2,800
607	Depreciation Expense	9,400
608	Interest Expense	1,400
609	Other Expenses	7,200

Required: (1) Prepare, in general journal form, the necessary closing entries for the year ended December 31, 19X1. (2) Prepare, in good form, the 19X1 income statement for Gatorberg Hospital.

P8–3. The following is the preadjusted trial balance of Grandtown Hospital at December 31, 19X1, the end of the hospital's current fiscal year:

Acct. No.		Dr.	Cr.
101	Cash	$37,500	
102	Temporary Investments	30,000	
103	Accrued Interest Receivable	-0-	
104	Accounts Receivable	120,000	
105	Allowance for Uncollectible Accounts		$ -0-

106	Inventory	$ 14,000	
107	Prepaid Insurance	3,600	
150	Land	25,000	
160	Building	250,000	
161	Accumulated Depreciation—Building		$ -0-
170	Equipment	140,000	
171	Accumulated Depreciation—Equipment		-0-
201	Accounts Payable		37,400
203	Accrued Interest Payable		-0-
204	Accrued Salaries and Wages Payable		-0-
205	Deferred Rental Income		2,700
250	Bonds Payable		150,000
301	Hospital Equity		395,700
302	Revenue and Expense Summary		-0-
401	Routine Services Revenue		171,200
402	Ancillary Services Revenue		110,300
403	Interest Income		-0-
404	Rental Income		-0-
406	Other Revenues		23,500
501	Charity Service	31,100	
502	Contractual Adjustments	22,700	
503	Bad Debts	-0-	
601	Salaries and Wages Expense	155,600	
602	Supplies Expense	33,100	
603	Utilities Expense	14,900	
604	Insurance Expense	-0-	
605	Repairs Expense	6,400	
607	Depreciation Expense	-0-	
608	Interest Expense	4,500	
609	Other Expenses	2,400	
	Totals	$890,800	$890,800

The following additional information is available:
1. The temporary investment consists of $30,000 (face value) of 8 percent bonds acquired by the hospital on November 1, 19X1. These bonds pay interest annually on November 1, commencing on November 1, 19X2.
2. Of the December 31, 19X1, accounts receivable, it is estimated that 14 percent will eventually prove uncollectible by reason of (a) charity service, 7 percent; (b) con-

tractual adjustments, 4 percent; and (c) bad debts, 3 percent.

3. A two-year insurance premium of $3,600 was paid in advance by the hospital on January 1, 19X1.

4. The hospital building, which was acquired on January 1, 19X1, has an estimated useful life of 50 years and a 20 percent salvage value.

5. The equipment, which was acquired on January 1, 19X1, has an estimated useful life of 12 years and a $20,000 salvage value.

6. On January 1, 19X1, the hospital issued $150,000 of 20-year, 6 percent bonds at face value. These bonds pay interest semiannually on January 1 and July 1, commencing July 1, 19X1.

7. Unpaid salaries and wages at December 31, 19X1, amount to $12,300.

8. The hospital received one year's rent of $2,700 in advance on June 1, 19X1.

Required: (1) Prepare a worksheet to develop financial statements in the manner illustrated in Figure 8–3. (2) Prepare, in good form, a complete set of financial statements for 19X1. (3) Prepare, in general journal form, the necessary adjusting entries at December 31, 19X1, for the year then ended. (4) Prepare in general journal form, the necessary closing entries on December 31, 19X1, for the year then ended.

Development of Interim Financial Statements

9

Up to now this book has dealt with the accounting process in annual terms: annual posting of transaction entries and annual financial statements. This chapter examines the procedures of accounting from a monthly point of view. The preparation of monthly adjusting entries and the development of a set of interim financial statements is the major objective. As mentioned earlier, interim financial statements are those prepared during the course of a hospital's fiscal year. The illustration presented in this chapter consists of preparation of an income statement for the month of September 19X1 and for the nine months ending September 30, 19X1. In addition, a September 30, 19X1, balance sheet will be prepared.

Interim financial statements are essential to the effective management of hospitals. Important managerial decisions are made during the course of a fiscal year that require the kinds of information provided by monthly income statements and balance sheets. In addition, many other types of accounting reports may be prepared weekly or daily (a cash report, for example). Certain of these special reports are illustrated later in this book. For now, you are concerned only with the routine income statements and balance sheets prepared at the end of each month.

Assume that a hypothetical Hiowa Hospital began its corporate existence on January 1, 19X1. Financial statements were prepared for 19X1 and 19X2, and the hospital is now in its third year of operations, 19X3. The 19X3 transactions have been journalized and posted through September 30. Monthly adjusting entries have been journalized and posted through August 31, and monthly financial statements have been prepared at the end of each month, January

Monthly Trial Balances

through August 19X3. It is now time to prepare financial statements for September 19X3 and for the nine months ended September 30, 19X3.

Hiowa Hospital's trial balances at August 31 and September 30, 19X3, are presented in Figure 9–1. Notice that the August 31 trial balance is an adjusted trial balance. It includes the adjusted balances, as of August 31, of all of the hospital's accounts. The equity balance is, of course, the opening (December 31, 19X2) equity balance because the books of the hospital have not been closed since December 31, 19X2.

This trial balance includes an eight-month accumulation of revenue, revenue deduction, and expense balances, adjusted through August 31, 19X3. In short, these are the figures used in Hiowa Hospital's August 31 balance sheet and in its income statement for the eight months ended August 31, 19X3. These statements are illustrated in Figures 9–2 and 9–3. (The income statement for the month of August 19X3 is not illustrated, although we assume the statement was prepared.)

Carefully note that Hiowa Hospital's trial balance for September 30, 19X3, is an *unadjusted* trial balance. The figures in this trial balance are those in the August 31 trial balance together with the effects of the September transactions of the hospital. In other words, this trial balance includes the unadjusted asset and liability balances as of September 30; the hospital equity balance as of December 31, 19X2; and the unadjusted revenue, revenue deduction, and expense balances at September 30, 19X3. So before financial statements can be prepared for September and for the nine months ended September 30, the September adjusting entries must be developed.

Developing the Adjusting Entries

September Adjusting Entries

You will have noticed that Hiowa Hospital's account titles and numbers are somewhat different from those used earlier in the Hoosier Hospital illustration. Some of these differences arise from an effort to simplify the illustration (a single account for depreciable plant assets, for example). Other changes were made to introduce new accounts and procedures. Although there is a degree of uniformity in charts of accounts from one hospital to another, there also may be considerable differences because of variations in size, organizational structure, and range of services, among other factors.

Accrued Interest Receivable

Hiowa Hospital's September 30 trial balance includes $60,000 of long-term investments (account 130). This consists of $60,000 (face

Acct. No.	Account Titles	Adjusted Trial Balance 8/31/X3 Dr.	Cr.	Unadjusted Trial Balance 9/30/X3 Dr.	Cr.
101	Cash	$ 30,900		$ 33,200	
102	Accrued Interest Receivable	800		800	
103	Accounts Receivable	84,000		87,100	
104	Allowance for Bad Debts		$ 8,400		$ 8,400
105	Inventory	9,800		11,300	
106	Prepaid Insurance	2,400		2,400	
130	Long-Term Investments	60,000		60,000	
150	Land	23,000		23,000	
160	Depreciable Plant Assets	187,500		187,500	
161	Accumulated Depreciation		20,000		20,000
201	Accounts Payable		18,200		19,400
202	Accrued Salaries and Wages Payable		4,600		-0-
203	Accrued Interest Payable		5,500		5,500
204	Deferred Rental Income		980		980
250	Bonds Payable		100,000		100,000
301	Hospital Equity		219,420		219,420
302	Revenue and Expense Summary		-0-		-0-
401	Inpatient Services Revenue		164,000		187,300
402	Outpatient Services Revenue		96,100		106,800
403	Interest Income		800		800
404	Rental Income		700		700
405	Other Revenues		46,300		52,200
501	Bad Debts	11,400		11,400	
502	Other Revenue Deductions	27,000		31,800	
601	Salaries and Wages Expense	160,000		176,400	
602	Supplies Expense	24,000		26,800	
603	Utilities Expense	16,000		18,100	
604	Insurance Expense	1,200		1,200	
605	Depreciation Expense	5,000		5,000	
606	Interest Expense	4,000		4,000	
607	Other Expenses	38,000		41,500	
	Totals	$685,000	$685,000	$721,500	$721,500

Figure 9–1 Hiowa Hospital Trial Balances, August 31 and September 30, 19X3

value) of 8 percent, 10-year corporate bonds purchased by the hospital at face value on July 1, 19X3. These bonds pay interest semiannually on July 1 and January 1, beginning on January 1, 19X4. The semiannual interest payments to the hospital will be $2,400 ($60,000 × 8 percent × 1/2). Thus, Hiowa Hospital is earning interest income of $400 per month ($2,400 ÷ 6) on these bonds.

Patient Service Revenues:			
Inpatient Services		$164,000	
Outpatient Services		96,100	
Gross Patient Service Revenue		260,100	
Less Revenue Deductions:			
Bad Debts	$11,400		
Other	27,000		
Total Revenue Deductions		38,400	
Net Patient Service Revenues			$221,700
Other Operating Revenues:			
Rent		700	
Other		46,300	
Total Other Operating Revenues			47,000
Total Operating Revenues			268,700
Less Operating Expenses:			
Salaries and Wages		160,000	
Supplies		24,000	
Utilities		16,000	
Insurance		1,200	
Depreciation		5,000	
Interest		4,000	
Other		38,000	
Total Operating Expenses			248,200
Operating Income			20,500
Add Nonoperating Income (Interest)			800
Net income			$ 21,300

On July 31 and August 31, Hiowa Hospital made an adjusting entry to accrue the monthly interest income:

Accrued Interest Receivable	102	$400	
Interest Income	403		$400

Monthly adjustment for accrual of
monthly interest income on corporate
bonds held as long-term investments.

Because this entry was made on July 31 and on August 31, Hiowa Hospital's August 31 trial balance includes $800 of accrued interest receivable and $800 of interest income. The September 30 (unad-

Assets			
Cash			$ 30,900
Accrued Interest Receivable			800
Accounts Receivable		$ 84,000	
Less Allowance for Bad Debts		8,400	75,600
Inventory			9,800
Prepaid Insurance			2,400
Total Current Assets			119,500
Long-Term Investments			60,000
Land		23,000	
Depreciable Plant Assets	$187,500		
Less Accumulated Depreciation	20,000	167,500	
Net Plant Assets			190,500
Total Assets			$370,000
Liabilities and Equity			
Accounts Payable		$ 18,200	
Accrued Salaries and Wages Payable		4,600	
Accrued Interest Payable		5,500	
Deferred Rental Income		980	
Total Current Liabilities			$ 29,280
Long-Term Debt (6% Bonds Payable, Due 19X8)			100,000
Total Liabilities			129,280
Hospital Equity, January 1[a]		219,420	
Add Net Income for 8 Months Ended August 31		21,300	
Hospital Equity, August 31			240,720
Total Liabilities and Equity			$370,000

[a]Change in equity balance shown within balance sheet in lieu of separate statement of hospital equity.

Figure 9–3 Hiowa Hospital Balance Sheet, August 31, 19X3

justed) trial balance, of course, includes the same figures because the September 30 adjustment has not yet been made, so the entry just shown must be repeated at September 30. This will be September 30, 19X3, adjusting entry (1). Notice that it has been entered on the worksheet in Figure 9–4. Later, the adjustment will be entered in Hiowa Hospital's journal.

The same adjusting entry will be made on October 31, November 30, and December 31 to produce a year-end balance of $2,400 in the Accrued Interest Receivable account. Then, when the interest is received in cash on January 1, 19X4, a transaction entry will be made to debit cash and credit the Accrued Interest Receivable account. As a result, the bond interest income is recognized monthly as it is *earned,* rather than at the time it is received in cash.

Recognizing Interest Income as It Is Earned

Acct. No.	Account Titles	Unadjusted Trial Balance, 9/30/X3 Dr.	Cr.	9/30/X3 Adjustments Dr.	Cr.	Adjusted Trial Balance, 9/30/X3 Dr.	Cr.	Income Statement Dr.	Cr.	Equity Statement Dr.	Cr.	Balance Sheet Dr.	Cr.
101	Cash	33,200				33,200						33,200	
102	Accrued Interest Receivable	800		(1) 400		1,200						1,200	
103	Accounts Receivable	87,100				87,100						87,100	
104	Allowance for Bad Debts		8,400		(2) 310		8,710						8,710
105	Inventory	11,300				11,300						11,300	
106	Prepaid Insurance	2,400			(3) 150	2,250						2,250	
130	Long-Term Investments	60,000				60,000						60,000	
150	Land	23,000				23,000						23,000	
160	Depreciable Plant Assets	187,500				187,500						187,500	
161	Accumulated Depreciation		20,000		(4) 625		20,625						20,625
201	Accounts Payable		19,400				19,400						19,400
202	Accrued Salaries and Wages Payable		-0-		(5) 3,100		3,100						3,100
203	Accrued Interest Payable		5,500		(7) 500		6,000						6,000
204	Deferred Rental Income		980	(6) 140			840						840
250	Bonds Payable		100,000				100,000						100,000
301	Hospital Equity		219,420				219,420				219,420		
302	Revenue and Expense Summary		-0-										
401	Inpatient Services Revenue		187,300				187,300		187,300				
402	Outpatient Services Revenue		106,800				106,800		106,800				
403	Interest Income		800		(1) 400		1,200		1,200				
404	Rental Income		700		(6) 140		840		840				
405	Other Revenues		52,200				52,200		52,200				
501	Bad Debts	11,400		(2) 310		11,710		11,710					
502	Other Revenue Deductions	31,800				31,800		31,800					
601	Salaries and Wages Expense	176,400		(5) 3,100		179,500		179,500					
602	Supplies Expense	26,800				26,800		26,800					
603	Utilities Expense	18,100				18,100		18,100					
604	Insurance Expense	1,200		(3) 150		1,350		1,350					
605	Depreciation Expense	5,000		(4) 625		5,625		5,625					
606	Interest Expense	4,000		(7) 500		4,500		4,500					
607	Other Expenses	41,500				41,500		41,500					
	Totals	721,500	721,500	5,225	5,225	726,435	726,435	320,885	348,340			405,550	405,550
	Net Income for 9 Months Ended 9/30/X3							27,455		-0-	27,455		
	Totals							348,340	348,340	246,875	246,875		
	Hospital Equity, 9/30/X3									246,875	246,875		246,875

Figure 9–4 Hiowa Hospital Worksheet to Develop Financial Statements, Nine Months Ended September 30, 19X3

At the end of each month since the year began, Hiowa Hospital has been making an adjusting entry to maintain a balance in its Allowance for Bad Debts account (number 104) equal to 10 percent of month-end accounts receivable. This is an accounting policy that assumes that 10 percent of the accounts receivable balance will prove to be bad debts. As mentioned before, there are other methods of accounting for bad debts, but this is the method we will use for our present purposes.

Bad Debts

As specific accounts are determined to be worthless, the accounts are written off by a debit to the Allowance for Bad Debts account. To illustrate, let us assume that the account had a credit balance of $6,000 to start the 19X3 year. At the end of each month from January through August, an adjusting entry has been made to adjust the account credit balance to 10 percent of receivables. A summary of the eight entries follows as a single entry:

Writeoff of Worthless Accounts

Bad Debts	501	$11,400	
Allowance for Bad Debts	104		$11,400
Adjustments of allowance account to 10% of month-end receivables.			

We assumed, however, that the year began with a $6,000 credit balance in the account. The eight adjusting entries added $11,400 to the account, so why is the August 31 balance only $8,400? It might appear to you that the August 31 balance should be $17,400 ($6,000 + $11,400).

In an unspecified number of journal entries during the first eight months of 19X3, Hiowa Hospital has written off $9,000 of worthless accounts. A summary of these entries is shown here as a single entry:

Allowance for Bad Debts	104	$ 9,000	
Accounts Receivable	103		$ 9,000
Writeoff of uncollectible receivables during first eight months of 19X3.			

Thus, between January 1 and August 31, the Allowance for Bad Debts account (which began with a $6,000 credit balance) has been credited with a total of $11,400 and debited for a total of $9,000. The August 31 balance of the account therefore is $8,400 (that is, $6,000 + $11,400 − $9,000). The August 31 debit balance of the bad debts account is of course the amount recorded during the first eight months of 19X3, or $11,400 (see the August 31 trial balance in Figure 9–4).

The balances in the Bad Debts and the Allowance for Bad Debts accounts have not changed since August 31. This is because the September 30 adjusting entry has not yet been made and because we assume that no accounts have been written off during September. The required September 30 adjusting entry is as follows:

Bad Debts	501	$310	
Allowance for Bad Debts	104		$310
Adjustment to increase allowance account to 10% of September 30, 19X3, accounts receivable:			
Allowance balance, 9/30	$8,400		
Desired balance (10% of $87,100)	8,710		
Required increase	$ 310		

This gives the Allowance for Bad Debts account a credit balance of $8,710, which is the desired 10 percent of September 30 receivables. This is entry (2) on the worksheet illustrated in Figure 9–4.

Prepaid Insurance   Assume a single comprehensive insurance policy on which Hiowa Hospital paid a two-year premium of $3,600 in advance on January 1, 19X3. This means that insurance expense is $150 per month ($3,600 ÷ 24 months). Assuming that the payment of the premium was recorded as a debit to Prepaid Insurance (account 106), the following adjusting entry has been made at the end of each of the eight months starting January 31:

| Insurance Expense | 604 | $150 | |
| Prepaid Insurance | 106 | | $150 |

Adjustment for monthly expiration of
prepaid insurance premium.

Because this entry has been made eight times, the trial balance for
August 31 shows $1,200 of insurance expense and $2,400 of prepaid
insurance ($3,600 − $1,200). This adjustment is repeated on September 30 as entry (3) in Figure 9–4.

Hiowa Hospital purchased all of its depreciable assets on January 1,
19X1, for $187,500. Let us say that these assets (buildings and
equipment) have a composite useful life of 25 years, but no salvage
value is expected. This means that depreciation expense on a
straight-line basis is $7,500 annually ($187,500 ÷ 25), or $625 per
month ($7,500 ÷ 12). So, Hiowa Hospital has been making the
following monthly adjusting entry:

Depreciation

| Depreciation Expense | 605 | $625 | |
| Accumulated Depreciation | 161 | | $625 |

Adjustment for monthly
depreciation.

Thus, the August 31 trial balance shows $5,000 ($625 × 8 months)
of depreciation expense. The accumulated depreciation balance,
however, includes all the depreciation recorded since the assets were
acquired: depreciation for 12 months in 19X1, 12 months in 19X2,
and 8 months in 19X3. This is a total of 32 months, or $20,000
($625 × 32) of accumulated depreciation at August 31, 19X3.

This depreciation adjustment also must be made at September
30. This is entry (4) in Figure 9–4. The entry will be repeated every
month until the assets are sold or otherwise retired from use by the
hospital.

Repeating the Depreciation
Adjustment Each Month

On August 31, Hiowa Hospital obviously made an adjusting entry
for $4,600 of accrued salaries and wages (refer to the August 31 trial
balance account 202). That entry charged $4,600 of salaries and
wages to expense and credited $4,600 to the accrued liability
account. When these salaries and wages were paid in early Septem-

**Accrued Salaries and
Wages Payable**

ber, the liability was eliminated. This is why no balance appears in the Accrued Salaries and Wages Payable account in the September 30 trial balance.

Now assume that, during the latter part of September, Hiowa Hospital employees earned $3,100 of salaries and wages that have not yet been paid. The required September 30, 19X3, adjusting entry is as follows:

Salaries and Wages Expense	601	$3,100	
Accrued Salaries and Wages			
Payable	202		$3,100
Adjustment for accrued payroll at			
September 30, 19X3.			

Use of Reversing Entries

This entry appears on the worksheet in Figure 9–4 as entry (5). As explained in Chapter 5, reversing entries sometimes are employed in connection with certain adjustments relating to accrued expenses. Hiowa Hospital, for example, might have made a September 1 reversing entry for the $4,600 adjustment of August 31. Similarly, the $3,100 adjustment just shown may be reversed on October 1. Whether or not reversing entries are made, however, the interim statements are not affected; the adjusted figures will be the same.

Deferred Rental Income

Assume that a private enterprise began operating a gift shop in the hospital on April 1, 19X3. At that time, Hiowa Hospital received one year's rent ($1,680) in advance. The hospital's rental income, then, is $140 per month ($1,680 ÷ 12). Assuming that the $1,680 was credited to Deferred Rental Income (account 204) at the time it was received, the hospital has been making a monthly adjustment of $140 to Rental Income (account 404) for five months (April through August). The monthly adjusting entry has been:

Deferred Rental Income	204	$ 140	
Rental Income	404		$ 140
Adjustment to record rental			
income earned during the month.			

Because this entry has been made five times, the August 31 trial balance shows a balance of $700 in the Rental Income account. The

Deferred Rental Income balance, for the same reason, is $980 ($1,680 − $700).

Now, at September 30, the same adjusting entry is required again. Figure 9–4 includes this rental income adjustment as entry (6).

Hiowa Hospital issued $100,000 of 6 percent, 12–year bonds at face value on October 1, 19X2. These bonds pay interest annually on October 1, commencing October 1, 19X3. At the end of each month, starting October 31, 19X2, Hiowa Hospital has been making the following adjusting entry for the monthly accrual of interest expense on these bonds:

Interest Expense	606	$500	
Accrued Interest Payable	203		$500
Adjustment for monthly accrual of			
interest on bonds payable:			
$100,000 × 6% × 1/12 = $500			

This entry has been made 11 times (October 19X2 through August 19X3) to produce an August 31 trial balance figure of $5,500 in Accrued Interest Payable. However, the August 31 balance of the Interest Expense account is only $4,000, because the remaining $1,500 of interest was charged to expense in 19X2. That $1,500 was interest expense for October, November, and December of 19X2, and the Interest Expense account balance was eliminated from the hospital's ledger by a December 31, 19X2, closing entry.

This $500 adjustment for interest expense must be made again at September 30, 19X3. This adjustment appears in Figure 9–4 as entry (7).

This completes all of the September 30, 19X3, adjustments required for Hiowa Hospital. The worksheet (Figure 9–4) for the first nine months of 19X3 is now completed, and a set of interim financial statements can be prepared.

Based on the information assembled on the worksheet (Figure 9–4), an interim income statement for the nine months ended September 30, 19X3, along with an income statement for the month of Sep-

	Month Ended 9/30/X3	Nine Months Ended 9/30/X3
Gross Patient Service Revenues:		
Inpatient Services	$ 23,300	$187,300
Outpatient Services	10,700	106,800
Total Gross Patient Service Revenues	34,000	294,100
Less Revenue Deductions:		
Bad Debts	310	11,710
Other	4,800	31,800
Total Revenue Deductions	5,110	43,510
Net Patient Service Revenues	28,890	250,590
Other Operating Revenues:		
Rent	140	840
Other	5,900	52,200
Total Other Operating Revenues	6,040	53,040
Total Operating Revenues	34,930	303,630
Less Operating Expenses:		
Salaries and Wages	19,500	179,500
Supplies	2,800	26,800
Utilities	2,100	18,100
Insurance	150	1,350
Depreciation	625	5,625
Interest	500	4,500
Other	3,500	41,500
Total Operating Expenses	29,175	277,375
Operating Income	5,755	26,255
Add Nonoperating Income (Interest)	400	1,200
Net Income	$ 6,155	$ 27,455

tember 19X3, can be prepared. Figure 9–5 shows the interim
income statement. The dollar amounts for the September income
statement are obtained simply by subtracting the eight-month
income statement figures from the nine-month income statement
figures. To obtain the salaries and wages expense for September, for
example, the $160,000 expense figure in the income statement for
the eight months ended August 31 (Figure 9–2) is subtracted from
the $179,500 expense figure in the income statement for the nine
months ended September 30, 19X3. In actual practice, the monthly
amounts are obtained by summarizing the transactions of each

	9/30/X3	8/31/X3
Assets		
Cash	$ 33,200	$ 30,900
Accrued Interest Receivable	1,200	800
Accounts Receivable (net of allowance for bad debts of $8,710 at September 30 and $8,400 at August 31)	78,390	75,600
Inventory	11,300	9,800
Prepaid Insurance	2,250	2,400
Total Current Assets	126,340	119,500
Long-Term Investments	60,000	60,000
Land	23,000	23,000
Depreciable Plant Assets (net of accumulated depreciation of $20,625 at September 30 and $20,000 at August 31)	166,875	167,500
Net Plant Assets	189,875	190,500
Total Assets	$376,215	$370,000
Liabilities and Equity		
Accounts Payable	$ 19,400	$ 18,200
Accrued Salaries and Wages Payable	3,100	4,600
Accrued Interest Payable	6,000	5,500
Deferred Rental Income	840	980
Total Current Liabilities	29,340	29,280
Long-Term Debt (6% Bonds Payable)	100,000	100,000
Total Liabilities	129,340	129,280
Hospital Equity, January 1	219,420	219,420
Add Net Income:		
For Nine Months Ended September 30	27,455	
For Eight Months Ended August 31		21,300
Hospital Equity	246,875	240,720
Total Liabilities and Equity	$376,215	$370,000

Figure 9–6 Hiowa Hospital Balance Sheets, September 30 and August 31, 19X3

month alone, thus providing an automatic verification of the change in year-to-date totals.

Figure 9–6 presents the Hiowa Hospital's September 30, 19X3, balance sheet, with the necessary figures taken from the worksheet (Figure 9–4). The August 31 balance sheet also is included so that comparative financial data is reported. Income and other statements, of course, also can be presented in comparative form. Later in this book, we will get into the managerial analysis and interpretation of comparative financial statements.

Providing for Comparative Data

Entry No.	Accounts and Explanations	Acct. No.	Dr.	Cr.
1	Accrued Interest Receivable	102	400	
	Interest Income	403		400
	Adjustment for accrual of monthly interest income on corporate bonds held as long-term investments.			
2	Bad Debts	501	310	
	Allowance for Bad Debts	104		310
	Adjustment to increase allowance account to 10% of month-end receivables.			
3	Insurance Expense	604	150	
	Prepaid Insurance	106		150
	Adjustment for monthly expiration of prepaid insurance premium.			
4	Depreciation Expense	605	625	
	Accumulated Depreciation	161		625
	Adjustment for monthly depreciation.			
5	Salaries and Wages Expense	601	3,100	
	Accrued Salaries and Wages Payable	202		3,100
	Adjustment for accrued payroll.			
6	Deferred Rental Income	204	140	
	Rental Income	404		140
	Adjustment to record rental income earned during the month.			
7	Interest Expense	606	500	
	Accrued Interest Payable	203		500
	Adjustment for monthly accrual of interest on 6% bonds payable.			

Figure 9–7 Hiowa Hospital 19X3 Journal (September 30 Adjusting Entries)

Journalizing and Posting Adjusting Entries

After the interim financial statements have been prepared, the accountant returns to the journal and records the September 30, 19X3, adjusting entries as shown in Figure 9–7. These journal entries then are posted to the ledger accounts (not shown here). When the postings are completed, Hiowa Hospital's ledger account balances will agree with the figures in the adjusted trial balance columns of the worksheet. During the following month (October 19X3), the procedures previously described for September are repeated. As a final point, notice that the books are not closed in the interim accounting process; the books are closed annually on the last day of the fiscal year.

Questions

Q9–1. What are interim financial statements?

Q9–2. Why are interim financial statements prepared?

Q9–3. Hart Hospital's long-term investments consist of $90,000 (face value) of 8 percent, 15-year bonds purchased by the hospital at face value on January 1, 19X1. These bonds pay interest semiannually on January 1 and July 1. Hart Hospital's accounting period is the calendar year. What amounts should be reported in the hospital's adjusted trial balance at November 30, 19X1, for interest income and accrued interest receivable?

Q9–4. Hello Hospital, whose accounting period is the calendar year, began 19X1 with a $10,000 credit balance in its Allowance for Bad Debts account. At the end of each month of the year, an adjusting entry is made to adjust the allowance account credit balance to 10 percent of receivables. Also at the end of each month of the year, an entry is made to write off accounts receivable deemed to be worthless (bad debts). Indicate the presentation of receivables in Hello Hospital's balance sheet at March 31, 19X1, given the following data:

	January	February	March
Accounts receivable at end of month[1]	$128,000	$151,000	$147,000
Accounts written off at end of month	8,000	11,000	15,000

Q9–5. On January 1, 19X1, Hope Hospital paid a three-year insurance premium of $6,480 in advance. This premium payment was recorded as a debit to prepaid insurance.
   a. What amount should be reported as prepaid insurance in the hospital's preadjusted trial balance at August 31, 19X1?
   b. What amount should be reported as insurance expense in the hospital's income statement for the nine months ended September 30, 19X1?
   c. What amount should be reported as prepaid insurance in the hospital's balance sheet at October 31, 19X1?

Q9–6. Happy Hospital paid $145,700 of salaries and wages during the month of May 19X1. The hospital's balance sheets reported accrued salaries and wages payable as follows:

[1]Prior to monthly writeoffs.

April 30, 19X1 $31,200
May 31, 19X1   37,800

What amount should be reported as salaries and wages expense in the hospital's income statement for the month ended May 31, 19X1?

Q9–7. If a hospital prepares interim financial statements, how often must adjusting entries be made? How often must closing entries be made?

Q9–8. A private enterprise began operating a gift shop in Hope Hospital on May 1, 19X1. At that time, the hospital received a year's rent ($3,000) in advance. The $3,000 was credited to deferred rental income. Assuming that the hospital prepares monthly statements, make the necessary adjusting entry at September 30, 19X1.

Q9–9. Hillside Hospital issued $300,000 of 6 percent, 15-year bonds at face value on April 1, 19X1. These bonds pay interest semiannually on April 1 and October 1, commencing October 1, 19X1. The hospital's fiscal year ends December 31. What amounts should be reported in the hospital's adjusted trial balance at November 30, 19X1, for bond interest expense and accrued bond interest payable?

Q9–10. Harmless Hospital purchased all its depreciable equipment on January 1, 19X1, for $800,000. This equipment has an estimated useful life of 12 years and an estimated salvage value of 10 percent. The hospital's fiscal year ends on December 31. What amounts should be reported in the hospital's preadjusted trial balance at May 31, 19X3, for depreciation expense and accumulated depreciation?

Exercises   E9–1. Hype Hospital provides you with the following information:

	10/31/X1	11/30/X1
Prepaid rent expense	$1,000	$2,000
Accrued rent receivable	3,000	4,000
Deferred rental income	5,000	6,000
Accrued rent payable	7,000	8,000

During November, $40,000 of rent was paid and $50,000 of rent was received in cash.

Required: What should the November 19X1 income statement report as rent expense and rental income?

E9–2. Hipp Hospital provides you with the following information:

	10/31/X2	11/30/X2
Accrued interest receivable	$4,100	$3,900
Prepaid interest	6,400	5,700
Accrued interest payable	3,200	3,600
Deferred interest income	4,800	5,300

The hospital's November income statement reports $25,000 of interest income and $30,000 of interest expense.

Required: (1) What was the amount of interest received in cash during November? (2) What was the amount of interest paid in cash during November?

E9–3. Helping Hospital provides you with the following accounts drawn from its adjusted general ledger at October 31, 19X1:

Accounts Receivable		Allowance for Uncollectible Accounts	
240,000	450,000	9,500	24,000
500,000	9,500		13,550

The hospital's fiscal year ends September 30. Uncollectible accounts are estimated at 10 percent of accounts receivable.

Required: Identify each of the dollar amounts in each of these ledger accounts.

E9–4. Highest Hospital provides you with the following accounts drawn from its adjusted general ledger at October 31, 19X1:

Inventory		Accounts Payable	
55,000	100,000	110,000	60,000
95,000			95,000

The hospital's fiscal year ends September 30.

Required: Identify each of the dollar amounts in each of these ledger accounts.

P9–1. Hohum Hospital's adjusted trial balance at March 31, 19X6, and its unadjusted trial balance at April 30, 19X6, are shown here:

Problems

Acct. No.		Adjusted Trial Balance March 31, 19X6		Unadjusted Trial Balance April 30, 19X6	
		Dr.	Cr.	Dr.	Cr.
101	Cash	$ 30,300		$ 25,400	
102	Accrued Interest Receivable	1,800		1,800	
103	Accounts Receivable	80,000		86,000	
104	Allowance for Bad Debts		$ 8,000		$ 1,400
105	Inventory	11,000		10,300	
106	Prepaid Insurance	3,675		3,675	
130	Long-Term Investments	90,000		90,000	
150	Land	15,000		15,000	
160	Depreciable Plant Assets	400,000		400,000	
161	Accumulated Depreciation		63,000		63,000
201	Accounts Payable		21,600		23,900
202	Accrued Salaries and Wages Payable		4,700		-0-
203	Accrued Interest Payable		2,400		2,400
204	Deferred Rental Income		2,340		2,340
250	Bonds Payable		160,000		160,000
301	Hospital Equity		355,235		355,235
302	Revenue and Expense Summary		-0-		-0-
401	Inpatient Services Revenue		81,400		115,200
402	Outpatient Services Revenue		56,100		72,900
403	Interest Income		1,800		1,800
404	Rental Income		780		780
405	Other Revenues		12,120		16,020
501	Bad Debts	3,300		3,300	
502	Other Revenue Deductions	11,500		14,900	
601	Salaries and Wages Expense	90,600		120,300	
602	Supplies Expense	15,100		21,700	
603	Utilities Expense	10,200		14,500	
604	Insurance Expense	525		525	
605	Depreciation Expense	3,000		3,000	
606	Interest Expense	2,400		2,400	
607	Other Expenses	1,075		2,175	
	Totals	$769,475	$769,475	$814,975	$814,975

The hospital's fiscal year ends December 31. Additional information is available as follows:

1. Long-term investments consist of $90,000 (face value) of 8 percent, 10–year bonds purchased by the hospital on January 1, 19X6. The bonds pay interest semiannually on January 1 and July 1, commencing July 1, 19X6.

2. A two-year insurance premium of $4,200 was paid in advance on January 1, 19X1.

3. Depreciable plant assets, all of which were acquired on January 1, 19X1, have an estimated useful life of 30 years and a 10 percent salvage value.

4. On January 1, 19X6, the hospital issued $160,000 of 6 percent, 15-year bonds at face value. These bonds pay interest annually on January 1, commencing January 1, 19X7.

5. A year's rent of $3,120 was received in advance on January 1, 19X6.

6. At the end of each month, the allowance for bad debts is adjusted to a credit balance equal to 10 percent of month-end accounts receivable.

7. Unpaid salaries and wages at April 30, 19X6, totaled $3,400.

Required: (1) Prepare a worksheet to develop financial statements for the four months ended April 30, 19X6, in the manner illustrated in Figure 9–4. (2) Prepare, in good form, income statements for the month of April 19X6 and for the four months then ended, in the manner illustrated in Figure 9–5. (3) Prepare, in good form, balance sheets at April 30 and March 31, 19X6, in the manner illustrated in Figure 9–6. (4) Prepare, in general journal form, all necessary adjusting entries for the month ended April 30, 19X6.

P9–2. Highcare Hospital's adjusted trial balance at May 31, 19X4, and its unadjusted trial balance at June 30, 19X4, are shown here (the hospital's fiscal year ends December 31):

Acct. No.		Adjusted Trial Balance May 31, 19X4		Unadjusted Trial Balance June 30, 19X4	
		Dr.	Cr.	Dr.	Cr.
101	Cash	$ 38,400		$ 16,640	
102	Accrued Interest Receivable	800		800	
103	Accounts Receivable	95,000		106,500	
104	Allowance for Bad Debts		$ 7,600		$ 300
105	Inventory	10,800		12,300	
106	Prepaid Insurance	3,420		3,420	
130	Long-term Investments	60,000		75,000	
150	Land	14,000		14,000	
160	Depreciable Plant Assets	480,000		480,000	
161	Accumulated Depreciation		82,250		82,250
201	Accounts Payable		19,700		24,100
202	Accrued Salaries and Wages Payable		3,900		-0-
203	Accrued Interest Payable		2,000		2,000
204	Deferred Rental Income		2,160		2,160
250	Bonds Payable		200,000		200,000
301	Hospital Equity		356,810		356,810
302	Revenue and Expense Summary		-0-		-0-
401	Inpatient Services Revenue		100,200		128,700
402	Outpatient Services Revenue		78,400		93,500
403	Interest Income		800		800
404	Rental Income		720		720
405	Other Revenues		12,880		15,100
501	Bad Debts	2,900		2,900	
502	Other Revenue Deductions	12,600		15,700	
601	Salaries and Wages Expense	101,400		122,300	
602	Supplies Expense	16,100		19,800	
603	Utilities Expense	11,200		13,900	
604	Insurance Expense	900		900	
605	Depreciation Expense	10,250		10,250	
606	Interest Expense	5,000		5,000	
607	Other Expenses	4,650		7,030	
	Totals	$867,420	$867,420	$906,440	$906,440

The following additional information is available:

1. Long-term investments consist of $60,000 (face value) of 8 percent, 15-year bonds purchased by the hospital on April 1, 19X4, with interest payable annually on April 1, and $15,000 (face value) of 8 percent, 10–year bonds purchased by the hospital on June 1, 19X4, with interest payable annually on June 1.

2. A two-year insurance premium was paid in advance on January 1, 19X4.

3. On January 1, 19X1, the hospital purchased $450,000 of depreciable plant assets having an estimated useful life of 15 years and an estimated salvage value of 20 percent. On May 1, 19X4, the hospital purchased additional depreciable plant assets at a cost of $30,000 (estimated useful life of 8 years and a 20 percent salvage value).

4. A year's rent was received in advance on March 1, 19X4.

5. On April 1, 19X2, the hospital issued $200,000 of 6 percent, 10-year bonds at face value. These bonds pay interest semiannually on April 1 and October 1.

6. At the end of each month, the allowance for bad debts is adjusted to a credit balance equal to 8 percent of month-end accounts receivable.

7. Unpaid salaries and wages at June 30, 19X4, totaled $4,100.

Required: (1) Prepare a worksheet to develop financial statements for the six months ended June 30, 19X4, in the manner illustrated in Figure 9–4. (2) Prepare, in good form, income statements for the month of June, 19X4, and for the six months then ended, in the manner illustrated in Figure 9–5. (3) Prepare, in good form, balance sheets at June 30 and May 31, 19X4, in the manner illustrated in Figure 9–6. (4) Prepare, in general journal form, all necessary adjusting entries for the month ended June 30, 19X4.

Expansion of the Chart of Accounts

10

Illustrations in the preceding chapters were based on a highly simplified chart of accounts suitable to an introductory discussion of the fundamentals of bookkeeping. Having accomplished this, we now must expand the chart of accounts to permit the introduction of more realistic accounting techniques and procedures. The expanded chart of accounts we develop in this chapter will serve as a basis for the discussion in the next four chapters, but we will make additional refinements at appropriate points throughout the remainder of this book. By the end of your study of this textbook, you will have been exposed to a substantially complete chart of accounts such as one would find in actual practice in an average hospital of medium size.

The chart of accounts presented in this chapter conforms closely to the account classifications and numerical coding system recommended for hospitals by the American Hospital Association (AHA).[1] We will not attempt, however, to deal with all of the accounts listed in the AHA publication. Your attention will be directed only to a representative sample of those accounts. Although a degree of realism may be lost through limiting the number of accounts involved in our illustrations, your comprehension of the underlying principles and procedures will not be impaired by unnecessary details.

---

[1]American Hospital Association, *Chart of Accounts for Hospitals* (Chicago: AHA, 1976). You are urged to read this important document in its entirety because its content can only be highlighted and summarized within these pages.

Figure 10–1 Hartful Hospital
Chart of Balance Sheet Accounts

Assets

Current Assets

1011	Cash—General Checking Account
1012	Cash—Payroll Checking Account
1014	Petty Cash Fund
1020	Temporary Investments
1029	Accrued Interest Receivable
1031	Inpatient Receivables—Inhouse
1032	Inpatient Receivables—Discharged
1044	Outpatient Receivables
1061	Allowance for Uncollectible Accounts—Bad Debts
1062	Allowance for Uncollectible Accounts—Contractual Adjustments
1066	Allowance for Uncollectible Accounts—Charity Service
1110	Inventories
1120	Prepaid Expenses
—	(Other accounts, as needed)

Property, Plant, and Equipment

1130	Land
1150	Buildings
1170	Equipment
1250	Accumulated Depreciation—Buildings
1270	Accumulated Depreciation—Equipment
—	(Other accounts, as needed)

Liabilities

Current Liabilities

2010	Notes Payable
2020	Accounts Payable
2031	Accrued Payroll
2035	FIT Withheld
2036	FICA Withheld and Accrued
2051	Accrued Interest Payable
2113	Deferred Rental Income
—	(Other accounts, as needed)

Noncurrent Liabilities

2190	Bonds Payable
—	(Other accounts, as needed)

Equity

2210	Hospital Equity
2219	Revenue and Expense Summary
—	(Other accounts, as needed)

The chart of balance sheet accounts employed by Hartful Hospital is shown in Figure 10–1. You are already acquainted with many of the accounts, but a number of changes and additions require brief explanations. A more thorough discussion of these accounts will appear in subsequent chapters. Segregation of the balance sheet accounts into self-balancing groups as required by fund accounting will be deferred to Chapter 15. The accounts described in the present chapter relate only to the general (unrestricted) fund.

Balance Sheet Accounts

In the AHA numerical coding system, the hospital's asset accounts are those numbered in the 1000 series. Any account having a 1 as the initial digit of its number is an asset account. When *fund accounting* (discussed in Chapter 15) is employed, the second digit is used to specify the fund in which the asset is located.

Asset Accounts

The general fund designators are the second digits 0, 1, or 2. The third and fourth digits of the account number specify the primary subclassification of assets. Consider, as an example, account 1011:

General Fund Designators

Digit
Position

First   1 = Asset
Second 0 = General Fund
Third   1 = Cash
Fourth   1 = General Checking Account

In other words, all 101 accounts are general fund cash accounts; the fourth digit indicates the type of cash account. Similarly, all 103 accounts are general fund asset accounts for inpatient receivables; the fourth digit is used to indicate whether the receivables relate to inhouse or discharged patients.

Meaning of the Third and Fourth Digits

The AHA system also provides for the use of a fifth and even a sixth digit, depending on individual hospital requirements, for a secondary subclassification of asset accounts. You need not be concerned, however, with this additional detail. Our discussion is limited, at this point, to the four-digit primary account number. Beginning in the next chapter, however, all asset account numbers will have five digits to be consistent with the five-digit revenue and expense account numbers. The fifth digit of all asset account num-

Uses of the Fifth and Sixth Digits

bers will always be 0 (for example, 1011.0, 1012.0, and so on), but this is *only* for the purposes of our discussion.

Notice that there are two cash checking accounts. Account 1011 is Hartful Hospital's general checking account, into which all cash receipts are deposited. All hospital disbursements, other than employees' individual payroll checks, are made by checks drawn against this account. Account 1012 is used only for payroll checks, and will be discussed in Chapter 13. The procedures relating to the uses of account 1014, account 1020, and account 1029 are topics for discussion in Chapter 16.

Hartful Hospital employs three accounts for receivables from patients. As services are rendered to inpatients, account 1031 is debited; it is credited when payments are received from patients prior to their discharge from the hospital. The account also is credited (and account 1032 debited) for the unpaid balances of patients' accounts at the time of discharge. All subsequent collections on these accounts are credited to account 1032. Account 1044 is debited for services provided to outpatients and is credited for all collections received on outpatients' accounts. These accounts for receivables are general ledger control accounts; they show the total amount due collectively from patients in each of the three classifications.

Information as to the amounts due from individual patients is developed and maintained in separate subsidiary ledgers to be illustrated subsequently in Chapter 12. At frequent intervals, the sum of the individual account balances in each subsidiary ledger will need to be reconciled to the balance reflected by the related general ledger control account.

Uncollectible Accounts   Also notice that the chart provides for a classification of the allowance for uncollectible accounts into three separate accounts according to the nature or type of the corresponding revenue deductions. Account 1066, for example, will reflect the amount of receivables estimated to prove eventually uncollectible by reason of charity service that has been rendered to financially indigent patients. Similar allowance accounts are maintained for estimated contractual adjustments and for estimated bad debts. All of these accounts, although listed in the asset classification, will carry credit balances. They are contraasset accounts. Detailed consideration is given to these accounts in Chapters 12 and 16.

In view of the explanations previously provided in this book, it is not necessary at this time to comment further on the remaining asset accounts. You will find additional coverage of these accounts

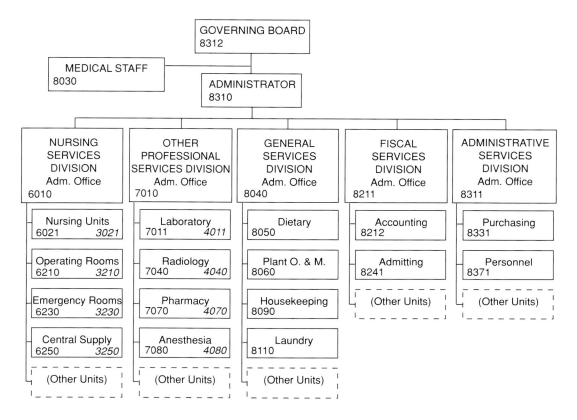

Figure 10-2 Hartful Hospital Organization Chart

in later chapters. Account 1110 (inventories), for example, will be attended to in Chapter 17, and the accounts for property, plant, and equipment will be treated fully in Chapter 18. Discussions of other asset accounts not included in Figure 10–2 will also be provided at appropriate points in subsequent chapters.

The liability and equity accounts are numbered in the 2000 series. The liability accounts are numbered 2000 through 2199; the equity accounts are numbered 2200 through 2299. (These numerical codings will be altered somewhat with the introduction of fund accounting in Chapter 15.) As was true for the asset accounts, fifth and sixth digits are available for a secondary subclassification of the liability and equity accounts whenever additional detail is required by the individual hospital. The present discussion, however, is confined to the four-digit primary account numbers. But, beginning with the next chapter, all liability and equity account numbers

Liability and Equity Accounts

will consist of five digits in order to be consistent with the five-digit revenue and expense account numbers. The fifth digit of all liability and equity account numbers will always be 0 (for example, 2010.0, 2020.0, 2031.0, and so on), but this is *only* for the purposes of our discussion.

Most of Hartful Hospital's liability and equity accounts have been discussed earlier. The two accounts you have not previously encountered are 2035 and 2036, the payroll tax accounts. The nature and use of these accounts will be described fully in Chapters 13 and 17, and you need not be concerned with them now. Of course, hospitals typically maintain liability and equity accounts that are not included in Figure 10–1; we shall add these accounts to our discussion at suitable times.

Income Statement Accounts

Hartful Hospital's organizational structure is presented in condensed form in Figure 10–2. Notice that the hospital activity is organized into five basic divisions, each having an administrative office. The managing officer of each division often has the title of director ("Director of Nursing Services," for example) or vice-president ("Vice-President for Fiscal Services," for example). These divisional managers report to the hospital's chief executive officer (president or administrator) to whom they are responsible for the activities organized within their particular divisions.

Figure 10–2 provides a representative sample of the types of services (or departments) included in each division. It is not feasible in this book to deal with a larger number of organizational units. Moreover, you should be aware that a single "box" in the sample organizational chart may represent two or more separately organized units. "Nursing Units," for example, may be organized somewhat as follows:

> Medical and Surgical Acute Care Units
> Pediatric, Acute
> Psychiatric, Acute
> Obstetric, Acute
> Newborn Nursery, Acute
> Intensive Care
> Cardiac Care
> Other

The significance of this, in terms of the design of the chart of accounts, is that a separate revenue and expense account must be provided for each nursing care unit. Only by accumulating and reporting revenues and expenses by individual organizational units can a financial evaluation of the performance of each unit be made by the hospital's management.

As another example, consider the box labeled "Accounting." This function may be organized into several different units:

General Accounting
Budgets and Costs
Payroll Accounting
Accounts Payable
Patient Accounting
Other

Although there are no revenues directly associated with these units, the expenses of each unit should be separately accumulated in the accounts. In the interest of brevity, however, this does not appear in our Hartful Hospital illustrations.

In addition to recognizing that the illustrative organization chart in Figure 10–2 is greatly condensed, you also should not regard the chart as indicative of how all hospitals are, or should be, organized. No two hospitals are exactly alike; hospitals differ in size, range of services, management philosophy, and other important ways. These differences have an effect on the manner in which hospitals are organized. What may be a sound organizational pattern for one hospital may not be satisfactory for another.

The important point to recognize is that, however a particular hospital is organized, the hospital's chart of income statement accounts should be designed to conform to that hospital's organizational structure. The basic principle of *responsibility accounting* is that each organizational unit (division, department, or section) of the hospital is a responsibility center, performing an activity or function, and headed by an individual responsible for attaining its mission. Each of these individuals is a decision maker who has a significant degree of control over the amounts of resources used in his or her center. Because all centers incur expenses, every center is an expense (or cost) center. Some centers also generate revenues through the provision of patient services for which a specific charge is made; these centers also are referred to as *revenue centers*. Housekeeping, for example, is an expense center but not a revenue center; radiology, however, is both an expense center and a revenue center.

Under responsibility accounting, the revenue and expense accounts are classified in a manner that permits revenues to be recorded according to the centers responsible for generating them and expenses to be recorded according to the centers responsible for their incurrence. Each center is charged only for those expenses that can be directly associated with the activities of that center, however, and over which the center manager has decision-making authority. All other expenses, as you will soon see, are recorded in a special "unassigned" expense classification.

Hartful Hospital's chart of income statement accounts appears in condensed form in Figure 10–3. Observe here that the classification of the income statement accounts conforms to Hartful Hospital's organizational pattern. This necessary relationship between a hospital's organizational structure and its chart of accounts is indicated by the placement of revenue and expense account numbers in the corresponding "boxes" in the organization chart as shown in Figure 10–2. As you can see, each of the organizational units has its own expense and (where applicable) revenue accounts. Each center is charged with the expenses it incurs and is credited with the revenues (if any) it generates. In this way, relevant expense and revenue data can be developed for the purpose of measuring and evaluating the performance of each center and its manager or supervisor.

Revenue Accounts

In the AHA numerical coding system, the first digit of revenue (and revenue deduction) accounts may be 3, 4, 5, or 9. Designations for this first digit are as follows:

First Digit	
3 =	Nursing Service Revenues
4 =	Other Professional Service Revenues
5 =	Other Operating Revenues; Deductions from Revenues
9 =	Nonoperating Revenues

When the first digit of a revenue account number is 3 or 4, the second, third, and fourth digits provide a classification of revenue

<table>
<tr><td colspan="2" align="center">Revenues</td></tr>
</table>

	Revenues
	Nursing Services
3021	Nursing Units
3210	Operating Rooms
3230	Emergency Rooms
3250	Central Supply
—	(Other accounts, as needed)
	Other Professional Services
4011	Laboratory
4040	Radiology
4070	Pharmacy
4080	Anesthesia
—	(Other accounts, as needed)
	Other Operating Revenue
5061	Cafeteria Sales
5155	Rental Income
5171	Purchase Discounts Earned
—	(Other accounts, as needed)
	Deductions from Revenue
5510	Bad Debts
5520	Contractual Adjustments
5540	Charity Service
—	(Other accounts, as needed)
	Nonoperating Revenue
9041	Unrestricted Contributions
9051	Interest Income
—	(Other accounts, as needed)
	Expenses
	Nursing Services
6010	Director's Administrative Office
6021	Nursing Units
6210	Operating Rooms
6230	Emergency Rooms
6250	Central Supply
—	(Other accounts, as needed)
	Other Professional Services
7010	Director's Administrative Office
7011	Laboratory
7040	Radiology
7070	Pharmacy
7080	Anesthesia
—	(Other accounts, as needed)

Figure 10–3 Hartful Hospital Chart of Income Statement Accounts

Other Services

| 8030 | Medical Staff |
| — | (Other accounts, as needed) |

General Services

8040	Director's Administrative Office
8050	Dietary
8060	Plant Operation and Maintenance
8090	Housekeeping
8110	Laundry
—	(Other accounts, as needed)

Fiscal Services

8211	Director's Administrative Office
8212	Accounting
8241	Admitting
—	(Other accounts, as needed)

Administrative Services

8310	Administrator's Office
8311	Director's Administrative Office
8312	Governing Board
8331	Purchasing
8371	Personnel
—	(Other accounts, as needed)

Unassigned Expenses

8510	Depreciation
8610	Insurance
8690	Interest
8710	Employee Benefits
—	(Other accounts, as needed)

by specific organizational units. Account number 3250, for example, designates the following:

Digit		
First	3	= Revenues—Nursing Services
Second	2	
Third	5	= Central Supply
Fourth	0	

In other words, 250 is the numerical code for the central supply department or function. Similarly, 011 is the code for laboratory, 040 is the designation for pharmacy, and so on.

When a particular service is organized into several subordinate units, as is often true of the laboratory department, the account numbering system provides for a numbering scheme such as the following:

Account No.	
	Laboratory Services
4011	Chemistry
4012	Hematology
4013	Histology
4016	Autopsy
4018	Immunology
.	.
.	.
.	.
4025	Blood Bank

Even when the laboratory is a single organizational unit, this series of accounts may be used to obtain a classification of laboratory revenues by type of service or examination.

As another example of the use of the second, third, and fourth digits for revenue accounts, observe the following account classifications for the types of revenues derived from Acute Care Nursing Units:

Account No.	
	Acute Care Nursing Units
3021	Medical and Surgical—Unit 1
3022	Medical and Surgical—Unit 2
.	.
.	.
.	.
3026	Medical and Surgical—Unit 6
3051	Pediatric—Unit 1
3052	Pediatric—Unit 2
3060	Psychiatric Unit
3080	Obstetric Unit
3090	Newborn Nursery

Although our Hartful Hospital illustration will not include this much detail, it is important to keep in mind that detailed revenue information of this kind is essential in actual practice.

When the first digit of a revenue (revenue deduction) account is 5 or 9, the second, third, and fourth digits are used mainly to classify the revenue (or revenue deduction) by type.

Fifth Digit to Classify Patient Service Revenues

The AHA system also calls for the use of a fifth digit in connection with revenue accounts in the 3000 and 4000 series. This fifth digit is employed to classify these patient service revenues by type of patient. The patient classifications may be handled as follows:

Fifth Digit	
0	Inpatient—Acute
1	Inpatient—Long-term
2	Outpatient—Emergency
3	Outpatient—Referred
4	Outpatient—Clinic
5	Day Care
6	Home Health Care
7 } 8 } 9 }	Other Classifications

A sixth digit may be used to subclassify further revenues in whatever manner may be desired by the individual hospital. Presumably, this classification could be related to the financial status of the patient (source of payment), the type of hospital accommodation (private, semiprivate, or ward), and so on.

Three-Digit Suffix to Classify Revenues by Functional Units

Finally, the AHA system also provides for seventh, eighth, and ninth digits to be used as a three-digit suffix to classify revenues by functional units for purposes of uniform reporting. If you have a particular interest in this procedure, you will want to refer to Chapter 6 of the AHA's *Chart of Accounts for Hospitals* manual. For our present purposes, you should only be concerned with the four-digit revenue account numbers that are seen in Hartful Hospital's chart of accounts. Beginning with the next chapter, however, we will add a fifth digit to all patient service revenue account numbers; those in the 3000 and 4000 series. This fifth digit will indicate the following:

Fifth
Digit

1 = Inpatient Revenues
2 = Outpatient Revenues

In this way, patient service revenues will be classified by type of patient. All other revenue accounts (those in the 5000 and 9000 series) always have 0 as a fifth digit.

In the AHA numerical coding system, the first digit of the expense accounts may be 6, 7, 8, or 9. Designations for this first digit follow:

Expense Accounts

First
Digit

6 = Nursing Service Expenses
7 = Other Professional Service Expenses
8 = Other Services Expenses
9 = Nonoperating Expenses

When the first digit of an expense account number is 6, 7, or 8, the second, third, and fourth digits provide a classification of expense by organizational units. Account number 6250, for example, designates the following:

Digit
Position

First   6 = Expenses—Nursing Services
Second 2 ⎫
Third   5 ⎬ = Central Supply
Fourth 0 ⎭

As noted earlier in the discussion of revenue accounts, 250 is the numerical code for the central supply department or function. Thus, the Central Supply revenue account is account 3250; the Central Supply expense account is account 6250. A similar procedure is followed for all other organized units that incur expenses and generate revenues.

In situations in which a particular service is organized into several subordinate units, as is often true of the laboratory department, the account numbering system for expense accounts parallels that of the revenue accounts in a scheme such as the one in the following:

Expense Account No.		Revenue Account No.
	Laboratory Services	
7011	Chemistry	4011
7012	Hematology	4012
7013	Histology	4013
7016	Autopsy	4016
7018	Immunology	4018
.	.	.
.	.	.
.	.	.
7025	Blood Bank	4025

As another example of the use of the second, third, and fourth digits as codes for the various organizational units, observe the following account classifications for expenses and revenues related to the Acute Care Nursing Units:

Expense Account No.		Revenue Account No.
	Acute Care Nursing Units	
6021	Medical and Surgical—Unit 1	3021
6022	Medical and Surgical—Unit 2	3022
.	.	.
.	.	.
.	.	.
6026	Medical and Surgical—Unit 6	3026
6051	Pediatric—Unit 1	3051
6052	Pediatric—Unit 2	3052
6060	Psychiatric Unit	3060
6080	Obstetric Unit	3080
6090	Newborn Nursery	3090

The Hartful Hospital illustrations presented in later chapters do not include this much detail, but you should keep in mind that detailed expense information of this kind is required in actual practice.

When the first digit of an expense account number is 9, the second, third, and fourth digits are used to classify the expense by major type. You may have noticed that Hartful Hospital's chart of accounts does not include any expense accounts in the 9000 series. Later points in this book introduce a number of expense items that may be recorded in this "nonoperating expense" classification.

For expense accounts in the 6000, 7000, and 8000 series, the AHA numbering system provides fifth and sixth digits to be used as indicators for the natural classification of expenses in each organizational unit of the hospital. The natural (or object of expenditure) classification may be as follows:

Fifth and Sixth Digits for Natural Classifications

Fifth and Sixth Digits	Major Categories
.00	Salaries and Wages
.15	Employee Benefits
.25	Professional Fees—Medical
.30	Other Professional Fees
.35	Supplies and Materials, Special Department
.45	General Supplies
.54	Purchased Services
.65 ⎫	
. ⎬ Other Direct Expenses	
.	
.99 ⎭	

Within each of the preceding major categories, detailed classifications should be maintained to indicate job classifications, kinds of benefits, types of fees, types of supplies, and so on. A sufficient number of digits is available to permit such breakdowns in each category.

The Hartful Hospital illustrations to follow in the next several chapters do not include this detailed use of the fifth and sixth digits. Instead, this text uses only a fifth digit for expense center accounts. The designation of this fifth digit will be as follows:

Fifth
Digit
  .1 = Salaries and Wages
  .2 = Supplies and Other Expense

Thus, account 6250.1, for example, will indicate Central Supply—Salaries and Wages. Account 6250.2 will designate Central Supply—Supplies and Other Expense. The fifth digit will have the same meaning in each expense center.

As was noted earlier in connection with revenue accounts, the AHA system also provides for the use of seventh, eighth, and ninth digits for expense accounts. These digits may be used as a three-digit suffix to the basic account numbers for purposes of uniform or functional reporting to external parties. For the moment, however, you need not concern yourself with this matter.

Handling Unassigned Expenses

Several accounts are provided for Hartful Hospital's unassigned expenses. These expenses are general in nature and, in the regular accounting routine, are not charged or assigned to specific departmental expense centers. The reason for this is that, for the most part, these expenses are not controllable by individual department managers and supervisors. In the periodic cost-finding procedure, however, the unassigned expenses are allocated to the various expense centers to determine the full costs of providing departmental services. Cost-finding procedures will be dealt with in detail in Chapter 23.

Chapter 11 incorporates Hartful Hospital's chart of accounts into a journal and ledger system. It is important, therefore, to master the materials presented in this chapter before you move on to the next chapter. Detailed applications of Hartful Hospital's chart of accounts also are encountered in Chapters 12, 13, and 14.

Questions

Q10–1. What is your understanding of the term *responsibility accounting*?

Q10–2. What is a responsibility center? Give an example.

Q10–3. Distinguish between an expense center and a revenue center. Give an example of each.

Q10–4. What are *unassigned expenses*? Give four examples.

Q10–5. Why do you think the American Hospital Association publishes a *Chart of Accounts for Hospitals* manual?

Q10–6. The AHA chart of accounts manual contains an account numbered 1031. Explain briefly what each digit of this account number means.

Q10–7. The following account appeared in the ledger of Hartful Hospital on May 31, 19X3:

Account Number 2020			
5/31	49,351	5/1	46,877
		5/31	52,308
			(49,834)

Briefly identify each of the figures in the account.

Q10–8. The AHA chart of accounts manual contains an account numbered 3230. Explain briefly what the digits of this account number mean.

Q10–9. In connection with revenue accounts in the 3000 and 4000 series, the AHA chart of accounts manual provides for the use of a fifth digit. For what purpose is this fifth digit employed?

Q10–10. In the AHA chart of accounts manual, the first digit of expense account numbers may be either 6, 7, 8, or 9. Briefly explain the meaning of each of these initial digits.

Q10–11. The AHA chart of accounts manual contains an account numbered 8212. Explain briefly what the digits of this account number mean.

Q10–12. In connection with expense accounts in the 6000, 7000, and 8000 series, the AHA chart of accounts manual provides for the use of fifth and sixth digits. For what purpose are these fifth and sixth digits employed?

Q10–13. In the AHA chart of accounts manual, the first digit of revenue account numbers may be either 3, 4, 5, or 9. Briefly explain the meaning of each of these initial digits.

Q10–14. In the account numbering system set forth in the AHA chart of accounts manual, how can you distinguish between a liability account number and a hospital equity account number?

Special Journals and Ledgers

11

In the preceding chapters, all transactions were recorded in one journal: the general journal. All postings of these transaction entries were made to one ledger: the general ledger. Charges to patients for services rendered were debited to a single accounts receivable account; purchases of supplies on account from suppliers were credited to a single accounts payable account. We rather conveniently ignored the need for maintaining a continuous record of the amounts due from each patient or due to each supplier.

These procedures were followed in earlier chapters only to simplify the introductory explanation of the accounting process. In actual practice, using a single journal and ledger is not feasible. The necessity for keeping receivables records for individual patients and records of payables according to individual creditors cannot be avoided. In this chapter, and in the next three, you will have an opportunity to study a multijournal, multiledger system as it would be maintained manually (in handwritten or typewritten form). The system overcomes the inefficiency of the single journal and ledger procedure, and provides the detailed information required for hospital receivables and payables.

The illustrated system assumes that the accounting records are maintained manually. This assumption is made only for pedagogical reasons. All hospitals, including smaller ones, have mechanized or electronic accounting systems because the volume of transactions prohibits the use of methods that are entirely manual. But your time is not wasted in a study of the manual system illustrated here, because in essence all systems fulfill the same functions. You will learn how an accounting system works, machine-oriented or not.

Overview of the System

The system of special journals and ledgers described in this chapter and explored in detail in the next three chapters includes

- A general journal
- Six special journals
- A general ledger
- Two special (subsidiary) ledgers

The five-digit numerical coding scheme for the accounts involved in this system was outlined in the previous chapter.

Recording Transactions

Figure 11–1 summarizes the flow of transaction data through the system. As transactions occur, documentary evidences—charge tickets, purchase orders, cash receipt slips, bank deposit slips, and other business papers—are accumulated. These source documents serve as a basis for transaction entries in the journal system. A separate journal is maintained for each major type of transaction. The cash receipts journal, for example, records all of the hospital's cash receipt transactions, the cash disbursements journal is used to record all cash disbursements, and so on. This permits a division and specialization of labor within the accounting function. In a large organization, for example, a different accounting employee may be assigned to each journal. Therefore, transactions are likely to be recorded in a more accurate and efficient manner than would be possible using only one journal.

Thus, as daily transactions are completed, they are recorded by transaction entries in the appropriate journal. These entries accumulate in the journals day by day over a period of a month. At the end of each month, the accumulated entries in each special journal are totaled, and the totals are posted to the hospital's general ledger; individual daily entries are not posted to the general ledger accounts. For example, daily entries are made in the cash receipts journal to record debits to cash. These numerous individual debits are totaled at the end of the month, and only the total is posted to the general ledger cash account. This greatly reduces the number of individual postings to be made to the general ledger accounts and eliminates much of the detail that the general ledger otherwise would contain.

Accounts Receivable and Accounts Payable Subsidiary Ledgers

Certain daily postings, however, are made to the subsidiary ledgers. Two of the subsidiary ledgers maintained by Hartful Hospital are identified in Figure 11–1. One of these is the accounts receivable subsidiary ledger, sometimes referred to simply as the "patients' ledger" or "receivables ledger." It consists of a ledger account for each patient. These accounts receive daily debit postings from the revenue journal, and daily credit postings come from the cash receipts journal. (Occasional debit and credit postings also may

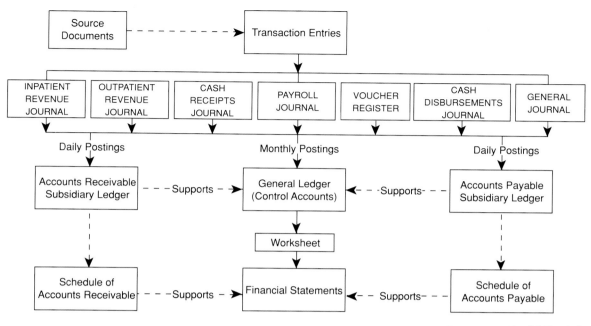

Figure 11–1 Hartful Hospital Journal and Ledger System

arise from certain transaction entries made in the general journal.) In this way, a continuous daily balance is maintained in each patient's account.

The total of these individual balances is reconciled monthly against the balances of the accounts receivable "control" accounts (accounts 1031.0, 1032.0, and 1044.0) in the general ledger. In addition, a schedule of individual subsidiary ledger balances can be prepared in support of the total of accounts receivable as reported in the month-end balance sheet. These procedures will be described more fully in Chapter 12.

The other subsidiary ledger seen in Figure 11–1 is the accounts payable subsidiary ledger, often called simply the "payables ledger." This ledger consists of a separate ledger account for each supplier of goods and services purchased by the hospital. These accounts receive daily credit postings from the voucher register and daily debit postings from the cash disbursements journal. In this way, a continuous daily balance is maintained in each supplier's account. The total of the individual subsidiary ledger balances is reconciled monthly with the accounts payable control account (account 2020.0) in the general ledger. A schedule of these subsidiary ledger balances can be prepared at the end of each month to support the accounts payable total reported in the month-end balance sheet. These procedures will be described more fully in Chapter 14.

Payroll Ledger   Another subsidiary ledger maintained by Hartful Hospital is the payroll subsidiary ledger, more often called the "employees' individual earnings record." This ledger is used in connection with the payroll journal and is discussed at length in Chapter 13. Subsidiary ledgers for inventories and plant assets are described and illustrated at subsequent points in this book.

Journal System

Hartful Hospital's journal system is based on the following classification of the business transactions of the hospital:

1. Charges to inpatients for services rendered
2. Charges to outpatients for services rendered
3. Cash receipts
4. Purchases of supplies and services
5. Payroll
6. Cash disbursements
7. All other transactions

In the system described here, as noted earlier, a separate journal is maintained for each of these seven major types of transactions.

Inpatient Revenue Journal

The inpatient revenue journal, illustrated in Figure 11–2, is used only to record those transactions that result in charges to inpatients for hospital services provided to them. No other type of transaction should be recorded in this journal, nor should inpatient revenue transactions be recorded in any of the other journals. As hospital services are rendered to inpatients, source documents—census reports and charge tickets, for example—are prepared. Copies of these documents are sent to the hospital accounting offices, where they are turned over to the employee who maintains the inpatient revenue journal. This person uses the source documents as the basis for daily journal entries that debit patients' accounts receivable and credit the various patient service revenue accounts. The details of this procedure are provided in Chapter 12.

Posting Totals to General Ledger   These daily entries in the inpatient revenue journal are not posted to the hospital's *general* ledger. Instead, at the end of the month, each column of the journal is totaled, and the totals (except for the sundry debits and credits columns) are posted to the general ledger accounts indicated. Entries in the sundry columns must be individually posted, but entries in these columns will not be frequent or numerous.

Daily postings, however, are made to the accounts receivable subsidiary ledger. These postings consist of debits to individual

19X1 Date	(✓)	Inpatient Receivables Dr.	Nursing Units	Operating Rooms	Emergency Rooms	Central Supply	Other Units	Other Units	Laboratory	Radiology	Pharmacy	Anesthesia	Other Units	Account Numbers	Dr.	Cr.
Totals		Debit 1031.0	Credit 3021.1	Credit 3210.1	Credit 3230.1	Credit 3350.1	Credit	Credit	Credit 4011.1	Credit 4040.1	Credit 4070.1	Credit 4080.1	Credit			

Note: Column group headers — Nursing Service Revenue Credits spans (Nursing Units, Operating Rooms, Emergency Rooms, Central Supply, Other Units, Other Units); Other Professional Service Revenue Credits spans (Laboratory, Radiology, Pharmacy, Anesthesia, Other Units); Sundry Debits and Credits spans (Account Numbers, Dr., Cr.)

Figure 11–2 Inpatient Revenue Journal

patients' accounts for the services rendered to them each day. Naturally, steps must be taken to ensure that the total of these debit postings for each day equals the total debit to accounts receivable entered in the journal for that day. Again, you will find the details of this posting procedure explained in Chapter 12.

Outpatient Revenue Journal

The outpatient revenue journal, illustrated in Figure 11–3, is used only to record transactions that result in charges to outpatients for hospital services provided to them. No outpatient revenue transactions should be recorded in any of the other journals, nor should any other type of transaction be recorded in this journal. We will assume, for our present purposes, that all services rendered to outpatients at Hartful Hospital are passed through the Outpatient Receivables account (account 1044.0). This procedure is followed even though payment is received from many outpatients at the time services are rendered to them. The alternative procedure, followed when outpatient services can be provided on a cash basis, is to bypass the receivables account and debit cash directly (crediting the appropriate outpatient revenue accounts). This alternative procedure generally should be discouraged, however, because it tends to weaken internal control over outpatient revenues and cash receipts.

As hospital services are rendered to outpatients, source documents (charge tickets) are prepared in the service-rendering departments. (These departments do not receive cash; outpatients pay for the services at a centralized cash-receiving station as they enter or leave the hospital.) The departments enter the charge tickets in outpatient service logs or reports. Copies of the logs, along with copies of the related charge tickets, are routed to the hospital's accounting offices where they are turned over to the accounting employee who is responsible for maintaining the outpatient revenue journal. These documents are used as the basis for debiting outpatient receivables and crediting the appropriate revenue accounts.

At the end of the month, the journal columns are footed, and the totals are posted to the general ledger. Daily postings of charges to outpatients are made to the accounts receivable subsidiary ledger. You will see the details of the process of journalizing and posting outpatient revenue transactions in Chapter 12. The procedure is much the same as for inpatient revenues.

Cash Receipts Journal

Hartful Hospital's cash receipts journal is illustrated in Figure 11–4. It is used to record all cash receipts from whatever source. As was noted earlier, the hospital has a centralized cashiering location. As cash is received, either by mail or over the counter, a cash receipt

19X1 Date	(✓)	Outpatient Receivables Dr.	Nursing Service Revenue Credits				Other Professional Service Revenue Credits					Sundry Debits and Credits		
			Operating Rooms	Emergency Rooms	Central Supply	Other Units	Laboratory	Radiology	Pharmacy	Anesthesia	Other Units	Account Numbers	Dr.	Cr.
Totals		Debit 1044.0	Credit 3210.2	Credit 3230.2	Credit 3250.2	Credit	Credit 4011.2	Credit 4040.2	Credit 4070.2	Credit 4080.2	Credit			

Figure 11-3 Outpatient Revenue Journal

19X1 Date	Cash Receipt Slip Nos.	Cash Dr.	Revenue Deduction Debits			Accounts Receivable Credits			Other Credits		Sundry Debits and Credits		
			Contractual Adjustments	Charity Services	Other	Inpatients		Outpatients	Cafeteria Sales	General Contrbns.	Account Numbers	Dr.	Cr.
						Inhouse	Discharged						
Totals		Debit 1011.0	Debit 5520.0	Debit 5540.0	Debit	Credit 1031.0	Credit 1032.0	Credit 1044.0	Credit 5061.0	Credit 5155.0			

Figure 11-4 Cash Receipts Journal

slip is prepared for each item. All cash receipts are deposited intact daily. Copies of the bank deposit slips, along with copies of the related cash receipt slips, are sent to the hospital's accounting offices each day. Here, the employee in charge of the cash receipts journal uses the source documents to record debits to cash and credits to the receivables accounts.

The journal columns are footed at the end of each month, and the totals are posted to the indicated general ledger accounts. Daily postings are made to the accounts receivable ledger to give individual patients credit for the payments received from them or on their behalf from their third-party sponsors. Details of the procedure of journalizing and posting of cash receipts appear in Chapter 12. We also will examine internal control principles and practices with respect to hospital revenues and cash receipts.

Payroll Journal

The payroll journal employed by Hartful Hospital is illustrated in Figure 11–5. This journal is used to record the salaries and wages earned by hospital employees during each pay period. As you can see, the journal provides columns for the recording of gross pay, payroll taxes and other withholdings, and the net payroll. The necessary data for the payroll journal entries are compiled from information provided by departmental time reports, personnel department records, time clock cards, and other source documents, as will be explained in detail in Chapter 13.

Once the net payroll (assume a figure of $116,492) is determined and credited to the Accrued Payroll Liability account (account 2031.0), individual paychecks are written and issued to hospital employees. The checks are drawn against the hospital's Payroll Checking account (account 1012.0), but no entry is made to credit that account. Instead, the amount of the net (accrued) payroll is vouchered through the accounts payable account in the voucher register as follows:

Accrued Payroll	2031.0	$116,492	
Accounts Payable	2020.0		$116,492

The debit closes the Accrued Payroll account (which previously was established with a credit from the payroll journal) and sets up the amount of the net payroll as an account payable.

Drawing the Payroll Funds

Then, a single check is written against the General Checking account (account 1011.0) and is recorded in the cash disbursements journal as follows:

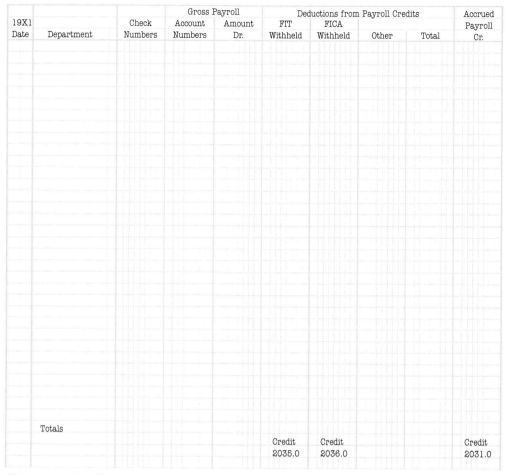

| 19X1 Date | Department | Check Numbers | Gross Payroll | | Deductions from Payroll Credits | | | | Accrued Payroll Cr. |
			Account Numbers	Amount Dr.	FIT Withheld	FICA Withheld	Other	Total	
	Totals								
					Credit 2035.0	Credit 2036.0			Credit 2031.0

Figure 11–5 Payroll Journal

| Accounts Payable | 2020.0 | $116,492 | |
| Cash | 1011.0 | | $116,492 |

Thus, the Payroll Checking account is never debited or credited, nor does it ever have a ledger balance (other than perhaps a nominal balance). The $116,492 check drawn on the general checking account, of course, is deposited to the payroll checking account at the hospital's bank. When the individual paychecks are cashed by employees, the Payroll Checking account is automatically cleared to a zero balance. This procedure removes the large volume of paychecks from the general checking account, thereby facilitating the reconciliation of that account with the monthly bank statement. Another illustration of these procedures will be provided in Chapter 14.

All postings from the payroll journal are made on a monthly basis. Hartful Hospital, however, does maintain (as required by law) an "employees' individual earnings record," which in effect is a subsidiary payroll ledger. We will examine this record in Chapter 13.

Hartful Hospital follows an accounting policy that requires that all disbursements be vouchered through accounts payable. In other words, an entry such as the following is prohibited by the system:

Voucher Register

Dietary—Supplies and Other			
Expenses	8050.2	$1,387	
Cash	1011.0		$1,387

This disbursement or any other disbursement requires the preparation of a document known as a *voucher*. The vouchering of proposed disbursements includes the auditing of invoices and the securing of authorizations. Once an item is vouchered and approved for payment, the voucher register entry is as follows:

Dietary—Supplies and Other			
Expense	8050.2	$1,387	
Accounts Payable	2020.0		$1,387

Thus, before a check is written, an investigation is made of the proposed disbursement, and (if approved) a credit is made to a liability account (accounts payable). When the check is written, an entry is made in the cash disbursements journal, as follows:

Accounts Payable	2020.0	$1,387	
Cash	1011.0		$1,387

This procedure, known as a *voucher system,* provides a high order of accounting control over hospital disbursements. A major portion of Chapter 14 will be devoted to a description of the voucher system employed by Hartful Hospital.

Entering Vouchers

Figure 11–6 illustrates Hartful Hospital's voucher register, which also may be called an "accounts payable" or "purchases journal." As invoices and bills are received by the hospital, they are vouchered (processed for payment) by accounting employees. The vouchers, along with the underlying documents (purchase orders and receiving reports, for example), are turned over to the person who maintains the voucher register. This person enters the vouchers in the register, recording debits to the various accounts indicated by the column headings. In each case, the credit is to accounts payable.

At the end of the month, the column totals are posted to the general ledger accounts. Daily postings are made to the accounts payable subsidiary ledger to maintain a daily record of the amounts due to individual hospital creditors. This procedure is described more fully in Chapter 14.

Cash Disbursements Journal

Hartful Hospital's cash disbursements journal is illustrated in Figure 11–7. This journal, which also is known as a "cash payments journal" or "check register," is used to record all hospital disbursements for whatever purpose. Vouchered items, as they become due for payment, are sent to the hospital's disbursing officer; that is, the individual who has authority to sign checks drawn on the hospital's checking account. This person, if satisfied as to the propriety of the disbursements, signs and mails the related checks. The paid voucher, along with attached underlying documents, is returned to the accounting office where the person in charge of the cash disbursements journal records the disbursements by debits to accounts payable and credits to cash. The paid vouchers are then placed in a file that should be retained for the period of time specified. Chapter 14 illustrates these procedures in more detail.

Posting the Cash Disbursements

Monthly postings are made to the general ledger of the column totals in the cash disbursements journal. Daily debit postings are made to the accounts payable subsidiary ledger.

General Journal

The general journal used by Hartful Hospital is shown in Figure 11–8. You are already well acquainted with this journal. It is important that you now understand, however, that in a multijournal system the general journal is used sparingly. In Hartful Hospital's system, the general journal is used only to record those transactions

19X1 Date	Accounts Payable Credits	Payroll-Related Debits				Adm. Office	Nursing Service Expense Debits				Other Professional Service Expense Debits					Medical Staff Expense
		(✔)	Accrued Payroll	FIT Withheld	FICA W/H & Accrued		Nursing Units	Operating Rooms	Emergency Rooms	Central Supply	Adm. Office	Laboratory	Radiology	Pharmacy	Anesthesia	
Totals	Credit 2020.0		Debit 2031.0	Debit 2035.0	Debit 2036.0	Debit 6010.2	Debit 6021.2	Debit 6210.2	Debit 6230.2	Debit 6250.2	Debit 7010.2	Debit 7011.2	Debit 7040.2	Debit 7070.2	Debit 7080.2	Debit 8030.2

Figure 11-6 Voucher Register

General Services Expense Debits					Fiscal Services Expense Debits			Administrative Services Expense Debits					Sundry Debits and Credits		
Adm. Office	Dietary	Plant O. & M.	House-keeping	Laundry	Adm. Office	Accounting	Admitting	Administra-tor's Office	Adm. Office	Governing Board	Purchasing	Personnel	Account Numbers	Dr.	Cr.
Debit 8040.2	Debit 8050.2	Debit 8060.2	Debit 8090.2	Debit 8110.2	Debit 8211.2	Debit 8212.2	Debit 8241.2	Debit 8310.2	Debit 8311.2	Debit 8312.2	Debit 8331.2	Debit 8371.2			

Figure 11-6 Voucher Register (*continued*)

19X1 Date	Description	Check Numbers	Cash Cr.	Purchases Discounts Cr.	Accounts Payable Dr.	Dr.	Account Numbers	Sundry Debits and Credits Dr.	Cr.
	Totals								
			Credit 1011.0	Credit 5171.0	Debit 2020.0	Debit			

Figure 11–7 Cash Disbursements Journal

for which a special journal has not been provided. It will be used mainly for adjusting and closing entries. Most transaction entries will be recorded in the six specialized journals.

Ledger System

If Hartful Hospital maintained only a general ledger, that ledger would have to contain a separate account for each patient and each hospital creditor. As you can imagine, such a ledger would be immense, cumbersome, and unmanageable. For this reason, the individual accounts for hospital patients and creditors are removed from the general ledger and are established as subsidiary ledgers.

Figure 11–8 General Journal

19X1 Date	Accounts and Explanations	Account Numbers	Dr.	Cr.

The general ledger, however, does contain control accounts for patient receivables and accounts payable.

Balancing Subsidiary
Ledgers

As mentioned several times in the preceding discussion, the general ledger control accounts are posted monthly for the *accumulated totals* provided by the special journals; the subsidiary ledgers, however, are posted daily in the *individual amounts* of transactions. This requires that the subsidiary ledgers be balanced against, and reconciled with, the month-end balances of the related general ledger control accounts. This is an extremely important feature of a hospital's overall internal control system, as you will see in the chapters to follow.

Q11–1. What are the advantages of maintaining several special journals rather than a single general journal?

Q11–2. Distinguish between the general ledger and a subsidiary ledger. Name three types of subsidiary ledgers.

Q11–3. What is the purpose of having sundry debits and credits columns in a special journal? Describe the posting procedure for the amounts entered in these columns.

Q11–4. State two advantages of maintaining control accounts in the general ledger of a hospital.

Q11–5. How would you determine that a special journal "balances"?

Q11–6. "Whenever a debit posting is made to a general ledger control account, one or more credit postings of the same aggregate total must be posted to the related subsidiary ledger." Do you agree? Explain.

Q11–7. Why must transactions be posted to the subsidiary ledgers more frequently than to the general ledger?

Q11–8. Hartful Hospital employs the seven journals indicated in Figure 11–1. Indicate the name of the journal in which each of the following types of transactions would be recorded:
   a. Charges for services rendered to outpatients
   b. Purchase of supplies on account
   c. Payments made on accounts payable
   d. Charges for services rendered to inpatients
   e. Issuance of payroll checks to employees
   f. Cash collections received on patients' accounts
   g. Cash purchases of supplies
   h. Sale of long-term investments for cash
   i. Purchase of new equipment on account
   j. Receipt of interest income from temporary investments

Q11–9. Describe briefly the posting procedure for the revenue journals and the cash receipts journal.

Q11–10. An inpatient charge ticket for $60 was correctly recorded in the inpatient revenue journal, but the patient's account in the accounts receivable subsidiary ledger was incorrectly debited for only $6. How will this error be discovered?

Q11–11. Describe briefly the posting procedure for the payroll journal, voucher register, and the cash disbursements journal.

Q11–12. An invoice for the purchase of $150 of supplies was correctly recorded in the voucher register, but the supplier's account in the accounts payable subsidiary ledger was incorrectly credited for $510. How will this error be discovered?

Q11–13. Hartful Hospital provides many outpatient services on a cash basis. In such cases, would it be appropriate to bypass the outpatient revenue journal and record the transaction directly in the cash receipts journal only to debit cash and credit outpatient revenue? Explain your opinion.

Q11–14. What is the purpose of the check ($\checkmark$) column in the inpatient revenue journal?

Q11–15. Describe briefly the use of the imprest Payroll Checking account (account number 1012).

Q11–16. In the accounting system described in this chapter, is an entry such as the following possible?

Laboratory—Supplies Expense	$259	
Cash		$259

    To record cash purchase of supplies for the laboratory department.

Explain your answer.

Q11–17. The following is a list of general ledger accounts. For each account, name the journals from which debit and credit postings normally would be received.
a. Pharmacy Revenues
b. Accounts Receivable—Outpatients
c. Accounts Receivable—Inpatients
d. Cafeteria Sales
e. Bank Loans Payable

Q11–18. The following is a list of general ledger accounts. For each account, name the journals from which debit and credit postings normally would be received.
a. Cash—General Checking Account
b. Pharmacy—Supplies Expense
c. Pharmacy—Salaries and Wages
d. Equipment
e. Accounts Payable

Q11–19. The following is a list of general ledger accounts. For each account, name the journals from which debit and credit postings normally would be received.
a. Operating Room Revenues
b. Notes Payable
c. General Contributions
d. Deductions from Revenues—Charity Service
e. Accrued Payroll

Q11–20. The following is a list of general ledger accounts. For each account, name the journals from which debit and credit postings normally would be received.
a. Prepaid Expense—Insurance
b. Temporary Investments
c. Allowance for Uncollectible Accounts
d. Land
e. Hospital Equity

Revenues, Receivables, and Cash Receipts

12

This chapter explains the basic procedures involved in recording revenues, receivables, and cash receipts. The discussion and illustrations relate to our hypothetical Hartful Hospital whose chart of accounts was outlined in Chapter 10, and whose journal and ledger system was introduced in Chapter 11. Although the procedures here are similar to those found in actual practice, you should recognize that there is no "ideal" system that is completely applicable to all hospitals. You should not assume, therefore, that the procedures followed by Hartful Hospital are precisely identical to those of any particular "real-life" hospital. The discussion will, however, give you an excellent understanding of the accounting requirements as well as an insight into certain methods that have been developed to meet those requirements. These observations also apply to the materials of Chapters 13 and 14.

Recording Inpatient Revenues

The greatest share of hospital revenues generally is derived from the services rendered to inpatients. These services are of two major types: (1) the daily room, board, and routine nursing services and (2) the other professional, or ancillary services. The accounting objective is to make a prompt and accurate record, on the accrual basis and at the hospital's established rates, of all services rendered, regardless of the amounts (if any) the hospital expects to collect for those services. As a matter of fact, hospitals usually collect less than their full, established service rates, but this has no effect on the amount of revenue to be recorded when services are rendered to patients. Any differences between gross revenues (measured at established rates) and collectible revenues are recorded as revenue deductions. This procedure permits a monetary measurement of earned revenues, "lost" revenues, and collectible revenues.

**Daily Inpatient
Services**

Uses of the Inpatient's
Ledger Card

As a person enters the hospital as an inpatient, several different forms are completed. An illustration of one of these forms is presented in Figure 12–1. It is a multipart form, one part of which is sent to the accounting office where it serves as the patient's individual subsidiary ledger card. It is important that information obtained in the admitting process allow for proper classification of the patient (and the related revenues and receivables) according to financial status, medical category, and so forth.

During the period of stay, the inpatient's ledger card is charged for the services provided, and the appropriate revenue accounts will be credited. The accounting and control systems must provide detailed written evidence of all hospital services provided as well as documentation of the attending physician's authorizations. This evidence appears in the patient's charts, maintained at the nursing stations, and in supporting source documents that are kept in the accounting department. As you will see shortly, the ledger card will be credited for payments received from or on behalf of the patient. And, in many cases, noncash credits for charity and contractual adjustments may be made to the ledger card. On the patient's discharge, the medical documents are filed in the medical records department; the financial documents are retained in the accounting department for billing and collection purposes.

A major portion of the charges to inpatients arise from the provision of room, board, and normal nursing services. These services sometimes are referred to as *routine services* or *daily patient services*. In any event, these charges (and revenues) are compiled from information obtained from the daily census report. Forms and procedures differ, but the determination of charges and revenues for daily patient services basically is a matter of multiplying occupied rooms (beds) by established daily charges for those accommodations. In the Hartful Hospital system, a "day rate service sheet" is used as a combination of census report and revenue-charge summary. This form, shown in Figure 12–2, consists of a preprinted listing of each room and bed in the hospital. It is classified by nursing unit, including an indication of the daily charge for each type of accommodation.

The sheet is pretotaled for 100 percent occupancy. As a part of the midnight census, a line is drawn through the listing of each unoccupied bed. The total revenue represented by these unoccupied accommodations is computed and deducted from the 100 percent-occupancy figures. This produces the gross earned revenues for the day as well as the charge to each patient's ledger card. The objective is to secure a high degree of assurance that the census of patients is

Hartful Hospital

37

LAST FIRST M.I. MAIDEN

DATE	ROOM NO.	BEDS	RATE	DAYS

PATIENT HOSP. NO.
STREET PHONE
CITY & STATE MAR. STATUS

| BLUE CROSS CASE NO. | TOTAL DAYS | |
| | BASIC | SUPPL. |

SEX & AGE BIRTHDATE BIRTHPLACE
ADM. DATE TIME SOC. SEC. NO.
I.D. NO. STATE INS. OR HIS. NO.

COMPLETE FINAL DIAGNOSIS

☐ A DISCHARGED ☐ B STILL HOSPITALIZED ☐ C EXPIRED

EFF. DATE INS. PAID THRU DISCHARGE DATE & TIME
GROUP NO. KIND OR OCCUPATION
FATHER'S NAME BENEFIT CODE RACE
NEAREST REL. MOTHER'S MAIDEN NAME
RESP. PARTY RELATION ADDRESS
EMPLOYER RELATION ADDRESS
ATTN. PHY. OCCUPATION ADDRESS
PREV. ADM. YR. RELIGION CHURCH M ☐ F ☐
ADM. DIAGNOSIS PASTOR ADDRESS
BABY BIRTHDATE

MED ☐ SUR ☐ PED ☐ OB ☐ EMERG ☐ URG ☐ ELEC ☐

SERVICE CHARGES

MISCELLANEOUS SERVICE		SUPPLIES (2)	X-RAY (3)	LAB-PATH (4)	DRUGS (5)	NURSERY (6)	ROOM, FOOD & NURSING (7)	DATE	CREDITS CASH UNLESS CODED		BALANCE	
CODE	AMOUNT								AMOUNT	CODE		
	(1)	SUPPLIES	X-RAY	LAB PATH	DRUGS	NURSERY	ROOM, FOOD & NURSING	TOTAL	CREDITS		BALANCE	
TOTAL CHARGES												

SUMMARY OF BILLING

BASIC												
SUPPL												
PATIENT'S PORTION											PATIENT'S PORTION	

LEDGER COPY

Figure 12–1 Inpatient Ledger Card

accurate, that debits are made to patients' accounts, and that credits are made to revenue accounts in the correct amounts for all daily service provided.

Most services rendered to patients must be ordered by a physician. Such orders are written in the patient's chart by attending physicians and prescribe all necessary patient services. The services so

Other Professional (Ancillary) Services

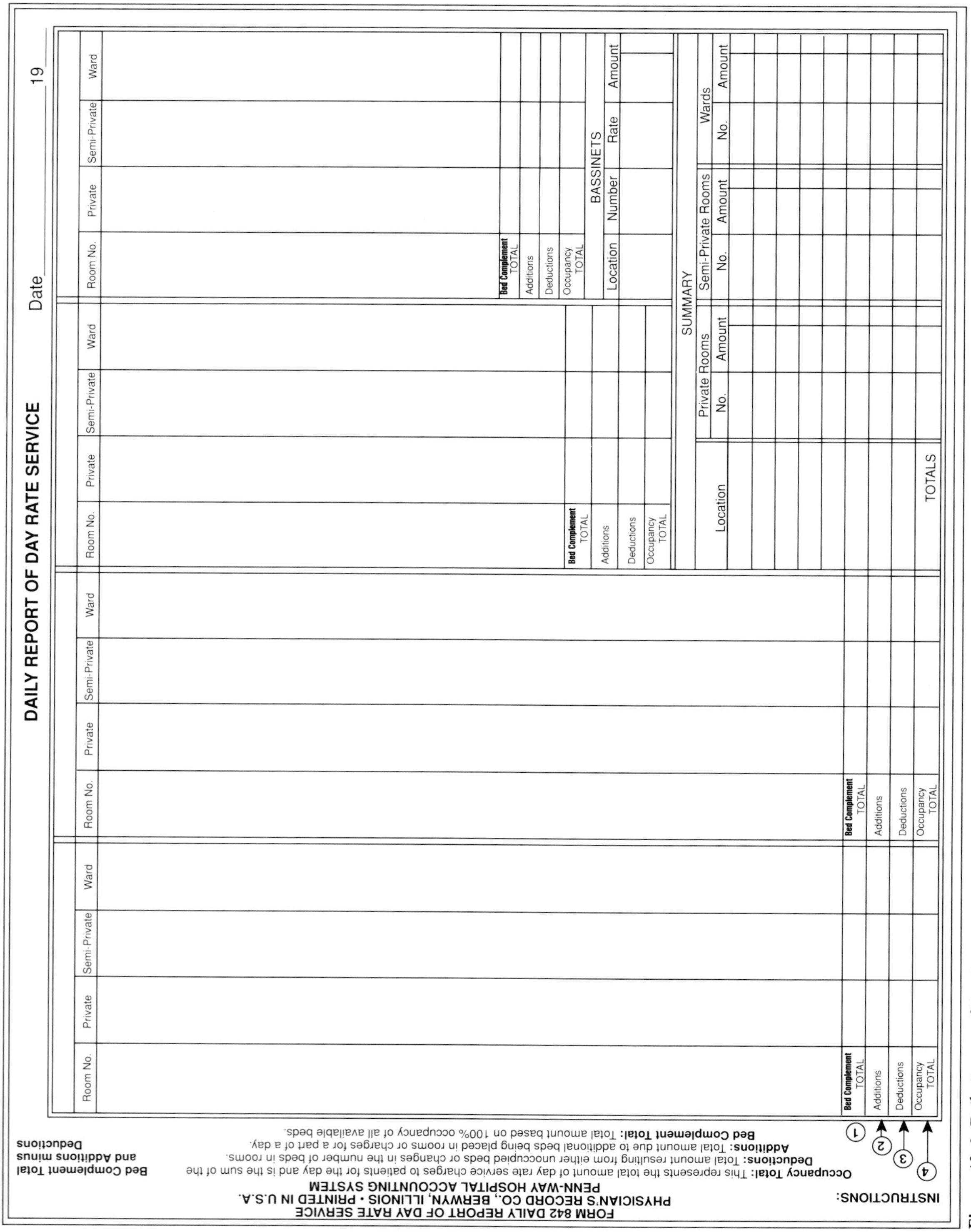

DAILY REPORT OF DAY RATE SERVICE

Date ________ 19___

Room No.	Private	Semi-Private	Ward
Bed Complement TOTAL			
Additions			
Deductions			
Occupancy TOTAL			

BASSINETS			
Location	Number	Rate	Amount

SUMMARY

Location	Private Rooms No.	Private Rooms Amount	Semi-Private Rooms No.	Semi-Private Rooms Amount	Wards No.	Wards Amount
TOTALS						

INSTRUCTIONS:

FORM 842 DAILY REPORT OF DAY RATE SERVICE
PHYSICIAN'S RECORD CO., BERWYN, ILLINOIS • PRINTED IN U.S.A.
PENN-WAY HOSPITAL ACCOUNTING SYSTEM

(4) **Occupancy Total:** This represents the total amount of day rate service charges to patients for the day and is the sum of the Bed Complement Total and Additions minus Deductions

(3) **Deductions:** Total amount resulting from either unoccupied beds or changes in the number of beds in rooms.

(2) **Additions:** Total amount due to additional beds being placed in rooms or charges for a part of a day.

(1) **Bed Complement Total:** Total amount based on 100% occupancy of all available beds.

Figure 12–2 Daily Report of Day Rate Service

LABORATORY

Walk ☐
Chair ☐
Bed ☐

Check If Patient
Is Leaving Today ....m.   ☐
★ If this is a CREDIT, check
here and also circle amount   ☐

N 99999

Patient's
Name —————————————————————————————

Room No. ——————————

If OUT-Patient
Address ———————————————————————

Age ——————————

Requested by Dr. ———————————————— Date   19

Adm.	Repeat	EXAMINATION OR TEST REQUESTED	CHARGE★	
		Blood Count —Complete ☐ R.B.C.☐ W.B.C.☐ Hb.☐ Diff.☐		
		Urinalysis—Voided ☐ Catheterized ☐ Time Collected _____.M.		
		Kahn ☐ Kline☐ Kolmer ☐ Mazzini ☐ Wassermann ☐ _____		
		Special Tests, etc. (Specify) _____		

Medical, etc. ☐ Surgical ☐ Operation Scheduled for—Date_____19_____Time_____.M.

Remarks_____Signed_____

1 **Please Send 1st and 2nd Copies
to Laboratory**

**Number Checked Off   ☐
on Control Sheet**

**Posted to   ☐
Patient's Account**

Figure 12–3 Requisition-Charge Ticket

prescribed are requisitioned by nurses or other nursing station personnel acting under the nurses' supervision. To obtain adequate accounting control over the charges and revenues arising from these services, therefore, the full cooperation of all nursing personnel is essential.

As various ancillary services are required for patients, nursing station personnel prepare requisition-charge tickets such as the one illustrated in Figure 12–3. A separate set of tickets may be used for each type of service. Each ticket may be prenumbered, and charge tickets for each service may be of different colors to aid with identification and sorting.

Preparing and Processing
Requisition-Charge Tickets

The charge tickets often are prepared in triplicate. The original and duplicate copies go to the professional department that renders the service; the triplicate copy remains at the nursing station. The ticket gives the professional department the authority to render the prescribed service. Periodically during each day, the original copies of the charge tickets are collected from the professional departments and are taken to the hospital's accounting offices; the duplicates remain with the professional department. The charge

19X1 Date		(✔)	Inpatient Receivables Dr,	Nursing Service Revenue Credits					
				Nursing Units	Operating Rooms	Emergency Rooms	Central Supply	Other Units	Other Units
5	5	✔	14,645	6,250	900	450	1,100		
	Totals		453,995	187,500	26,100	14,400	34,100		
			Debit 1031.00	Credit 3021.1	Credit 3210.1	Credit 3230.1	Credit 3250.1	Credit	Credit

Figure 12–4 Inpatient Revenue Journal

tickets are usually priced either in the professional departments or in the accounting office.

Each day, an accounting employee sorts the charge tickets by color (department). Each color group is then totaled to determine the day's revenue for each departmental service. The same tickets are re-sorted according to individual patient so that appropriate charges can be made to the appropriate patient's ledger card. Naturally a reconciliation must be made to ascertain whether the total debits to the ledger cards equal the total of all tickets and whether the total credits to the various revenue accounts equal the total of all tickets. In some systems, a worksheet is prepared to summarize the charge tickets and make the necessary daily reconciliations.

Other Professional Service Revenue Credits					Sundry Debits and Credits		
Laboratory	Radiology	Pharmacy	Anesthesia	Other Units	Account Numbers	Dr.	Cr.
1,820	2,135	1,040	950				
56,420	88,835	24,960	21,680				
Credit 4011.1	Credit 4040.1	Credit 4070.1	Credit 4080.1	Credit			

Figure 12–4 Inpatient Revenue Journal (*continued*)

Whatever the data collection system, daily journal entries must be made to record debits to the inpatient receivables control accounts and credits to the various revenue accounts. We will assume that Hartful Hospital uses the day rate service sheet and requisition-charge tickets to generate the necessary data. These data are journalized in the inpatient revenue journal as indicated in Figure 12–4. This is merely a sample entry to illustrate the manner in which a day's inpatient revenues may be recorded. A similar entry is made each day of the month. You will have to imagine that all 31 lines of the journal are filled. Assume that the 31 daily entries add to the column totals shown in the journal.

Inpatient Revenue Journal

Summarizing Charges

It is assumed here that a daily worksheet summary of the day rate service sheet and all charge tickets is prepared in the accounting office. The total of the day rate service sheet and the total of the charge tickets together make up the total $14,645 debit to Inpatient Receivables (account 1031.0) for May 5, 19X1. Similarly, an analysis of the day rate service sheet and of the charge tickets provides the totals credited to each revenue center account for the same day. Each day's entry should be cross-footed to check whether the total of credits equals the amount of the debit to inpatient receivables.

Thus, a daily summary of charges and revenues is entered on a single line of the journal. When this procedure is followed, an indication of charge ticket numbers in the journal is not feasible. This requires the retention of the worksheet or other form on which the summary totals were determined, as well as retention of the day rate service sheets and charge tickets in appropriate files. In this way the necessary "audit trails" (paperwork proofs) are provided for the hospital's internal and external auditors. In other words, the system must facilitate the auditors' tracing of journal entries to source documents and must provide safeguards against either the omission of transactions or the recording of the same transaction more than once. An alternative would be to journalize the charge tickets individually, but this often is not feasible in a manual system because of the large number of charge tickets issued each day.

Notice the sundry debit and credit columns on the far right-hand side of the journal. These columns are provided for occasional debits or credits that may be required but for which appropriate separate columns have not been included in the journal. The journal should be designed so that the use of these sundry columns will rarely be necessary.

As these daily summaries of charges and revenues are entered in the journal, daily postings of charges are made to the inpatients' subsidiary ledger cards on the basis of the information provided by the day rate service sheet and the individual charge tickets sorted according to patient name, hospital number, or room number. The total of these debit postings, of course, must equal the total debited to inpatient receivables in the journal. When this equality has been established, a check mark ($\checkmark$) is placed in the journal column provided beside the date.

No daily postings are made to the general ledger accounts. At month-end, however, the various columns of the journal are totaled and cross-footed to ensure that the total of the debit columns equals the total of the credit columns. Each column total is then posted to the appropriate general ledger account as indicated at the foot of each column.

As noted earlier, the Hartful Hospital procedure is a manual system; it is described here in simplified terms to illustrate certain principles more easily. Even a small hospital, however, will find that the use of posting machines, other accounting equipment, or computers is necessary due to the great volume of account activity.

Recording Outpatient Revenues

Charges and revenues for departmental services to outpatients also may be determined in much the same way as was described for inpatient revenue accounting. A charge ticket is originated—either at a centralized outpatient reception desk or in the professional departments providing the outpatient services. In some cases, the outpatient charge tickets are summarized by personnel of the service-rendering department in daily service logs. A copy of this log, along with copies of related charge tickets, is collected daily by the accounting department. On the basis of these documents, a daily summary of outpatient charges and revenues is prepared and entered on a single line of the outpatient revenue journal as illustrated in Figure 12–5 for May 5, 19X1. The worksheet on which this summary was developed, the logs, and the charge tickets should be retained to provide an appropriate audit trail.

Daily postings are made of charges to outpatient subsidiary ledger cards. Again, a special column (✔) is provided in the journal to indicate that the individual debit postings to the ledger cards equal the total debited to the outpatient receivables column in the journal. At month's end, the various columns are totaled, and the totals are posted to the general ledger accounts. Entries in the sundry columns, however, must be posted individually.

Recording Cash Receipts

An immediate written record should be made of all cash receipts. In many hospital accounting systems, this record is generated through the preparation of a cash receipt slip such as the one illustrated in Figure 12–6. Cash receipts are of two types: mail receipts and over-the-counter receipts. Two employees may be assigned responsibility for opening incoming mail. Working together, they extract the cash items from the mail and list these items on a mail remittance report. One copy of the report is sent directly to the accounting department, one copy (with the cash items) goes to cashiering, and one copy is retained by the mail openers.

19X1 Date	(✓)	Outpatient Receivable Dr.	Nursing Service Revenue Credits				Other Professional Service Revenue Credits					Account Numbers	Sundry Debits and Credits	
			Operating Rooms	Emergency Rooms	Central Supply	Other Units	Laboratory	Radiology	Pharmacy	Anesthesia	Other Units		Dr.	Cr.
5 5	✓	2,160	1500	4800	290		470	510	210	50				
Totals		64,800	3,900	9,000	5,700		17,040	21,630	5,880	1,650				
		Debit 1044.00	Credit 3210.2	Credit 3230.2	Credit 3250.2	Credit	Credit 4011.2	Credit 4040.2	Credit 4070.2	Credit 4080.2	Credit			

Figure 12-5 Outpatient Revenue Journal

```
┌─────────────────────────────────────────────────────────────────────┐
│                         ┌─ CASH RECEIPT ─┐                            │
│                                                                       │
│    GENERAL COMMUNITY HOSPITAL                                         │
│            STREET ADDRESS                              No. 10351       │
│            CITY, STATE, ZIP CODE                                      │
│                                                                       │
│    Patient's                                                          │
│    Name _____              │
│                                                                       │
│                                              Room No....              │
│                                                                       │
│                                                       $...            │
│    Received                                                           │
│    the Sum of_____and_____Dollars    │
│                                                      100              │
│    Cash □  Check □  Money Order □       GENERAL COMMUNITY HOSPITAL     │
│                                                                       │
│                                                                       │
│    Date          19                          By                      │
│                         └─ THANK YOU ─┘                               │
└─────────────────────────────────────────────────────────────────────┘
```

Figure 12–6 Cash Receipt Slip

Distributing Cash Receipt Slips

On receipt of the cash items from the incoming mail, the cashier issues a cash receipt slip for the total amount. One copy is given to the mail openers, one copy is sent to the accounting department, and one copy is retained by the cashier. For counter receipts, the cashier prepares individual cash receipt slips, again in triplicate. One copy is given to the patient, one copy is sent to the accounting department as a medium for postings to the patients' ledger, and one copy is filed permanently in numerical sequence. All cash items, both mail and counter receipts, should be carefully controlled and should be deposited daily and intact. Cash disbursements should never be made from cash receipts. A copy of the bank deposit slip is routed to the accounting office.

At the end of each day, the cash receipt slips are summarized and entered in the cash receipts journal. An accounting employee compares the cash receipt slips with the mail remittance report and with the duplicate bank deposit slip. The cash receipt slips, sorted by patient name, and the mail remittance report can be used to make the necessary credit postings to the individual patient's ledger card.

Hartful Hospital's cash receipts journal is illustrated in Figure 12–7. A sample entry for May 5, 19X1, has been included to indicate how the daily cash receipt transactions are recorded. If cash receipt slips are issued in several different numerical series concurrently, an indication of cash receipt slip numbers in the journal may

19X1 Date	Cash Receipt Slip Nos.	Cash Dr.	Revenue Deduction Credits Contractual Adjustments	Charity Service	Other	Account Receivable Credits Inpatients Inhouse	Discharged	Outpatients	Other Credits Cafeteria Sales	General Contrbns.	Sundry Debits and Credits Account Numbers	Dr.	Cr.
5	443-657	13,815	1,040	480		1,420	11,350	1,930	560	75			
Totals		477,500	31,600	14,400		43,020	401,850	57,900	18,480	2,250			
		Debit 1011.0	Debit 5520.0	Debit 5540.0	Debit	Credit 1031.0	Credit 1032.0	Credit 1044.0	Credit 5061.0	Credit 3155.0			

Figure 12–7 Cash Receipts Journal

not be practicable. When this is the case, either the slips must be journalized individually or a worksheet summary must be developed to provide an adequate audit trail.

The posting of entries from the cash receipts journal is the same as for the revenue journals. Daily postings are made to the patients' ledger; monthly postings of column totals are made to the general ledger.

Notice that the cash receipts journal includes columns for debits to the revenue deduction accounts. To describe how these columns are used, assume a discharged patient with an account balance of $1,250. On May 5, 19X1, $1,000 is received by the hospital from the patient's third-party sponsor in full payment of the account. The entry to be made by the hospital is as follows:

Debits to Revenue Deduction Accounts

Cash	1011.0	$1,000	
Contractual Adjustments	5520.0	250	
Inpatient Receivables—			
Discharged	1032.0		$1,250

It is assumed here that the $250 difference between the patient's hospital bill and the amount reimbursed by the third party is not, under the terms of the contract, recoverable from the patient.

Thus, in Hartful Hospital's system, debits are made to the revenue deduction accounts as patients' accounts are paid. Here the cash receipts journal is designed to provide columns for those debits. In other systems, however, a separate receivables adjustments and allowances journal or revenue deductions journal is employed to account for these items. But whatever the procedure may be, it is essential that all noncash credits to receivables be authorized and approved by a responsible hospital official who has no access to the hospital's cash receipts and receivables records. This is necessary to protect against a theft of cash receipts that may be covered up by unwarranted writeoffs of accounts receivable balances that were really paid.

The method used by Hartful Hospital in accounting for revenue deductions is satisfactory as an accounting routine. Care must be taken, however, to make sure that revenue deductions are recognized on the accrual basis. The deductions must be recognized in the same period as the related revenues. To accomplish this, an adjusting entry is required at the end of each period for which a balance sheet and income statement are prepared. To illustrate the procedure for contractual adjustments, let us assume that a hospital had $3.6 million revenues in 19X1 and that $600,000 of this total remains in accounts receivable at December 31, 19X1. In collecting the $3 million of accounts receivable during the year, assume that contractual adjustments totaling $150,000 were recorded. In other words, contractual adjustments averaged about 5 percent of receivables.

Adjusting Entry for Year-End Receivables

This means that the year-end accounts receivable probably include $30,000 (5 percent of $600,000) of unrecognized contractual adjustments. This $30,000 must be recognized as revenue deductions in 19X1, the year in which the related revenues are recorded. The required December 31, 19X1, adjusting entry is the following:

Contractual Adjustments	5520.0	$30,000
Allowance for Uncollectible Accounts— Contractual Adjustments	1062.0	$30,000

When the $600,000 of accounts receivable are collected in 19X2, the actual contractual adjustments on these accounts are recorded in accordance with the routine described for Hartful Hospital, without regard to the adjusting entry. A reversing entry (the reverse of the above adjusting entry) can be made by the hospital on January 1, 19X2, to avoid recording the same contractual adjustments twice (in 19X1 and 19X2). Or, if one prefers, the adjusting entry at the end of the first monthly reporting period in 19X2 can simply adjust to the appropriate balance at that time in the allowance for uncollectible accounts—contractual adjustments.

A similar procedure can be followed for revenue deductions arising from the provision of charity service. The treatment of bad debts, however, is generally somewhat different, and we will defer a discussion of this point to Chapter 16.

As you have seen, Hartful Hospital maintains three receivables control accounts in its general ledger. These accounts (with assumed May 1, 19X1, balances) are as follows:

1031.0	Inpatient Receivables—Inhouse	$110,000
1032.0	Inpatient Receivables—Discharged	800,000
1044.0	Outpatient Receivables	16,000

Hartful Hospital also maintains a separate patients' subsidiary ledger for each of these control accounts. Let us assume that the total of the individual debit balances in each subsidiary ledger at May 1, 19X1, agrees with the debit balance of the related general ledger control account at May 1, 19X1.

During the month of May, as entries were made in the revenue and cash receipt journals, daily postings of charges and credits were made to the patients' subsidiary ledgers. Month-end postings of journal column totals were made to the control accounts in the general ledger, as illustrated here:

Reconciling Control Accounts and Subsidiary Records

Month-End Postings to General Ledger

Inpatient Receivables—Inhouse				Inpatient Receivables—Discharged			
BB	110,000	CRJ	43,020	BB	800,000	CRJ	401,850
IRJ	453,995	GJ	412,975	GJ	412,975		
CB	108,000			CB	811,125		

Outpatient Receivables		
ORJ	64,800	
CB	22,900	

Posting references:

IRJ = Inpatient revenue journal
CRJ = Cash receipts journal
GJ = General journal
ORJ = Outpatient revenue journal
CB = Closing balance

All of the postings in this illustration are drawn from the journals shown previously in this chapter, except for postings from the general journal. Not mentioned earlier is the fact that as inpatients are discharged, Hartful Hospital makes entries in the general journal to transfer the unpaid account balances from the "inhouse" to the "discharged" classification of receivables. That is, during May, patients whose unpaid balances together totaled $412,975 were discharged from the hospital.

Now, after the month-end postings are made as indicated in the preceding T accounts, we have a May 31, 19X1, balance in each of the three receivables control accounts. The individual ledger-card balances in each of the three subsidiary ledgers are totaled. In the absence of accounting errors, the total of the inhouse inpatient receivables ledger should be $108,000. Similarly, the discharged inpatient receivables ledger cards should total $811,125, and the outpatient ledger cards should total $22,900.

Investigating Discrepancies

Whenever a subsidiary ledger does not reconcile with the corresponding control account, the situation should be thoroughly investigated, and the reasons for the discrepancy identified. Considering the importance of recording hospital receivables accurately and the availability of efficient data processing equipment, there simply is no excuse for a failure to make regular monthly reconciliations of accounts receivable controls and subsidiary ledgers.

You now have seen the Hartful Hospital accounting system as related to its revenue and cash receipt transactions. The next chapter deals with the payroll accounting procedures of the hospital.

Questions

Q12–1. State the basic objective of accounting for services rendered to inpatients and outpatients.

Q12–2. Describe briefly how the amounts to be charged to inpatients for services rendered to them generally are determined.

Q12–3. Describe briefly how the amounts to be charged to outpatients for services rendered to them generally are determined.

Q12–4. How often should postings be made from the inpatient and outpatient revenue journals? Explain.

Q12–5. Describe briefly how the daily amounts to be debited to cash and credited to patients' accounts receivable generally are determined.

Q12–6. How often should postings be made from the cash receipts journal? Explain.

Q12–7. Lyst Hospital's general ledger contained the following receivables control account balances at October 31:

Inpatient Receivables—Inhouse	$ 57,000
Inpatient Receivables—Discharged	216,000
Outpatient Receivables	19,000

The inpatient receivables column in the November inpatient revenue journal totaled $98,000, and the outpatients receivables column of the November outpatient revenue journal totaled $34,000. The receivables columns of the November cash receipts journal provided the following totals:

Inpatient Receivables—Inhouse	$ 11,400
Inpatient Receivables—Discharge	107,600
Outpatient Receivables	32,300

The November general journal contained a number of entries that transferred a total of $101,900 in inpatient receivables from the inhouse account to the discharged account. If you prepared adding machine tape totals of the individual patients' ledger card balances at November 30, what total would you expect to find in each of the following subsidiary ledgers?

a. Inpatient Receivables—Inhouse
b. Inpatient Receivables—Discharged
c. Outpatient Receivables

Q12–8. Inpatient Joe Lane received the following services on November 7, 19X1:

Daily patient service (room and board)	$125
Operating room	750
Central supply	124
Laboratory	116
Pharmacy	79
Anesthesia	225
Telephone (long-distance calls)	34

Explain how you would enter this information in the journal and ledger system described in this chapter.

Q12–9. On October 12, 19X1, Loud Hospital borrowed $50,000 from a local bank by issuance of a 120-day, 9 percent note. Explain how you would enter this transaction in the hospital's cash receipts journal.

Q12-10. Lana Lowe, when admitted to Lawson Hospital, was classified as a charity service patient. Lana was admitted on June 1 and was discharged from the hospital on June 8. Services rendered to her during this period totaled $3,672 at the hospital's established rates. What entries should be made by Lawson Hospital to record the services rendered to Lana and to give recognition to the fact that nothing will be collected for those services? Indicate the names of the journals in which these entries will be made.

Q12-11. What are some of the basic features of a good system of internal control over revenues and cash receipts?

Q12-12. Lamp Hospital's daily patient service (routine service) charge is $85 per day for a semiprivate accommodation. On August 29, 19X1, daily patient service charges were correctly entered in the inpatient revenue journal but, in posting to the receivables subsidiary ledger, one patient's account was inadvertently charged for only $58. How might this error be detected?

Payroll Accounting Procedures

13

The discussion presented in this chapter deals with some of the basic accounting principles and practices relating to the hospital payroll. You may be aware that employee compensation accounts for more than 50 percent of the operating expenses of a hospital. That the majority of expense is related to employee compensation, however, should not be surprising in view of these factors:

- The hospital is largely a personal-service, labor-intensive business that generally requires two to three employees per patient.
- The hospital necessarily must employ many highly skilled specialists and professional people who command relatively high salaries.
- The nature and importance of healthcare services is such that high-quality, adequately paid personnel should be employed.
- Competition from industrial and commercial businesses for such personnel has led to an increased general level of compensation.

Like any other business, the hospital also is subject to minimum wage laws, a variety of payroll taxes, and other governmental regulations that have added significant amounts to employee compensation costs. In addition, the unionization of hospital workers and the emergence of employee pension plans are two relatively recent developments that have had a major impact on salaries, wages, and other employee benefits.

It seems clear, therefore, that particular emphasis must be given in hospitals to personnel management and labor cost control. Among other things, this emphasis requires the development of accurate and reliable information about payroll and payroll-related costs through sound accounting methods and practices. This chapter continues the Hartful Hospital illustration to give you an opportunity to study some of the procedures hospital accounting departments follow for employee compensation costs. If your interest in this topic goes beyond the scope of this chapter, you will find a more advanced discussion of payroll accounting and management in the author's *Hospital Financial Accounting: Theory and Practice.*[1]

Compilation of Gross Payrolls

Mechanisms for Recording Employee Hours

Hartful Hospital, like most hospitals, maintains a centralized personnel department whose basic functions include recruitment and orientation of new employees and maintenance of permanent personnel records. In addition to the many records that must be kept for tax purposes, the personnel department keeps a complete, up-to-date employment history or service file for all employees. The centralization of these functions and records localizes responsibility, promotes efficiency, and facilitates control over the size, quality, productivity, and cost of the hospital labor force.

The personnel department, in cooperation with the accounting department of the hospital, should develop and administer a clear-cut procedure for recording and reporting the time worked by all employees. Some hospitals use time clocks for this purpose; others use manually prepared time reports or time cards such as the one illustrated in Figure 13–1. In either case, the department head or supervisor signs and approves the time records before they are sent to the accounting department for processing.

It is essential for time records to be complete and accurate in recording attendance and hours worked. The records should also fully comply with the provisions of the Internal Revenue Code, Fair Labor Standards Act, and other laws imposing various requirements on employers. Time records also should be designed to facilitate the computation of the payroll and the development of the necessary labor statistics. Analyses of the payroll in terms of hours as well as dollars are extremely important to financial management in hospitals.

Compiling the gross payroll is not particularly difficult. Accounting employees independent of the timekeeping function examine all time cards for hourly employees to determine that the records have been properly executed and approved and that the hours worked by each employee have been correctly computed. Hours must then be multiplied by authorized rates of pay. If overtime hours have been worked, a separate calculation is required.

[1]L. Vann Seawell, *Hospital Financial Accounting: Theory and Practice,* Second Edition (Chicago: HFMA, 1987).

Name_____											Month_____ 19_____			

Emp. No. or Dept. _____ Floor _____ Position _____

	DATES *	ON	OFF	Hrs.	ON	OFF	Hrs.	ON	OFF	Hrs.	TOTAL HOURS	Employees DO NOT WRITE IN THIS SPACE		
*Cross Out Column of Dates Which Does Not Apply	1 16											TOTAL ☐Hours ☐Days		
	2 17											Rate per ☐Hour ☐Day		
	3 18											Total Cash Compensation		
	4 19											Other Compensation		
	5 20													
	6 21													
	7 22											TOTAL EARNINGS		
	8 23											Deductions:		
	9 24											Withholding Tax		
	10 25													
	11 26													
	12 27													
	13 28													
	14 29											TOTAL DEDUCTIONS		
	15 30													
	31											AMOUNT OF CHECK		

CODE: A—Absent, deduct   S—Sick, deduct
AN—Absent, no deduction   Ⓢ Sick, no deduction   TOTAL   ☐ Hours
V—Vacation, no deduction   ☐ Days

SUPERVISOR

Time and Salary Computation

Figure 13–1 Employee Time Record

Employee benefits such as paid vacations, paid holidays, and sick leave also affect computation of gross earnings.

To illustrate, assume that a particular employee is paid $6 per hour for a regular workweek of 40 hours. This employee's gross earnings for a week during which he or she worked 48 hours ordinarily would be $288 (48 hours × $6). The Fair Labor Standards Act (popularly known as the Wages and Hours Law) provides not only for a minimum hourly wage but also requires that time and a half be paid for hours in excess of 40 hours worked in a given week. The computation of the employee's earnings for the 48–hour week therefore becomes the following:

Example of Overtime Computation

Regular workweek (40 hours × $6)	$240
Overtime (8 hours × $6)	48
Overtime premium (8 hours × $3)	24
Gross earnings	$312

Application of the provisions of the Wages and Hours Law to the compensation of hospital employees is substantially more involved than indicated here, but we cannot pursue the matter further in this book. It is important to note, however, that good payroll accounting practice provides for the separate recording of overtime compensation because such information is useful in evaluating the utilization of personnel by department heads.

For salaried employees, the gross pay per period is a fixed amount that, once determined, does not vary until the salary is changed. All changes in salaries or in hourly rates should enter into the calculation of gross pay only when such changes are authorized in writing by the personnel department. The payroll clerk should not act on verbal orders. The time records kept for salaried personnel also should be properly executed, approved, and signed by department heads or supervisors.

Payroll Deductions

Payroll accounting is complicated greatly by the various deductions or withholdings that must be made from employees' gross earnings so as to determine the amounts in which paychecks should be written. Many withholding deductions are required by legislation enacted by federal, state, and local governments, which impose a number of taxes on salaries and wages paid to hospital personnel. Other withholding items arise in connection with group insurance, retirement plan, and savings plan agreements with employees. Some of these deductions are described here.

Income Taxes

The federal income tax program has operated on a pay-as-you-go basis for about 50 years. This payment system requires employers to withhold from employees' salaries and wages an amount approximating the income tax on those earnings. The amount, computed from tax withholding tables furnished by the government, varies according to the amount of taxable wages, the length of the payroll period, the employee's marital status, and the number of dependents (exemptions) claimed by the employee.

Tax Remittances and Reports

The income tax amounts so withheld by the hospital must be remitted to the government at times specified by law. For most hospitals, remittance must often be made within a few days following each pay period. This is accomplished by deposit of the withheld amounts in an authorized government depository (bank). In addition, a quarterly report must be filed to provide a summary of all wages paid and tax withheld during each quarter. Rather severe penalties and interest charges are imposed on employers who fail to withhold taxes and deposit taxes, or who fail to file payroll tax returns in the prescribed manner and at the specified time.

Most states and some large cities also levy income taxes. In such cases, hospitals often must withhold these taxes. Amounts withheld, as determined by formulas or tables, are remitted periodically to the governmental units in accordance with the particular laws.

The Federal Insurance Contributions Act (FICA), popularly known as social security, provides for a tax on employees' earnings to finance a federal program of old-age, survivors', disability, and healthcare benefits for workers and members of their families. Hospitals and their employees were at first exempt from this law as it was originally enacted in 1935, but the basic law has been amended many times to extend its coverage and to increase the tax rate, the amount of earnings subject to tax, and benefits provided. The 1965 amendment included enactment of the Federal Hospital Insurance Program, widely known as Medicare.

FICA (Social Security) Taxes

As is true of income tax, the FICA tax must be withheld by the hospital from taxable wage payments to employees. The 1935 act provided for a 1 percent tax on the first $3,000 of wages paid to each employee in any one year, but subsequent amendments to the law have increased both the tax rate and the base earnings (maximum annual earnings subject to tax) substantially. At this writing, the FICA tax is 7.65 percent of the first $53,400 of taxable wages paid to each employee. Earnings from $53,401 to $145,000 are taxed an additional 1.45 percent for Medicare hospital insurance. In other words, the maximum annual tax is $4,085.10 per employee earning $53,400 or less. This amount may be increased in the future by increasing the tax rate, base earnings, or both.

So, FICA taxes are withheld from employees' earnings just as are income taxes. Provisions of the FICA tax legislation, however, also require an equal contribution by the hospital. The employer must "match" the amount of FICA tax withheld from employees' wages. Thus, a tax is imposed on the hospital. To put it another way, the 1991 FICA tax was 15.3 percent; half was withheld from employees' earnings and half was paid by the hospital employer. Both the employer's and the employees' FICA taxes are remitted to the U.S. government at the same time as and together with the federal income tax (FIT) withholdings.

Employer's Matching FICA Payment

Entries for the withholding of FIT and FICA, and for the accrual of the hospital's share of FICA, are illustrated later in this chapter for Hartful Hospital, but a simpler example might be useful at this point. Assume that a single employee earns a salary of $2,000 per month, all of which is subject to tax. Assume a 15 percent FIT

Example of Hospital's Withholding Entries

rate and an 8 percent FICA tax rate. Monthly entries with respect to this particular employee are the following:

Salaries and Wages Expense	$2,000	
FICA Withheld and Accrued		$ 160
FIT Withheld		300
Accrued Payroll Liability		1,540
Accrual of payroll and withholding of related taxes.		
Accrued Payroll Liability	1,540	
Cash		1,540
Issuance of paycheck.		
Employee Benefits (expense)	160	
FICA Withheld and Accrued		160
Accrual of hospital's share of FICA.		
FICA Withheld and Accrued	320	
FIT Withheld	300	
Cash		620
Remittance of payroll taxes withheld and accrued.		

You should recognize that the matching FICA tax imposed on the hospital represents a significant expense. There also is the rather considerable clerical expense involved in computing and recording the withholdings, in preparing the many payroll tax reports, and in keeping the detailed payroll records required by these laws.

Other Deductions

In addition to the compulsory tax withholdings, a variety of other items may be withheld from salary and wage payments to employees. These withholding categories usually require the written consent of the employee. Other deductions include the following:

- Government savings bonds or other employee savings plan
- Premiums for health, accident, hospital, and life insurance
- Union membership dues
- Employee retirement plans
- Employee contributions to the Community Chest, United Fund, or other charities

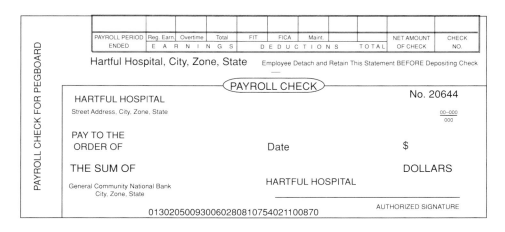

| PAYROLL PERIOD | Reg. Earn. | Overtime | Total | FIT | FICA | Maint. | | NET AMOUNT | CHECK |
| ENDED | E A R N I N G S | | | D E D U C T I O N S | | | T O T A L | OF CHECK | NO. |

Hartful Hospital, City, Zone, State   Employee Detach and Retain This Statement BEFORE Depositing Check

⟨ PAYROLL CHECK ⟩

HARTFUL HOSPITAL   No. 20644

Street Address, City, Zone, State   00–000 / 000

PAY TO THE
ORDER OF   Date $

THE SUM OF   DOLLARS

General Community National Bank   HARTFUL HOSPITAL
City, Zone, State

                                                                    AUTHORIZED SIGNATURE

01302050093006028081O754021100870

Figure 13-2 Employee Payroll Check

At specified intervals, the hospital must summarize these withholdings in appropriate reports and remit the amounts withheld to the proper agencies.

Recording the Payroll

On the basis of time cards, time reports, and other source documents that have been collected from the various departments, the payroll clerk is able to compute the gross pay of each employee for the pay period involved. The payroll tax deductions then are calculated for each employee by the application of tax rates and the use of tax tables. Other deductions are determined on the basis of written agreements and authorizations obtained from employees. A final step is the subtraction of total deductions from gross pay to arrive at net pay for each employee. All of these data then are entered on the face of the time card or other record for each employee.

Next, a payroll check is prepared for each employee in the net pay amount indicated on the employee's time card. A sample payroll check is illustrated in Figure 13-2. Notice that the upper portion is a stub that provides, for the employee's personal records, complete information as to gross earnings, deductions, and net pay.

Sample Payroll Check and Stub

The individual time cards (or carbon copies of the payroll checks), sorted by department, are now summarized to obtain departmental totals for gross pay, deductions, and net pay. These totals then are entered in the payroll journal, as indicated in Figure 13-3. (An alternative procedure is to list each employee's name and data in the journal individually, but this procedure may not be feasible.) The illustrative entry includes figures for the nursing

Recording Totals in the Payroll Journal

19X1 Date	Department	Check Numbers	Gross Payroll Account Numbers	Gross Payroll Amount Dr.	FIT Withheld	FICA Withheld	Other	Total	Accrued Payroll Cr.
5 31	Nursing Services:								
	Administrative Office	231–233	6010.1	2,750	550	165		715	2,035
	Nursing Units		6021.1	161,400					
	Operating Rooms		6210.1	8,200					
	Emergency Rooms		6230.1	6,400					
	Central Supply		6250.1	7,700					
	Other Professional Services:								
	Administrative Office		7010.1	3,800					
	Laboratory		7011.1	8,200					
	Radiology		7040.1	7,700					
	Pharmacy		7070.1	4,900					
	Anesthesia		7080.1	5,500					
	Medical Staff		8030.1	12,000					
	General Services:								
	Administrative Office		8040.1	2,000					
	Dietary		8050.1	9,400					
	Plant O. & M.		8060.1	6,200					
	Housekeeping		8090.1	7,500					
	Laundry		8110.1	6,800					
	Fiscal Services:								
	Administrative Office		8211.1	4,100					
	Accounting		8212.1	6,700					
	Admitting		8241.1	5,300					
	Administrator's Office		8310.1	5,250					
	Administrative Services:								
	Administrative Office		8311.1	2,200					
	Purchasing		8331.1	3,900					
	Personnel		8371.1	4,100					
	Totals			292,000	48,400	16,520		64,920	227,080
				Debit	Credit 2035.0	Credit 2036.0	Credit	Credit	Credit 2031.0

Figure 13-3 Payroll Journal

service administrative office only, with FIT and FICA withholdings assumed to be 20 percent and 6 percent, respectively. We also assume, for simplicity, that Hartful Hospital pays all of its employees once each month. The column totals shown in the journal therefore are totals for May 19X1. If the hospital paid its employees every two weeks or twice each month, a separate journal page would be used for each pay period.

Recording Matching
Payments in the General
Journal

As indicated in the payroll journal, May payroll withholdings were $48,400 for federal income taxes and $16,520 for FICA taxes. The hospital's matching share of FICA taxes for the month is recorded in the general journal by the following entry on May 31, 19X1:

Employee Benefits—FICA	8710.0	$16,520
FICA Withheld and		
Accrued	2036.0	$16,520
Accrual of hospital's share		
of FICA taxes on May		
payroll.		

Notice that the May net payroll of $227,080 is not credited to Cash (even though the payroll checks have already been written) but to the Accrued Payroll liability account (account 2031.0). As you will see in the next chapter, a single voucher is prepared in this amount and is entered in the hospital's voucher register as follows:

Accrued Payroll	2031.0	$227,080
Accounts Payable	2020.0	$227,080
Voucher for May payroll.		

Immediately following this, a check for $227,080 is drawn against the general checking account and is entered in the cash disbursements journal, as follows:

Entering Accrued Payroll in the Cash Disbursements Journal

Accounts Payable	2020.0	$227,080
Cash	1011.0	$227,080
Issuance of check for May		
payroll.		

This check is deposited in the hospital's payroll checking account, but no entry is made in the payroll checking account to record the deposit. The individual payroll checks, you remember, were drawn on the payroll checking account, but no entry was made to that account for those checks. When the payroll checks are cashed by employees, the payroll checking account automatically clears to the

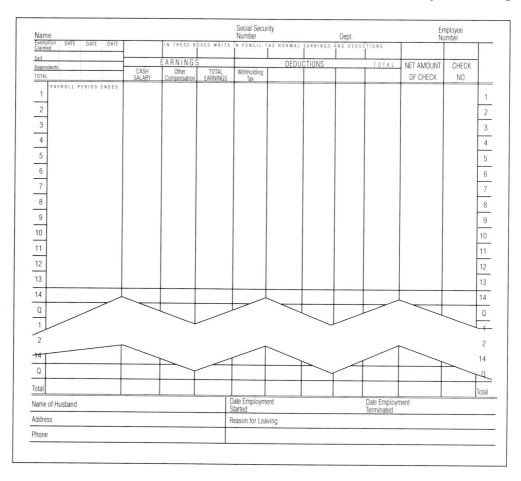

Figure 13–4 Employee's Individual Earnings Record

zero or imprest balance maintained in the account. This procedure removes a large volume of paychecks from general checking and simplifies reconciliation of the payroll checking account.

Posting Departmental Totals

Each departmental total in the gross pay column is posted at the end of the month to the general ledger salaries and wages expense accounts indicated. Other postings to the general ledger are of column totals. In addition to those in the general ledger, postings also must be made to the employees' individual earnings records that often take the form illustrated in Figure 13–4. This detailed record, which is required by tax laws and regulations, is in effect a subsidiary ledger supporting the departmental salaries and wages expense accounts.

The information in this subsidiary ledger is quite useful for preparing various quarterly and annual tax reports and other employment information forms.

The employees responsible for compilation of payrolls should neither sign nor distribute payroll checks. Once prepared, the unsigned checks should be examined by the disbursing authority, who should be satisfied as to their accuracy and authenticity. This may involve a check of certain computations on a sample basis and a comparison of payees and pay rates with independently controlled personnel records. (In many instances, these procedures are performed by the hospital's internal auditors.) Care particularly must be given to avoiding the following:

Safeguarding Payroll Funds

- Inclusion of nonexistent persons on the payroll of a department
- Issuance of any checks to former employees whose names have not been removed from the payroll
- Payment of incorrect rates of pay
- Payment for overtime hours when none were worked

If a mechanical check signer is employed, its use should be strictly controlled.

The distribution of payroll checks should be centralized, and procedures should be employed that ensure that employees receiving checks are properly identified. The method of distributing checks, as well as the person who distributes checks, should be changed occasionally. Unclaimed paychecks should not be returned to the payroll accounting unit but should be investigated and retained for a reasonable period of time by a person who is independent of the payroll functions. Checks that remain unclaimed beyond this period should be fully investigated for cause.

Donated Services

Hospitals sometimes receive services donated by various organizations whose members work without monetary compensation in certain areas of hospital activity. Donated services such as these should properly be recorded at fair market value only when (1) the donor and hospital have the equivalent of an employer-employee relationship and (2) there is an objective basis for determining the amounts that might otherwise have been paid for such services. Where these requirements are met, the determined amounts should be recorded as operating expenses with an offsetting credit to nonoperating revenues. The necessary entry (amount assumed) in general journal form is indicated here:

Salaries and Wages Expense—Donated Services	$28,400	
Nonoperating Revenues—		
Donated Services		$28,400
To record fair market value of services		
donated to the hospital.		

Services of a nonessential nature provided by guilds, auxiliaries, and similar organizations generally should not be recorded in the accounts.

Payroll-Related Costs

In addition to the basic earnings of hourly and salaried employees, a number of other related cost elements enter into hospital labor cost considerations. These elements include the previously discussed overtime earnings, vacation, holiday pay, sick pay, and the FICA taxes imposed on hospitals. Some other elements include unemployment taxes, workmen's compensation insurance, employee life and hospitalization insurance premiums, and pension plan costs. The total of these and other employee benefits constitutes a very substantial cost to the hospital (often 25 percent or more of total employee compensation).

Vacation Pay

After a specified period of employment, hospital employees generally are entitled to an annual vacation with full pay. Assuming a 2-week vacation each year, employees in effect are paid for 50 weeks of work over a 52-week period. The reality of the situation is that the vacation pay is earned by employees, and is incurred as a cost by the hospital, during the 50 working weeks. It is incorrect, therefore, to defer recognition of vacation pay as an expense until it is actually paid. Instead, vacation pay should be charged to expense in the periods during which it is earned by employees.

Example of Recording Vacation Pay Expense

To illustrate the necessary entries, let us assume that a hospital has 200 employees, each of whom earns $500 per week and is entitled to a two-week vacation each year. The proper weekly payroll entry for this group (disregarding withholdings) is as follows:

Salaries and Wages Expense (classified
    by departmental expense centers) $104,000
      Cash $100,000
      Accrued Vacation Pay Liability   4,000
    Accrual of weekly payroll,
    including earned vacation pay.

In other words, each employee earns $1,000 ($500 × two weeks) of vacation pay over the 50 weeks of work, or $20 per week. This means that $4,000 ($20 × 200 employees) should be charged to expense weekly with a corresponding accrual of the vacation pay liability. When vacations are taken, the liability account is debited and cash is credited.

In addition to FICA taxes, hospitals may also be subject to federal and state tax laws dealing with unemployment compensation. The gross federal unemployment tax (FUTA) is at this writing 6.2 percent of the first $7,000 of taxable wages paid to each employee during a given year, but a maximum 5.4 percent credit may be allowed for participation in a state unemployment tax (SUTA) program. Thus, the net federal tax is currently 0.8 percent. State tax laws vary, but we will assume a 5.4 percent rate.

    In any event, the hospital must accrue these taxes on each payroll by making an entry such as the following (assuming a $100,000 payroll):

Unemployment Taxes

Employee Benefits—FUTA (0.8% ×
    $100,000) $ 800
Employee Benefits—SUTA (5.4% ×
    $100,000)   5,400
      FUTA Taxes Payable $ 800
      SUTA Taxes Payable   5,400
    Accrual of payroll tax expenses.

Notice that these taxes are charged to the Employee Benefits account under the unassigned expense classification rather than to departmental expense centers. To charge these expenses to departments as a part of the normal accounting routine is troublesome and of little (if any) month-to-month value. These expenses are, how-

FUTA and SUTA Charged to Employee Benefits Account

ever, allocated to departmental expense centers in the cost-finding procedure at the end of the year.

Observe that the unemployment taxes are paid by the hospital; these taxes are not withheld from employees' wages. Periodically, as required by law, the hospital must submit unemployment tax reports and remit the taxes to the appropriate governmental agency.

Other Cost Elements   States have workmen's compensation laws that provide various benefits to disabled workers. In some cases, a tax is imposed on the employer, but more often the state laws establish standard benefits and allow hospitals to provide for such benefits through the purchase of appropriate insurance from a commercial insurance company. The premiums paid by the hospital are charged to expense (employee benefits).

Life, health, accident, disability, dental, and hospitalization insurance plans on a group basis often are established by hospitals on behalf of their employees. Participation in these group programs generally is voluntary, but the hospital frequently pays a substantial portion of the premiums as an employee benefit. Such payments by the hospital naturally are chargeable to expense in the employee benefits classification.

Increasing attention recently has been given to the establishment of pension and retirement plans for hospital employees. All or most of the costs of such programs frequently are paid by the hospital. A discussion of the rather complex accounting procedures involved, however, is beyond the scope of this book.

This concludes the discussion of payroll accounting. Having studied this and the materials on revenues and cash receipts in the preceding chapter, we can now begin our examination of Hartful Hospital's procedures for nonlabor expenses, accounts payable, and cash disbursements.

Questions   Q13-1. Give four reasons why employee compensation generally composes more than 50 percent of total operating expenses in hospitals.

Q13-2. An employee of Mount Hospital is paid $8.80 per hour for a normal work-week of 40 hours. During a given week, this employee worked a total of 50 hours. Compute the employee's earnings for that week, assuming time and a half for overtime work.

Q13–3. What is the current FICA tax rate? What is the maximum annual amount of FICA tax that is paid by an employee?

Q13–4. An employee of Monroe Hospital earns a salary of $4,000 per month, payable on the first day of the following month. Assume that the federal income tax withholding is 20 percent and that the FICA tax is 7 percent. With respect to this one employee, make the following necessary entries:

    a. Record the employee's gross earnings, tax deductions, and net pay for January 19X1.

    b. Accrue the hospital's share of FICA taxes as of January 31, 19X1.

    c. Record issuance of the paycheck on February 1, 19X1.

    d. Record remittance of January payroll taxes to the government.

Q13–5. Other than taxes, list five types of withholding deductions that often are made from hospital employees' paychecks.

Q13–6. Describe briefly the general procedures followed in computing the gross payroll in a hospital for a given pay period.

Q13–7. How should hospital accountants record donated services?

Q13–8. The fair market value of donated services received by Madison Hospital during April 19X1 was $31,400. Make the necessary entry at April 30, 19X1, to record these donated services.

Q13–9. Briefly describe the basic features of a good internal control system for a hospital payroll.

Q13–10. Lucky Hospital has 450 employees, each of whom earns $800 per week and is entitled to a two-week vacation each year. Disregarding withholding deductions, make the proper weekly payroll entry for this group of employees. Twenty of these employees take their vacations during the first two weeks of June. Make the necessary entry to record the paychecks issued to these 20 employees for the vacation period.

Q13–11. Liston Hospital's gross payroll for January 19X1 is $250,000. Assuming a 0.5 percent federal unemployment tax rate and a 2.5 percent state unemployment tax rate, make the necessary entry to accrue the hospital's unemployment tax expense for January 19X1.

Q13–12. As a part of the regular accounting routine, should unemployment taxes and the hospital's share of FICA taxes be charged to departmental cost center accounts? Explain.

Q13–13. Explain briefly how state workmen's compensation laws affect the hospital's payroll accounting.

Q13–14. Describe briefly the operation of an imprest payroll checking account. What are the advantages of such a system?

Q13–15. An employee of Lefferson Hospital is paid $10 per hour for a regular work-week of 40 hours. During a particular week, this employee worked 48 hours. Assume that the FICA tax is 8 percent and that 20 percent of the employee's gross pay is withheld for federal income taxes. Assume also that the federal unemployment tax is 2 percent and that the state unemployment tax is 5 percent. Make all necessary entries for this week.

Q13–16. Mason Hospital's payroll for the month ended May 31, 19X1, is summarized here:

Gross payroll	$462,000
FIT withheld	20%
FICA withheld	8%
FUTA rate	2%
SUTA rate	4%

Indicate how the May payroll would be entered in the journal and ledger systems described in Chapter 13.

Q13–17. What specific information would you expect to find on an employee's individual earnings record?

Q13–18. An employee of Moppup Hospital earns a salary of $1,000 per month, payable on the first day of the following month. Assume the following tax rates:

FIT	20%
FICA	8%
FUTA	2%
SUTA	5%

For this employee, make all necessary entries to record the March 19X1 payroll and related matters. Indicate the journal in which each entry should be made.

Expenses, Payables, and Cash Disbursements

14

In accounting for hospital expenses, considerable attention naturally is given to salaries, wages, and employee benefits. These costs added together typically represent more than 50 percent of total operating expenses. The remaining expenses, however, require the same careful attention by hospital accountants. Very substantial amounts are expended each year for supplies, utilities, other purchased services, insurance, interest, and other items. Effective management of these nonlabor costs requires the use of sound accounting procedures.

This chapter examines Hartful Hospital's accounting system as it relates to these expenses, along with the corresponding liabilities and cash disbursements. The discussion touches briefly on the purchasing and receiving functions, describing the voucher system and illustrating the use of the voucher register and the cash disbursements journal. In the last part of this chapter, you will also see a summary of postings from all of Hartful Hospital's journals to the general ledger accounts. This is provided in an effort to tie together the materials of Chapters 10 through 14.

Purchasing

Procurement of supplies and services is a function of major importance in hospitals. It cuts across all departmental lines and accounts for a significant percentage of the hospital's annual expenditures. The purchasing responsibility consists basically of acquiring required supplies and services of the appropriate quality, in the proper quantities, at the times needed, and at reasonable costs. Ideally, the purchasing function is centralized and performed by an organized purchasing department headed by an experienced purchasing agent. This tends to minimize waste and duplication through standardization of buying and use of the many supply

HARTFUL HOSPITAL
PURCHASE REQUISITION   PURCHASE ORDER NO. _____

DEPARTMENT _____ DATE _____ 19____
FLOOR OR DIVISION _____ DATE REQUIRED ____ 19____

TO ELIMINATE DELAY KINDLY FURNISH COMPLETE DESCRIPTION OF ARTICLE				
QUANTITY	UNIT	DESCRIPTION OF ARTICLE	(State Fully what Item is to be used for)	UNIT PRICE

REQUESTED BY   APPROVED BY

SEND ORIGINAL TO PURCHASING AGENT. DUPLICATE IS RETAINED BY STORE ROOM CLERK OR DEPARTMENT HEAD.

Figure 14–1 Sample of a Purchase Requisition

items required in the provision of hospital services. Limited authority to purchase certain products and services, however, sometimes must be given to selected department heads. In smaller hospitals, administrative personnel may do the buying personally or may carefully supervise and coordinate it.

Initiating Purchases with the Purchase Requisition

To set the wheels of purchasing in motion, the purchasing department must be made aware of the need to purchase. This may be accomplished through the preparation of a purchase requisition form such as the one illustrated in Figure 14–1. The form is generally executed by a department head or inventory storekeeper. A copy of the purchase requisition is sent to the purchasing department to inform that department of the items to be purchased; a duplicate copy is retained in a file as evidence that the request was made.

The purchasing department, noting that the purchase requisition is properly authorized, makes appropriate choices of quantity, price, and vendor, in accordance with prescribed administrative

PURCHASE ORDER	**HARTFUL HOSPITAL** ADDRESS CITY—STATE—ZIP CODE	**NO. 49793**			

THIS ORDER NUMBER MUST APPEAR
ON ALL CORRESPONDENCE, INVOICES,
PACKAGES AND SHIPPING PAPERS

DATE _____ 19 __

TO

DEPT. _____

SHIP VIA _____

F.O.B. _____

TERMS _____

DELIVERY
REQUIRED _____

QUANTITY	DESCRIPTION	PRICE	PER UNIT	AMOUNT

1

BY _____

Figure 14–2 Sample of a Purchase Order

policies. A purchase order, one form of which is presented in Figure 14–2, is then prepared to acquire the supplies or services desired. The purchase order generally is a multipart form with several copies, distributed as follows:

1. One copy of the purchase order is sent to the accounting department for subsequent use in invoice audit and approval for payment. The information also is useful in the budgeting of cash disbursements.
2. A second copy is sent to the requisitioning department and/or storekeeper as notification that the order has been placed. The originator of the purchase will match this copy with the retained copy of the purchase requisition to make sure that the purchasing department received and acted on all requisitions.

3. Two copies are sent to the vendor company. One copy is for the vendor's own use; the other is signed and returned to the hospital's purchasing department as an acknowledgment of the order and the vendor's intent to fill it.

4. In some systems, another copy of the purchase order is routed to the hospital's receiving department (or to the inventory storeroom, where the storekeeper performs the receiving function). This copy, however, generally should not provide information about quantities ordered.

5. A final copy is retained by the purchasing department in an unfilled orders file, which is carefully monitored to avoid delays in the acquisition of desired supplies and services.

When the vendor returns the acknowledgment copy of the purchase order to indicate its acceptance of the order on the terms specified, the purchasing department will match this document with the copy of the purchase order in the unfilled-orders file. The document will be retained in this file and is monitored until the purchasing department is notified of the receipt of the items purchased. An acknowledged purchase order constitutes a legal contract with the supplier, and all required information (including quantities, accurate description, price, and terms) therefore must be carefully indicated.

Receiving

On receipt of purchased supplies from vendors, the hospital's receiving department manager has the responsibility for counting, weighing, or otherwise measuring the quantities of goods received. The quality and condition of the goods are also checked. As a result of this process, a receiving report such as the one shown in Figure 14–3 is prepared. (In some systems, the packing slip, bill of lading, or a copy of the purchase order may serve this purpose.) After the incoming shipment has been examined in this way, the goods are moved into the hospital storerooms (or directed to the appropriate department). Supplies placed in the hospital's general storerooms remain there, under the storekeeper's control, until issued from the inventory for use in various service departments.

Preparing a Receiving Report

Thus, the receiving report is prepared as a record of the quantity of goods actually received. A copy of the receiving report is sent to the purchasing department, where it is used to clear the related purchase order from the unfilled-orders file. A second copy is routed to the accounting department to be used in subsequent invoice processing and approval for payment. Another copy follows

```
┌─────────────────────────────────────────────────────────────────┐
│                     HARTFUL HOSPITAL                              │
│                    RECEIVING REPORT          NO. _____       │
│                                                                   │
│                                          DATE _____ 19____      │
│                                                                   │
│  RECEIVED FROM_____   PURCHASE                 │
│  ADDRESS_____    ORDER NO. _____      │
│  ┌──────────┬────────┬─────────────────────────────────────────┐ │
│  │ QUANTITY │  UNIT  │       DESCRIPTION OF ARTICLE             │ │
│  ├──────────┼────────┼─────────────────────────────────────────┤ │
│  │          │        │                                         │ │
│  │          │        │                                         │ │
│  │          │        │                                         │ │
│  │          │        │                                         │ │
│  │          │        │                                         │ │
│  │          │        │                                         │ │
│  │          │        │                                         │ │
│  │          │        │                                         │ │
│  │          │        │                                         │ │
│  │          │        │                                         │ │
│  │          │        │                                         │ │
│  │          │        │                                         │ │
│  │          │        │                                         │ │
│  │          │        │                                         │ │
│  └──────────┴────────┴─────────────────────────────────────────┘ │
│                     RECEIVED OKAY_____         │
└─────────────────────────────────────────────────────────────────┘
```

Figure 14–3 Sample of a Receiving Report

the goods into the storeroom, and a final copy may be retained by the receiving department as a work record.

Recording Purchases

In due course, the vendor bills the hospital for the items purchased. When it arrives in the incoming mail, the invoice should be sent directly from the mailroom to the accounting department. In the accounting department, the three documents relating to the purchase—the purchase order, the receiving report, and the vendor's bill or invoice—are then matched. This comparison is made to ascertain the correctness of prices, quantities, invoice extensions (quantities times unit prices), and other matters.

In the voucher system employed by Hartful Hospital, a combination voucher/check is now prepared in duplicate and is attached to the other three documents to form what is called a *voucher*

Preparing the Voucher/Check and Voucher Package

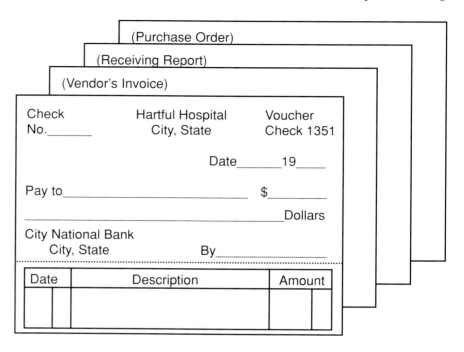

Figure 14-4 Components of the Voucher Package

package, as illustrated in Figure 14–4. The package is turned over to the accounting employee responsible for maintaining the hospital's voucher register.

Entering Information in the
Voucher Register
On the basis of the information contained in the approved voucher packages, the transactions are entered in the voucher register, as shown in Figure 14–5. Once these entries are made, the voucher packages are placed in a file of unpaid vouchers where they are retained until their respective due dates. This file functions as the accounts payable subsidiary ledger in some accounting systems. In other systems, postings are made to individual vendor or supplier accounts in much the same manner as described earlier for accounts receivable. In any case, the subsidiary record for accounts payable should be reconciled regularly with the control account for accounts payable in the general ledger.

Examine the sample entries in Figure 14–5's voucher register. On May 1, 19X1, for example, you see the entry to record a $450 voucher for the purchase of certain pharmaceuticals. This required a debit to the Pharmacy Supplies and Other Expense account (account 7070.2) and a credit to Accounts Payable (account 2020.0). The entry indicates how individual vouchers are journalized in the register. As an alternative, all the vouchers issued on a given day may be

The Voucher Register

19X1 Date	(✓)	Account Payable Cr.	Payroll-Related Debits — Accrued Payroll	FIT Withheld	FICA W/H & Accrued	Adm. Office	Nursing Service Expense Debits — Nursing Units	Operating Rooms	Emergency Rooms	Central Supply	Other Professional Service Expense Debits — Adm. Office	Laboratory	Radiology	Pharmacy	Anesthesia	Medical Staff Expense
5 1	✓ ✓	450												450		
2	✓	4,690					1,060					1,820	1,400			
10	✓	16,000														
31	✓	227,080	227,080													
31	✓	81,440		48,400	33,040											
Totals		458,600	227,080	48,400	33,040	2,100	23,120	4,600	3,900	9,800	1,700	4,100	4,700	7,460	2,200	1,748
		Credit 2020.0	Debit 2051.0	Debit 2035.0	Debit 2036.0	Debit 6010.2	Debit 6021.2	Debit 6210.2	Debit 6250.2	Debit 6250.2	Debit 7010.2	Debit 7011.2	Debit 7040.2	Debit 7070.2	Debit 7080.2	Debit 8030.2

Figure 14-5 The Voucher Register

Adm. Office	Payroll-Related Debits				Fiscal Services Expense Debits			Administra- tor's Office	Administrative Services Expense Debits				Sundry Debits and Credits		
	Dietary	Plant O. & M.	House- keeping	Laundry	Adm. Office	Accounting	Admitting		Adm. Office	Governing Board	Purchasing	Personnel	Account Numbers	Dr.	Cr.
	410												1170.0	16,000	
1,300	21,500	14,124	3,800	4,300	2,400	7,008	6,100	3,800	1,100	1,000	1,020	1,200		16,000	
Debit 8040.2	Debit 8050.2	Debit 8060.2	Debit 8090.2	Debit 8110.2	Debit 8211.2	Debit 8212.2	Debit 8241.2	Debit 8310.2	Debit 8311.2	Debit 8312.2	Debit 8331.2	Debit 8371.2			

Figure 14-5 The Voucher Register (*continued*)

summarized and entered on a single line of the register, as illustrated by the entry of May 2, 19X1. The sample entry of May 10, 19X1, relates to the purchase of an item of depreciable equipment. This entry demonstrates the use of the sundry debit and credit columns, and emphasizes the fact that all disbursements (no matter what the purpose) must be vouchered through accounts payable.

Notice also the voucher register entries of May 31, 19X1. Vouchering of the May payroll requires the preparation of (1) a voucher in the amount of $227,000 to record the amount to be transferred from the general checking account to the payroll checking account and (2) a voucher for $81,440 to record the liability to governmental agencies for payroll taxes withheld and accrued. Later, you will see entries in the cash disbursements journal to record payment of these vouchers. The following shows the payroll journal and general journal entries. Note that various departmental account numbers for salaries and wages expenses would appear in the account number column.

Payroll Journal

Salaries and Wages Expense		$292,000	
FIT Withheld	2035.0		$ 48,400
FICA Withheld and Accrued	2036.0		16,520
Accrued Payroll	2031.0		227,080
To record May payroll.			

General Journal

Employee Benefits—FICA	8710.0	$ 16,520	
FICA Withheld and Accrued	2036.0		$ 16,520
To record hospital's share of FICA taxes on May payroll.			

Just prior to their due dates, the approved voucher packages are removed from the file for unpaid vouchers and are sent to the hospital's treasurer or other disbursing authority. These voucher

Recording Cash Disbursements

19X1 Date	Description		Check Numbers	Cash Cr.	Purchases Discounts Cr.	Accounts Payable Dr.	Dr.	Sundry Debits and Credits		
								Account Numbers	Dr.	Cr.
5 9	Central Pharmaceutical Co.		2275	441	9	450				
31	Payroll Checking Account		2690	227,080		227,080				
31	Internal Revenue Service		2691	81,440		81,440				
	Totals			451,295	2,309	453,604				
				Credit 1011.0	Credit 5171.0	Debit 2020.0	Debit			

Figure 14–6 Cash Disbursements Journal

packages, with the unsigned check included, may be examined by the disbursing officer to confirm the propriety of the disbursements proposed. When the officer is satisfied, he or she signs the checks and mails them directly to the vendor. (Signed checks should not be returned to the accounting department for mailing.) All documents in the voucher packages then are indelibly stamped or perforated "PAID" to prevent their reuse in support of another disbursement. The packages then are returned to the accounting department to the person responsible for the cash disbursements journal. This employee now records the paid vouchers in this journal, as illustrated in Figure 14–6. After these entries are made, the voucher packages marked as paid are placed in a file for paid vouchers; here they are kept for the period specified by the hospital's record retention policies.

Observe the illustrative entries in the journal. Check number 2275, for example, was issued on May 9, 19X1, in payment of the $450 voucher seen earlier in the voucher register. Because a 2 percent discount was deducted and credited to the Purchases Discounts account, the check was written for only $441. On May 31, 19X1, check number 2690 was issued to transfer the amount of the net payroll for May from the general checking account to the payroll checking account. Check number 2691 was written for the remittance of May payroll taxes withheld and accrued. (All checks issued on a given day may be summarized and entered on a single line of the journal, rather then journalizing each individual check.)

Summary of Procedures for Recording Transactions

To summarize the Hartful Hospital illustration in the last five chapters, let us examine the general ledger postings from all journals and present the hospital's financial statements for the five months ended May 31, 19X1. The revenue and cash receipts journals were shown in Chapter 12, the payroll journal was illustrated in Chapter 13, and the voucher register and cash disbursements journal were provided in this chapter. Now, in Figure 14–7, Hartful Hospital's general journal for May is reproduced to indicate the adjusting entries that were necessary at the end of the month.

Tracing the Postings for Hartful Hospital

It is suggested that you trace all the postings from each of Hartful Hospital's journals to the general ledger accounts provided in Figure 14–8. The posting references are as follows:

Posting Reference	
BB	Balance, May 1, 19X1 (assumed)
IRJ	Inpatient revenue journal (Chapter 12)
ORJ	Outpatient revenue journal (Chapter 12)
CRJ	Cash receipts journal (Chapter 12)
PJ	Payroll journal (Chapter 13)
VR	Voucher register (Chapter 14)
CDJ	Cash disbursements journal (Chapter 14)
GJ	General journal (Chapter 14)
CB	Balance, May 31, 19X1

Figure 14–7 General Journal

19X1 Date	Accounts and Explanations	Account Numbers	Dr.	Cr.
5 31	Inpatient Receivables—Discharged	1032.0	412,975	
	Inpatient Receivables—Inhouse	1031.0		412,975
	To transfer unpaid account balances from inhouse to discharged receivables.			
31	Accrued Interest Receivable	1029.0	1,350	
	Interest Income	9051.0		1,350
	To accrue interest earned in May.			
	Deductions from Revenues—Bad Debts	5510.0	3,700	
31	Deductions from Revenues—Contractual Adjustments	5520.0	11,400	
	Deductions from Revenues—Charity Service	5540.0	6,600	
	Allowance for Uncollectible Accounts:			
	Bad Debts	1061.0		
	Contractual Adjustments	1062.0		
	Charity Service	1066.0		
	To adjust allowance accounts to correct balances.			
	Insurance Expense	8610.0	1,800	
31	Prepaid Expenses	1120.0		1,800
	To adjust for expiration of insurance premiums.			
	Depreciation Expense	8510.0	28,000	
31	Accumulated Depreciation—Buildings	1250.0		13,000
	Accumulated Depreciation—Equipment	1270.0		15,000
	To record depreciation expense for May.			
	Employee Benefits			
31	FICA Withheld and Accrued	8710.0	16,520	
	To accrue hospital's share of FICA taxes on May payroll.	2036.0		
	Interest Expense	8690.0	14,700	
31	Accrued Interest Payable	2051.0		14,700
	To accrue interest expense for May.			
31	Deferred Rental Income	2113.0	1,800	
	Rental Income	5155.0		1,800
	To record rental income earned in May.			

Cash—General Checking 1011.0

BB	180,000	CDJ	451,295
CFJ	447,500		

Cash—Payroll Checking 1012.0

Petty Cash Fund 1014.0

BB	500		

Temporary Investments 1020.0

BB	150,000		

Accrued Interest Receivable 1029.0

BB	5,400		
GJ	1,350		

Inpatient Receivables— Inhouse 1031.0

BB	110,000	CRJ	43,020
IRJ	453,995	GJ	412,975

Inpatient Receivables— Discharged 1032.0

BB	800,000	CRJ	401,850
GJ	412,975		

Outpatient Receivables 1044.0

BB	16,000	CRJ	57,900
ORJ	64,800		

Allowance for Bad Debts 1061.0

		BB	11,000
		GJ	3,700

Allowance for Contractual Adjustments 1062.0

		BB	56,000
		GJ	11,400

Charity Service 1066.0

		BB	28,000
		GJ	6,600

Inventories 1110.0

BB	96,000		

Prepaid Expense 1120.0

BB	14,000	GJ	1,800

Land 1130.0

BB	175,000		

Buildings 1050.0

BB	5,000,000		

Equipment 1170.0

BB	3,000,000		
VR	16,000		

Accumulated Depreciation— Buildings 1250.0

		BB	1,200,000
		GJ	13,000

Accumulated Depreciation— Equipment 1270.0

		BB	900,000
		GJ	15,000

Notes Payable 2010.0

		BB	80,000

Accounts Payable 2020.0

CDJ	453,604	BB	65,000
		VR	458,600

Accrued Payroll 2031.0

VR	227,080	PJ	227,080

FIT Withheld 2035.0

VR	48,400	PJ	48,400

FICA Withheld and Accrued 2036.0

VR	33,040	PJ	16,520
		GJ	16,520

Accrued Interest Payable 2051.0

		BB	18,300
		GJ	14,700

Deferred Rental Income 2113.0

GJ	1,800	BB	9,600

Bonds Payable 2190.0

		BB	2,400,000

Hospital Equity 2210.0

		BB	4,559,240

Revenue and Expense Summary 2219.0

Nursing Units— IP Revenues 3021.1

		BB	896,500
		IRJ	187,500

Operating Rooms— IP Revenues 3210.1

		BB	104,400
		IRJ	26,100

Operating Rooms— OP Revenues 3210.2

		BB	15,600
		ORJ	3,900

Emergency Rooms— IP Revenues 3230.1

		BB	57,600
		IRJ	14,400

Emergency Rooms— OP Revenues 3230.2

		BB	36,100
		ORJ	9,000

Figure 14–8 General Ledger Accounts

Figure 14–8 General Ledger Accounts (*continued*)

Central Supply— IP Revenues 3250.1			Central Supply— OP Revenues 3250.2			Laboratory— IP Revenues 4011.1		
	BB	136,400		BB	22,800		BB	225,680
	IRJ	34,100		ORJ	5,700		IRJ	56,420

Laboratory— OP Revenues 4011.2			Radiology— IP Revenues 4040.1			Radiology— OP Revenues 4040.2		
	BB	68,160		BB	355,340		BB	86,520
	ORJ	17,040		IRJ	88,835		ORJ	21,630

Pharmacy— IP Revenues 4070.1			Pharmacy— OP Revenues 4070.2			Anesthesia— IP Revenues 4080.1		
	BB	99,840		BB	23,520		BB	86,720
	IRJ	24,960		ORJ	5,880		IRJ	21,680

Anesthesia— OP Revenues 4080.2			Cafeteria Sales 5061.0			Rental Income 5155.0		
	BB	6,600		BB	83,920		BB	4,800
	ORJ	1,650		CRJ	18,480		GJ	1,800

Purchase Discounts 5171.0			Revenue Deductions— Bad Debts 5510.0			Revenue Deductions— Contractual Adjustments 5520.0		
	BB	9,240	BB	12,600		BB	126,400	
	CDJ	2,309	GJ	3,700		CRJ	31,600	
						GJ	11,400	

Revenue Deductions— Charity Service 5540.0			Nursing Services— Administrative Office—S&W 6010.1			Nursing Services— Administrative Office—S&E 6010.2		
BB	67,600		BB	11,200		BB	8,400	
CRJ	14,400		PJ	2,750		VR	2,100	
GJ	6,600							

Nursing Units— S&W 6021.1			Nursing Units— S&E 6021.2			Operating Rooms— S&W 6210.1		
BB	645,600		BB	92,480		BB	32,800	
PJ	161,400		VR	23,120		PJ	8,200	

Operating Rooms— S&E 6210.2			Emergency Rooms— S&W 6210.1			Emergency Rooms— S&E 6230.2		
BB	18,400		BB	25,600		BB	15,600	
VR	4,600		PJ	6,400		VR	3,900	

Central Supply— S&W 6250.1			Central Supply— S&E 6250.2			Other Professional Services Admin. Office— S&W 7010.1		
BB	30,800		BB	39,200		BB	15,200	
PJ	7,700		VR	9,800		PJ	3,800	

Figure 14–8 General Ledger Accounts (*continued*)

Other Professional Services
Admin. Office—
S&E   7010.2

BB	6,800
VR	1,700

Laboratory—
S&W   7011.1

BB	32,800
PJ	8,200

Laboratory—
S&E   7011.2

BB	16,400
VR	4,100

Radiology—
S&W   7040.1

BB	31,800
PJ	7,700

Radiology—
S&E   7040.2

BB	17,800
VR	4,700

Pharmacy—
S&W   7070.1

BB	19,600
PJ	4,900

Pharmacy—
S&E   7070.2

BB	29,800
VR	7,460

Anesthesia—
S&W   7080.1

BB	23,000
PJ	5,500

Anesthesia—
S&E   7080.2

BB	8,700
VR	2,200

Medical Staff
S&W   8030.1

BB	49,000
PJ	12,000

Medical Staff
S&E   8030.2

BB	6,800
VR	1,748

General Services Admin.
Office S&W   8040.1

BB	7,900
PJ	2,000

General Services Admin. Office
S&E   8040.2

BB	5,200
VR	1,300

Dietary S&W   8050.1

BB	37,600
PJ	9,400

Dietary S&E   8050.2

BB	86,000
VR	21,500

Plant O&M
S&W   8060.1

BB	24,800
PJ	6,200

Plant O&M
S&E   8060.2

BB	56,500
VR	14,124

Housekeeping
S&W   8090.1

BB	29,100
PJ	7,500

Housekeeping
S&E   8090.2

BB	15,200
VR	3,800

Laundry S&W   8110.1

BB	27,200
PJ	6,800

Laundry S&E   8110.2

BB	15,300
VR	4,300

Fiscal Services Admin. Office
S&W   8211.1

BB	16,500
PJ	4,100

Fiscal Services Admin. Office
S&E   8211.2

BB	9,600
VR	2,400

Accounting
S&W   8212.1

BB	26,800
PJ	6,700

Accounting S&E 8212.2

BB	31,300
VR	7,008

Admitting S&W 8241.1

BB	21,200
PJ	5,300

Admitting S&E 8241.2

BB	24,500
VR	6,100

Figure 14–8 General Ledger Accounts (*continued*)

Administrator's Office S&W 8310.1		Administrator's Office S&E 8310.2		Administrative Services Executive Office S&W 8311.1	
BB	20,600	BB	15,700	BB	8,900
PJ	5,250	VR	3,800	PJ	2,200

Administrative Services Executive Office S&E 8311.2		Governing Board S&E 8312.2		Purchasing S&W 8331.1	
BB	4,600	BB	15,600	BB	15,600
VR	1,100	VR	3,900	VR	3,900

Purchasing S&E 8331.2		Personnel S&W 8371.1		Personnel S&E 8371.2	
BB	4,100	BB	16,400	BB	4,700
VR	1,020	PJ	4,100	VR	1,200

Depreciation Expense 8510.0		Insurance Expense 8610.0		Interest Expense 8690.0	
BB	112,000	BB	5,900	BB	48,700
GJ	28,000	GJ	1,800	GJ	14,700

Employee Benefits 8710.0		General Contributions 9041.0		Interest Income 9051.0	
BB	66,300		BB	10,900		BB	5,400
GJ	16,520		CRJ	2,250		GJ	1,350

Financial Statements and Supporting Schedules

After all postings are made from the journals, a trial balance (not shown here) is taken of the general ledger account balances at May 31, 19X1. Let us assume that this trial balance indicates the necessary equality of debit and credit balances.

Using the May 31, 19X1, general ledger balances, we present Hartful Hospital's income statement for the five months ended May 31, 19X1, in Figure 14–9. Notice that certain totals contained in this statement are supported by a schedule of gross revenues from services to patients (Figure 14–10) and a schedule of operating expenses (Figure 14–11). You should examine this statement and accompanying schedules to acquaint yourself with both their format and content. You also will find it useful to trace some of the statement figures back to the general ledger accounts.

Figure 14–12 presents Hartful Hospital's balance sheet for May 31, 19X1. Carefully examine the format and content of this statement; also, try to trace some of the balance sheet figures back to the general ledger accounts. It is very important for you to have a good understanding of the flow of financial data from the journals, through the ledgers, and into the hospital's financial statements.

Gross Patient Service Revenues:		
Nursing Services		$1,550,100
Other Professional Services		1,190,475
Total (Schedule A)		2,740,575
Less Revenue Deductions:		
Bad Debts	$ 16,300	
Contractual Adjustments	169,400	
Charity Service	88,600	
Total Revenue Deductions		274,300
Net Patient Service Revenues		2,466,275
Other Operating Revenues:		
Cafeteria Sales	102,400	
Rental Income	6,600	
Purchases Discounts	11,549	
Total Other Operating Revenues		120,549
Total Operating Revenues		2,586,824
Less Operating Expenses:		
Nursing Services	1,150,050	
Other Professional Services	321,708	
General Services	381,724	
Fiscal Services	161,508	
Administrative Services (including $140,000 of depreciation and $63,400 of interest)	411,790	
Total Operating Expenses (Schedule B)		2,426,780
Operating Income		160,044
Add Nonoperating Revenues:		
General Contributions	13,150	
Interest Income	6,750	
Total Nonoperating Revenues		19,900
Net Income		$ 179,944

Figure 14–9 Hartful Hospital Income Statement, Five Months Ended May 31, 19X1

Schedule A	Inpatients	Outpatients	Total
Nursing Services:			
Nursing Units	$1,084,000		$1,084,000
Operating Rooms	130,500	$ 19,500	150,000
Emergency Rooms	72,000	45,100	117,100
Central Supply	170,500	28,500	199,000
Total Nursing Service Revenues	1,457,000	93,100	1,550,100
Other Professional Services:			
Laboratory	282,100	85,200	367,300
Radiology	444,175	108,150	552,325
Pharmacy	124,800	29,400	154,200
Anesthesia	108,400	8,250	116,650
Total Other Professional Service Revenues	959,475	231,000	1,190,475
Totals	$2,416,475	$324,100	$2,740,575

Schedule B	Salaries and Wages	Other Expenses	Total
Nursing Services:			
Administrative Office	$ 13,950	$ 10,500	$ 24,450
Nursing Units	807,000	115,600	922,600
Operating Rooms	41,000	23,000	64,000
Emergency Rooms	32,000	19,500	51,500
Central Supply	38,500	49,000	87,500
Total Nursing Services Expense	932,450	217,600	1,150,050
Other Professional Services:			
Administrative Office	19,000	8,500	27,500
Laboratory	41,000	20,500	61,500
Radiology	39,500	22,500	62,000
Pharmacy	24,500	37,260	61,760
Anesthesia	28,500	10,900	39,400
Medical Staff	61,000	8,548	69,548
Total Other Professional Services Expense	213,500	108,208	321,708

General Services:			
Administrative Office	9,900	6,500	16,400
Dietary	47,000	107,500	154,500
Plant Operation and Maintenance	31,000	70,624	101,624
Housekeeping	36,600	19,000	55,600
Laundry	34,000	19,600	53,600
Total General Services Expense	158,500	223,224	381,724
Fiscal Services:			
Administrative Office	20,600	12,000	32,600
Accounting	33,500	38,308	71,808
Admitting	26,500	30,600	57,100
Total Fiscal Services Expense	80,600	80,908	161,508
Administrative Services:			
Administrator's Office	25,850	19,500	45,350
Administrative Office	11,100	5,700	16,800
Governing Board		4,700	4,700
Purchasing	19,500	5,120	24,620
Personnel	20,500	5,900	26,400
Depreciation		140,000	140,000
Insurance		7,700	7,700
Interest		63,400	63,400
Employee Benefits		82,820	82,820
Total Administrative Services Expense	76,950	334,840	411,790
Total Operating Expenses	$1,462,000	$964,780	$2,426,780

Figure 14-11 Hartful Hospital Operating Expenses, Five Months Ended May 31, 19X1 (*continued*)

Figure 14–12 Hartful Hospital
Balance Sheet, May 31, 19X1

Assets			
Current Assets:			
Cash in Bank		$ 176,205	
Petty Cash		500	
Temporary Investments		150,000	
Accrued Interest Receivables		6,750	
Receivables from Patients	$942,025		
Less Allowance for Uncollectibles	116,700	825,325	
Inventories		96,000	
Prepaid Expenses		12,200	
Total Current Assets			$1,266,980
Property, Plant, and Equipment:			
Land		175,000	
Buildings		5,000,000	
Equipment		3,016,000	
Total		8,191,000	
Less Accumulated Depreciation		2,128,000	
Net Property, Plant, and Equipment			6,063,000
Total Assets			$7,329,980
Liabilities and Equity			
Current Liabilities:			
Notes Payable		$ 80,000	
Accounts Payable		69,996	
Accrued Interest Payable		33,000	
Deferred Rental Income		7,800	
Total Current Liabilities			$ 190,796
Bonds Payable			2,400,000
Total Liabilities			2,590,796
Hospital Equity, January 1, 19X1		4,559,240	
Add Net Income for Five Months Ended May 31, 19X1		179,944	
Hospital Equity, May 31, 19X1			4,739,184
Total Liabilities and Hospital Equity			$7,329,980

Questions

Q14–1. What is the purpose of a purchase requisition? Who prepares it? How many copies are usually made? To whom are the copies sent, and why?

Q14–2. What is the purpose of a purchase order? Who prepares it? How many copies are usually made? To whom are the copies sent, and why?

Q14-3. Describe briefly the purchasing function in hospitals.

Q14-4. Describe briefly the receiving function in hospitals.

Q14-5. What is the purpose of a receiving report? Who prepares it? How many copies are usually made? To whom are the copies sent, and why?

Q14-6. What documents generally are included in a voucher package?

Q14-7. Describe the voucher system as a means of internal control over cash disbursements by hospitals.

Q14-8. On September 6, 19X1, Newton Hospital purchased $2,500 of dietary supplies on account, terms 2/10, n/30. In other words, if the account is paid within 10 days after the invoice date, a 2 percent discount is given to the hospital. Otherwise, the full invoice amount ($2,500) is due and payable within 30 days following the invoice date. The invoice from the supplier is paid on September 15, 19X1. Indicate, in detail, how these transactions should be recorded in the hospital's voucher register, cash disbursements journal, accounts payable subsidiary ledger, and general ledger.

Q14-9. How often should postings be made from (a) the voucher register and (b) the cash disbursements journal? Explain why the frequency is needed.

Q14-10. Nearby Hospital purchased a new item of equipment for $45,000 on May 27, 19X1. The supplier's invoice was paid on June 10, 19X1. Indicate how these transactions should be recorded in the voucher register, cash disbursements journal, and general ledger of the hospital.

Problems

P14-1. The following is the adjusted trial balance for Northside Hospital as of May 31, 19X1 (the fiscal year ends June 30):

	Dr.	Cr.
1011.0 Cash—General Checking	$ 172,000	
1014.0 Petty Cash Fund	750	
1020.0 Temporary Investments	160,000	
1029.0 Accrued Interest Receivable	6,200	
1031.0 Inpatient Receivables—Inhouse	97,400	
1032.0 Inpatient Receivables—Discharged	831,500	

		Dr.	Cr.
1044.0	Outpatient Receivables	18,100	
1061.0	Allowance for Uncollectible Accounts—Bad Debts		$ 12,300
1062.0	Allowance for Uncollectible Accounts—Contractual Adjustments		53,700
1066.0	Allowance for Uncollectible Accounts—Charity Service		29,800
1110.0	Inventories	89,000	
1120.0	Prepaid Expenses	12,900	
1130.0	Land	155,000	
1150.0	Buildings	5,500,000	
1170.0	Equipment	2,800,000	
1250.0	Accumulated Depreciation—Buildings		1,075,000
1270.0	Accumulated Depreciation—Equipment		840,000
2010.0	Notes Payable		90,000
2020.0	Accounts Payable		73,400
2031.0	Accrued Payroll		-0-
2035.0	FIT Withheld		-0-
2036.0	FICA Withheld and Accrued		-0-
2051.0	Accrued Interest Payable		19,700
2113.0	Deferred Rental Income		7,800
2190.0	Bonds Payable		2,500,000
2210.0	Hospital Equity		4,934,350
2219.0	Revenue and Expense Summary		-0-
3021.1	Nursing Service Revenues—Inpatient Nursing Units		901,300
3210.1	Operating Rooms—Inpatient Revenues		98,200
3210.2	Operating Rooms—Outpatient Revenues		14,400
3230.1	Emergency Rooms—Inpatient Revenues		58,100
3230.2	Emergency Rooms—Outpatient Revenues		37,900
3250.1	Central Supply—Inpatient Revenues		140,500
3250.2	Central Supply—Outpatient Revenues		21,300
4011.1	Laboratory—Inpatient Revenues		231,600
4011.2	Laboratory—Outpatient Revenues		77,700
4040.1	Radiology—Inpatient Revenues		341,600
4040.2	Radiology—Outpatient Revenues		84,800
4070.1	Pharmacy—Inpatient Revenues		100,900

		Dr.	Cr.
4070.2	Pharmacy—Outpatient Revenues		22,600
4080.1	Anesthesia—Inpatient Revenues		87,500
4080.2	Anesthesia—Outpatient Revenues		5,900
5061.0	Cafeteria Sales		91,500
5155.0	Rental Income		5,200
5171.0	Purchase Discounts		8,700
5510.0	Deductions from Revenues—Bad Debts	14,800	
5520.0	Deductions from Revenues—Contractual Adjustments	131,300	
5540.0	Deductions from Revenues—Charity Service	59,900	
6010.1	Nursing Services Administrative Office—Salaries and Wages	12,300	
6010.2	Nursing Services Administrative Office—Other Expense	7,200	
6021.1	Nursing Units—Salaries and Wages	656,600	
6021.2	Nursing Units—Other Expense	87,200	
6210.1	Operating Rooms—Salaries and Wages	31,300	
6210.2	Operating Rooms—Other Expense	17,100	
6230.1	Emergency Rooms—Salaries and Wages	26,600	
6230.2	Emergency Rooms—Other Expense	14,500	
6250.1	Central Supply—Salaries and Wages	30,700	
6250.2	Central Supply—Other Expense	38,100	
7010.1	Other Professional Services Administrative Office—Salaries and Wages	14,900	
7010.2	Other Professional Services Administrative Office—Other Expense	7,700	
7011.1	Laboratory—Salaries and Wages	33,100	
7011.2	Laboratory—Other Expense	15,700	
7040.1	Radiology—Salaries and Wages	32,800	
7040.2	Radiology—Other Expense	16,900	
7070.1	Pharmacy—Salaries and Wages	20,100	
7070.2	Pharmacy—Other Expense	31,600	
7080.1	Anesthesia—Salaries and Wages	19,500	
7080.2	Anesthesia—Other Expense	9,700	
8030.1	Medical Staff—Salaries and Wages	52,900	
8030.2	Medical Staff—Other Expense	7,100	
8040.1	General Services Administrative Office—Salaries and Wages	8,500	
8040.2	General Services Administrative Office—Other Expense	4,800	

		Dr.	Cr.
8050.1	Dietary—Salaries and Wages	38,200	
8050.2	Dietary—Other Expense	91,700	
8060.1	Plant Operation and Maintenance—Salaries and Wages	23,000	
8060.2	Plant Operation and Maintenance—Other Expense	62,300	
8090.1	Housekeeping—Salaries and Wages	30,400	
8090.2	Housekeeping—Other Expense	14,300	
8110.1	Laundry—Salaries and Wages	25,500	
8110.2	Laundry—Other Expense	14,600	
8211.1	Fiscal Services Administrative Office—Salaries and Wages	15,300	
8211.2	Fiscal Services Administrative Office—Other Expense	8,200	
8212.1	Accounting—Salaries and Wages	25,900	
8212.2	Accounting—Other Expense	19,400	
8241.1	Admitting—Salaries and Wages	22,800	
8241.2	Admitting—Other Expense	17,500	
8310.1	Administrator's Office—Salaries and Wages	24,700	
8310.2	Administrator's Office—Other Expense	7,400	
8311.1	Administrative Services Office—Salaries and Wages	7,900	
8311.2	Administrative Services Office—Other Expense	3,700	
8312.2	Governing board—Other Expense	2,900	
8331.1	Purchasing—Salaries and Wages	14,600	
8331.2	Purchasing—Other Expense	5,400	
8371.1	Personnel—Salaries and Wages	17,300	
8371.2	Personnel—Other Expense	3,800	
8510.0	Depreciation Expense	115,600	
8610.0	Insurance Expense	6,100	
8690.0	Interest Expense	51,700	
8710.0	Employee Benefits	67,500	
9041.0	General Contributions		11,400
9051.0	Interest Income		6,300
		$11,983,450	$11,983,450

Required: (1) Prepare an income statement for the 11 months ended May 31, 19X1. (2) Prepare a balance sheet for May 31, 19X1. Support the income statement with separate schedules for gross revenues and operating expenses, as illustrated in Figures 14–10 and 14–11.

P14–2. Refer to the May 31, 19X1, trial balance provided in Problem 14–1 and assume the following column totals in Northside Hospital's special journals for June, 19X1:

1. Inpatient revenue journal:

		Dr.	Cr.
1031.0	Inpatient Receivables—Inhouse	$462,500	
3021.1	Nursing Units—Inpatient Revenues		$188,900
3210.1	Operating Rooms—Inpatient Revenues		27,200
3230.1	Emergency Rooms—Inpatient Revenues		15,100
3250.1	Central Supply—Inpatient Revenues		36,500
4011.1	Laboratory—Inpatient Revenues		57,300
4040.1	Radiology—Inpatient Revenues		89,600
4070.1	Pharmacy—Inpatient Revenues		25,700
4080.1	Anesthesia—Inpatient Revenues		22,200

2. Outpatient revenue journal:

		Dr.	Cr.
1044.0	Outpatient Receivables	$ 70,300	
3210.2	Operating Rooms		$ 4,200
3230.2	Emergency Rooms		9,700
3250.2	Central Supply		6,800
4011.2	Laboratory		18,300
4040.2	Radiology		23,100
4070.2	Pharmacy		6,400
4080.2	Anesthesia		1,800

3. Cash receipts journal:

		Dr.	Cr.
1011.0	Cash—General Checking	$494,100	
5520.0	Deductions from Revenues—Contractual Adjustments	29,700	
5540.0	Deductions from Revenues—Charity Service	14,800	
1031.0	Inpatient Receivables—Inhouse		$ 44,600
1032.0	Inpatient Receivables—Discharged		413,300
1044.0	Outpatient Receivables		58,400
5061.0	Cafeteria Sales		19,700
5155.0	General Contributions		2,600

4. Payroll journal:

		Dr.	Cr.
6010.1	Nursing Services—Administrative Office	$ 2,750	
6021.1	Nursing Units	159,200	
6210.1	Operating Rooms	7,900	
6230.1	Emergency Rooms	6,600	

		Dr.	Cr.
6250.1	Central Supply	7,300	
7010.1	Other Professional Services—		
	Administrative Office	3,900	
7011.1	Laboratory	8,400	
7040.1	Radiology	7,500	
7070.1	Pharmacy	5,100	
7080.1	Anesthesia	5,400	
8030.1	Medical Staff	12,000	
8040.1	General Services Administrative Office	2,000	
8050.1	Dietary	9,600	
8060.1	Plant Operation and Maintenance	6,100	
8090.1	Housekeeping	7,300	
8110.1	Laundry	7,100	
8211.1	Fiscal Services—Administrative Office	4,100	
9212.1	Accounting	6,800	
8241.1	Admitting	5,600	
8310.1	Administrator's Office	5,250	
8311.1	Administrative Services—Executive		
	Office	2,200	
8331.1	Purchasing	3,900	
8371.1	Personnel	4,100	
2035.0	FIT Withheld		$ 49,200
2036.0	FICA Withheld		17,300
2031.0	Accrued Payroll		223,600

5. Voucher register:

		Dr.	Cr.
2020.0	Accounts Payable		$461,500
2031.0	Accrued Payroll	$223,600	
2035.0	FIT Withheld	49,200	
2036.0	FICA Withheld and Accrued	34,600	
6010.2	Nursing Services—Administrative Office	1,800	
6021.2	Nursing Units	22,500	
6210.2	Operating Rooms	4,700	
6230.2	Emergency Rooms	4,100	
6250.2	Central Supply	9,300	
7010.2	Other Professional Services—		
	Administrative Office	1,400	
7011.2	Laboratory	4,500	
7040.2	Radiology	4,800	
7070.2	Pharmacy	7,600	
7080.2	Anesthesia	2,100	
8030.2	Medical Staff	1,300	
8040.2	General Services—Administrative Office	1,100	
8050.2	Dietary	23,400	

		Dr.	Cr.
8060.2	Plant Operation and Maintenance	12,200	
8090.2	Housekeeping	3,600	
8110.2	Laundry	4,200	
8211.2	Fiscal Services—Administrative Office	2,100	
8212.2	Accounting	6,300	
8241.2	Admitting	5,800	
8310.2	Administrator's Office	2,300	
8311.2	Administrative Services—Executive Office	900	
8312.2	Governing Board	1,000	
8331.2	Purchasing	800	
8371.2	Personnel	1,300	
1170.0	Equipment	25,000	

6. Cash disbursements journal:

		Dr.	Cr.
1011.0	Cash—General Checking		$448,600
5171.0	Purchases Discounts		2,700
2020.0	Accounts Payable	$451,300	

In addition to the special journal information just given, you are provided with the following general journal entries made by Northside Hospital during June, 19X1:

	Account Numbers	Dr.	Cr.
Inpatient Receivables—Discharged	1032.0	$410,600	
Inpatient Receivables—Inhouse	1031.0		$410,600
Transfer unpaid account balances from inhouse to discharged receivables.			
Accrued Interest Receivable	1029.0	1,400	
Interest Income	9051.0		1,400
Accrual of interest earned in May.			
Deductions from Revenues:			
Bad Debts	5510.0	3,900	
Contractual Adjustments	5520.0	12,400	
Charity Service	5540.0	7,300	
Allowance for Uncollectible Accounts:			
Bad Debts	1061.0		3,900
Contractual Adjustments	1062.0		12,400
Charity Service	1066.0		7,300
Adjustment of allowance accounts to correct balances.			

	Account Numbers	Dr.	Cr.
10 Insurance Expense	8610.0	1,600	
Prepaid Expenses	1120.0		1,600
Adjustment for expiration of insurance premiums.			
11 Depreciation Expense	8510.0	31,400	
Accumulated Depreciation:			
Buildings	1250.0		14,300
Equipment	1270.0		17,100
Depreciation expense for June.			
12 Employee Benefits	8710.0	17,300	
FICA Withheld and Accrued	2036.0		17,300
Accrual of hospital's share of FICA taxes on June payroll.			
13 Interest Expense	8690.0	15,800	
Accrued Interest Payable	2051.0		15,800
Accrual of interest expense for June.			
14 Deferred Rental Income	2113.0	1,400	
Rental Income	5155.0		1,400
Adjustment for rental income earned in June.			

Required: (1) Establish the May 31, 19X1, balances in general ledger accounts. (2) Make all necessary postings from the special journals and the general journal to the general ledger accounts. (3) Prepare an adjusted trial balance at June 30, 19X1. (4) Prepare an income statement for the year ended June 30, 19X1. (5) Prepare a balance sheet at June 30, 19X1.

Principles of Fund Accounting

15

In addition to the revenue received from patients and third parties for healthcare services provided by the hospital, many hospitals also receive contributions, donations, gifts, grants, and endowment resources. Certain of these resources might be available, at the discretion of the governing board, for the financing of the regular day-to-day operating activities of the hospital. Let us assume, for example, that a person gives Hartful Hospital $25,000 in cash and says to the hospital, "Use this money however you wish!" There is no stipulation or restriction by the donor about the specific purpose for which the money is to be used. In cases such as this, regardless of the amount involved, the resources are classified as *unrestricted resources.* Although the receipt of such resources must be recorded by the hospital as nonoperating revenue (account 9041.0, General Contributions), the resources may be used to acquire plant assets, to pay operating expenses, or for any other purpose determined by the governing board.

Other donated resources received by hospitals, however, may be restricted by donors to specific uses and purposes such as construction of new hospital buildings, purchase of new equipment, or the financing of hospital charity work, research, and educational activities. Such resources are not available for any purpose other than that specified by the donor. Let us assume, for example, that an individual gives Hartful Hospital $25,000 in cash and says to the hospital, "Use this money to purchase new equipment for your radiology department." In all such cases, regardless of the amount involved, the resources are classified as *restricted resources.* The resources must be employed or expended by the hospital precisely as indicated by the donors.

There is both a legal and a moral obligation on the part of the hospital to comply fully with donors' restrictions and stipulations. Failing to observe the stated wishes of donors or not providing a proper accounting for the use or disposition of donor-restricted resources may give rise to very serious legal penalties.

Maintaining Separate
Unrestricted and Restricted
Accounts

Aside from the legal obligation to fulfill donors' requirements, there is also an administrative or managerial need to maintain in the accounting records a careful distinction between unrestricted and restricted resources. A hospital's managers, in making their financing and investing decisions, must have information regarding which resources are available for any general operating purpose and which resources are limited to particular donor-restricted purposes. Otherwise, unauthorized and even illegal use might be made of donated resources. Furthermore, donors often require from the hospital a periodic accounting for the use of the donated resources.

The system of fund accounting has evolved in response to these stewardship (fiduciary) accountability requirements. It is the objective of this chapter to give you an opportunity to learn the basic principles of the fund accounting system. Because many not-for-profit hospitals employ fund accounting procedures, the materials in this chapter deserve your attention. The discussion, however, will be at an introductory level. A more advanced treatment of the subject may be found in the author's *Hospital Financial Accounting: Theory and Practice* (Chicago: HFMA, 1987).

Nature of Fund Accounting

Fund accounting may be defined as a system of accounting in which the resources (and related obligations) of a hospital are segregated in the accounting records into self-balancing sets of accounts ("funds") for the purpose of carrying on specific activities or attaining particular objectives in accordance with legal and other restrictions. The hospital itself is the primary accounting entity. In a fund accounting system, however, this primary entity is broken down into a number of subordinate accounting entities: funds.

In view of this rather complex definition, perhaps your understanding of fund accounting will be enhanced if you consider a simple example. Take a moment to examine Figure 15–1, a condensed balance sheet for an assumed Community Hospital.

This balance sheet could be quite misleading about the financial position of Community Hospital, however, if there were donor or other externally imposed restrictions on the hospital's use of certain of its assets. Assuming there are such restrictions, a revised

Assets	$8,500
Liabilities	$2,500
Hospital equity	6,000
Total liabilities and hospital equity	$8,500

Figure 15–1 Community Hospital Balance Sheet, September 30, 19X1

balance sheet is shown in Figure 15–2 as it would appear in accordance with the principles of fund accounting and reporting.

Clearly, this revised balance sheet provides a much different impression of Community Hospital's financial position. We see that of the $8,500 of assets, only $4,000 are unrestricted and available for general operating purposes. These are the only assets that can be used to pay the $1,900 of liabilities reported in the unrestricted fund. The other $4,500 of hospital assets are restricted by donors to particular uses, whatever they may be. So, the column in Figure 15–2 that totals all funds really has no particular significance to the hospital's creditors. It is included only to indicate the relationship between Figures 15–1 and 15–2.

Reporting Resources Available to Pay Particular Liabilities

Thus, in fund accounting, assets and related liabilities are segregated in the hospital's accounts and reports into unrestricted and restricted "funds," depending on the absence or presence of donor or other externally imposed restrictions. In this context, *funds* does not mean *cash,* but simply a self-balancing group of related accounts. Notice that funds, unrestricted and restricted, consist of equal debits (assets) and credits (liabilities and equity). This equality is maintained throughout all operations in the fund accounting process.

Observe that Community Hospital has a single unrestricted fund. In fund accounting, there is one (and only one) unrestricted fund. On the other hand, the hospital has three restricted funds. Restricted resources, as you will shortly see, are classified according to the three major types of restrictions that are externally imposed on donated resources.

Maximum of One Unrestricted Fund

An extremely important point to recognize here is that the term *restricted* should be used only to refer to resources that are externally restricted. That is, when we speak of restricted funds, we are referring to a self-balancing set of accounts containing resources whose use has been restricted by persons or other entities external to the hospital. The hospital's governing board, by its actions, can *designate* certain assets to particular uses, but the board does not have the power to restrict their use in terms of the hospital's legal relationships with its creditors.

Restrictions from External Sources Only

	Unrestricted Fund	Restricted Funds			Total All Funds
		Fund A	Fund B	Fund C	
Assets	$4,000	$1,000	$2,000	$1,500	$8,500
Liabilities	$1,900	$ 200	$ 400	$ -0-	$2,500
Hospital equity	2,100	800	1,600	1,500	6,000
Total liabilities and equity	$4,000	$1,000	$2,000	$1,500	$8,500

Figure 15–2 Community Hospital Balance Sheet, September 30, 19X1

Restricted Funds Versus Board-Designated Assets

The board can make whatever designations it wishes for internal management purposes, but, if donors do not restrict the use of resources they contribute to the hospital, the board cannot do it for the donors. Moreover, what the board can do, it can undo. So, this text does not refer to "board-restricted funds." When the board earmarks certain assets for a specific purpose, the term *board-designated assets* describes the situation. Assets that are so designated, however, are unrestricted assets and must be reported as a part of the hospital's unrestricted fund.

Note that many hospitals have established separately incorporated foundations. A foundation seeks and receives donations on behalf of the hospital. Eventually, the donated resources are transferred from the foundation to the hospital, but an in-depth discussion of this topic is beyond the scope of this book.

Types of Funds

Fund accounting, as it is employed by hospitals, uses two major categories of funds: unrestricted and restricted. There is only one unrestricted fund, but restricted funds are classified into three major types: (1) specific purpose funds, (2) plant replacement and expansion funds, and (3) endowment funds. Let us now briefly examine the nature and content of each of these types of funds.

Unrestricted Fund

An unrestricted fund (often called *general fund*) is maintained by all hospitals using fund accounting. This fund includes all hospital resources, with related obligations, that are not restricted by any external authority or donor. All of the resources of this fund are available for general operating activities at the discretion of the hospital's governing board. In addition, the accounts of the unrestricted fund include all the revenues and expenses to be reported in the hospital's income statement.

Think back to the extended Hartful Hospital illustration of the last five chapters; all of the accounts were unrestricted fund accounts. The chart of accounts presented in Chapter 10 is, except for a few accounts to be added in this and later chapters, a chart of accounts for Hartful Hospital's unrestricted fund.

Some hospitals receive substantial amounts of resources by donation. If no strings are attached by donors, such resources are recorded in the unrestricted funds regardless of any action that might be taken by the hospital's governing board. It must be presumed that if the donor wished to restrict the use of the resources, the donor would do so at the time of donation. If no such restrictions are made by the donors, the governing board cannot do it for the donors because such board actions would not be proper or legally binding.

Restricted Funds

A majority of donated resources, however, generally are restricted in some way by donors. These resources are of three major types:

Majority of Donations
Carry Restrictions

- Resources restricted for specific operating purposes
- Resources restricted for acquisition of plant assets
- Resources restricted as endowments

These resources are recorded in three types of restricted funds. A chart of accounts for each of these three types of restricted funds (and some additional unrestricted fund accounts) is presented in Figure 15–3.

The account numbering system closely conforms to the system prescribed in the American Hospital Association's *Chart of Accounts for Hospitals*. Account numbers are constructed according to the following system:

1. The first digit of account numbers for restricted funds is either 1 or 2, with the following designations:

First Digit
1 = Asset accounts
2 = Liability and equity accounts

| | Account Numbers | | | |
	Plant Replacement and Expansion Fund	Specific Purpose Fund	Endowment Fund	Unrestricted Fund
Assets:				
Cash—General Checking Account	1511.0	1611.0	1711.0	
Investments	1520.0	1620.0	1720.0	
Accrued Income Receivable	1529.0	1629.0	1729.0	
Pledges Receivable	1581.0	1681.0	1781.0	1081.0
Allowance for Uncollectible Pledges	1582.0	1682.0	1782.0	1082.0
Due from Unrestricted Fund	1591.0	1691.0	1791.0	
Due from Plant Replacement and Expansion Fund		1692.0	1792.0	1092.0
Due from Specific Purpose Fund	1593.0		1793.0	1093.0
Due from Endowment Fund	1594.0	1694.0		1094.0
Other Assets	1593.0	1630.0	1730.0	
Liabilities and Fund Balances:				
Due to Unrestricted Fund	2581.0	2681.0	2781.0	
Due to Plant Replacement and Expansion Fund		2682.0	2782.0	2082.0
Due to Specific Purpose Fund	2583.0		2783.0	2083.0
Due to Endowment Fund	2584.0	2684.0		2084.0
Fund Balance	2511.0	2611.0	2711.0	
Transfers from Unrestricted Fund	2512.1			
Transfers from Plant Replacement and Expansion Fund				2212.2
Transfers from Specific Purpose Fund				a
Transfers from Endowment Fund	2512.4	1612.4		a
Donated Resources Received	2513.1	2613.1	2713.1	
Investment Income	2513.2	2613.2		
Investment Gains and Losses	2513.3	2613.3	2713.3	
Transfers to Unrestricted Fund	2514.1	2614.1		
Transfers to Plant Replacement and Expansion Fund				2214.2

ªSee text discussion later in this chapter.

Figure 15-3 Hartful Hospital Chart of Accounts—Restricted Funds Including Additional Unrestricted Fund Accounts

Restricted Funds Have Asset, Liability, and Equity Accounts Only

Notice that all accounts of restricted funds are asset, liability, or equity accounts. There are no revenue or expense accounts for the restricted funds, although it can be argued that the use of such accounts would be logical and useful.

2. The second digit of account numbers for restricted funds is 5, 6, or 7, with the following designations:

Second Digit

5	=	Plant replacement and expansion fund accounts
6	=	Specific purpose fund accounts
7	=	Endowment fund accounts

Thus, the second digit of these account numbers identifies the type of restricted fund to which the account is related.

3. The third and fourth digits provide a primary subclassification of the accounts by specific type of asset, liability, or equity.

The AHA manual also provides for the use of fifth and sixth digits where needed by individual hospitals. We will limit restricted fund account numbers, for our present purposes, to five digits.

Specific Purpose Funds.   Resources that are restricted by donors for purposes other than plant asset acquisitions or endowments are recorded in a specific purpose fund. Assume, for example, that Hartful Hospital receives $25,000 in cash from a donor who restricts the use of the resources to a specific purpose such as charity service, research activities, or education programs conducted by the hospital. The specific purpose fund entry uses the following general format:

Specific Purpose Fund Transaction Entries

Cash	1611.0	$25,000	
Donated Resources			
Received	2613.1		$25,000
Receipt of resources donor-			
restricted to			
[educational programs].			

Once recorded as specific purpose funds, these resources remain restricted funds until such time as the specified purposes are completed by appropriate activity in the unrestricted fund, such as rendering charity service to indigent patients, performing research work, or providing educational programs.

As expenditures are made for the donor-specified purposes by the unrestricted fund, periodic transfers of the previously restricted resources are made to the unrestricted fund from the appropriate specific purpose fund. Assuming that the $25,000 is transferred to the unrestricted fund to finance educational programs, the necessary entries are as follows:

Specific Purpose Fund

Transfers to Unrestricted Fund	2614.1	$25,000	
Cash	1611.0		$25,000
Transfer of resources to unrestricted fund to finance educational programs.			

Unrestricted Fund

Cash	1011.0	$25,000	
Transfers from Restricted Funds for Educational Programs	5021.0		$25,000
Resources received from specific purpose fund to finance educational programs.			

Notice that the account (5021.0) credited in the unrestricted fund is a revenue account in the "other operating revenues" category. Because expenditures for educational programs are recorded as unrestricted fund expenses, this credit accomplishes an appropriate matching of revenues and expenses. Similar procedures would be followed for transfers related to charity service and research activities.

Until transfers such as these are made, however, the resources of the specific purpose funds should be prudently invested. Income and gains on these temporary investments should be credited to the proper specific purpose fund accounts (for example, accounts 2613.2 and 2613.3). At the end of each fiscal year, these accounts (as well as accounts 2612.4, 2613.1, and 2614.1) should be closed to the specific purpose Fund Balance (account 2611.0).

Plant Replacement and Expansion Fund Transaction Entries

Plant Replacement and Expansion Funds. Cash and other restricted resources received from donors and other external authorities for the acquisition of plant assets are included in the plant replacement and expansion fund. Assume, for example, that a donor gives the hospital $80,000 for the purchase of a new item of radiological equipment. The entry in a plant replacement and expansion fund is as follows:

Cash	1511.0	$80,000	
Donated Resources			
Received	2513.1		$80,000
Receipt of resources			
donor-restricted to			
purchase of plant assets.			

Until the equipment is purchased using the resources of the unrestricted fund, this $80,000 remains in the plant replacement and expansion fund. The $80,000 should be placed in some form of income-producing investment. Income and gains on such investments should be credited to accounts 2513.2 and 2513.3. At the end of the year, these accounts (along with accounts 2512.1, 2512.4, 2513.1, and 2514.1) are closed to the plant replacement and expansion fund balance account (account 2511.0).

When the equipment is purchased by the unrestricted fund, $80,000 (plus any net investment income) is transferred to the unrestricted fund. The entries to record the transfer are the following:

Plant Replacement and Expansion Fund

Transfers to Unrestricted Fund	2514.1	$80,000	
Cash	1511.0		$80,000
Transfer of resources to			
unrestricted fund to finance			
purchase of equipment for			
radiology department.			

Unrestricted Fund

Cash	1011.0	$80,000	
Transfers from Plant			
Replacement and			
Expansion Fund	2212.2		$80,000
Receipt of resources			
from plant replacement and			
expansion fund to finance			
purchase of equipment.			

The credit in the unrestricted fund is made to a temporary unrestricted fund balance account, not a revenue account. Plant assets, including those that are purchased with previously restricted resources, are not recorded in the plant replacement and expansion fund but in the unrestricted fund.

In some instances, a hospital receives pledges from donors to contribute money for future purchases of plant assets. The receipt of such pledges should be recorded in the plant replacement and expansion fund as follows:

Pledges Receivable	1581.0	$40,000	
Allowance for			
Uncollectible Pledges	1582.0		$ 4,000
Donated Resources			
Received	2513.1		36,000
Receipt of pledges			
(estimated to be 90%			
collectible) donor-restricted			
to the acquisition of plant			
assets.			

A similar procedure is followed for the receipt of pledges relating to other funds. Figure 15–3 indicates the relevant accounts used in the other funds.

Another important point concerns the procedure to be followed when plant assets are donated in kind to a hospital. Assume, for example, that a donor gives the hospital an item of equipment having a fair market value of $80,000 (rather than giving the hospital $80,000 with which to purchase the equipment). Where this occurs, no entry is made in the plant replacement and expansion fund. Instead, the following entry is made in the unrestricted fund:

Equipment	1170.0	$80,000	
Value of Donated Plant			
Assets	2213.0		$80,000
Receipt of donated			
equipment at fair market			
value.			

The account credited is not a revenue account but a temporary unrestricted fund balance account. A donation of plant assets in kind is assumed to be a contribution to the permanent capital of the hospital and is not reported as revenue in the income statement.

Endowment Fund. *Endowments* consist of contributed resources that, by donor restriction, are not to be expended but are to be held intact for the production of income. Assume, for example, that Hartful Hospital receives $100,000 from a donor who specifies that the money is to be invested in securities and held as an endowment of the hospital. The endowment fund entries are the following:

Endowment Fund
Transaction Entries

Cash	1711.0	$100,000	
Donated Resources			
Received	2713.1		$100,000
Receipt of resources to be			
held as an endowment.			
Investments	1720.0	$100,000	
Cash	1711.0		$100,000
To record the investment			
of endowment funds			
received.			

At the year's end, account 2713.1 (along with account 2713.3) is closed to the endowment fund balance account (2711.0).

Income from investments of endowment funds may be donor restricted or immediately available for general operating purposes. If the income is restricted by the donor to specific operating purposes, for example, this income should not be recorded in the endowment fund but should be recorded directly in the appropriate specific purpose fund as follows (amount is assumed):

Cash	1611.0	$7,500	
Transfers from Endowment			
Fund	2612.4		$7,500
Receipt of income earned on			
endowment fund investments			
and donor restricted to specific			
operating purposes.			

If the income is donor restricted to the acquisition of plant assets, the income should be recorded directly in the plant replacement and expansion fund through accounts 1511.0 and 2512.4 in the manner illustrated earlier.

On the other hand, the income earned on endowment fund investments may not be donor restricted in any way. In these cases, the income should be recorded directly in the unrestricted fund as follows:

Cash	1011.0	$7,500	
Unrestricted Income from			
Endowment Fund	9055.0		$7,500
Receipt of unrestricted income			
from endowment fund			
investments.			

Notice that the credit in the unrestricted fund is to a revenue account to be reported as nonoperating revenues in the hospital's income statement.

Thus, investment income on endowment funds is directly recorded in a fund other than the endowment fund. It is not correct to record the income initially in the endowment fund and later to transfer it to another fund. Gains and losses on endowment fund investments, however, generally are recorded in the endowment fund (account 2713.3) on the theory that gains and losses follow the endowment fund principal rather than the endowment fund income.

Financial Statements

To illustrate the effect of fund accounting on the financial statements of the hospital, we provide a set of statements for Hartful Hospital for the year ended December 31, 19X1 (dollar amounts assumed). In addition to the income statement and balance sheet, a statement of changes in fund balances is introduced to provide an analysis and summary of all changes that took place in the various fund balances during the year.

Income Statement

Hartful Hospital's income statement for 19X1 is presented in Figure 15–4 in condensed form. Although this statement is virtually identical in format and content to the income statement illustrated

Patient Service Revenues:		
Nursing Services		$3,565,282
Other Professional Services		2,738,130
Gross Patient Service Revenues		6,303,412
Less Revenue Deductions:		
Bad Debts	$ 53,790	
Contractual Adjustments	389,620	
Charity Service (net of specific purpose gifts of $34,000)	194,920	
Total Revenue Deductions		638,330
Net Patient Service Revenues		5,665,082
Other Operating Revenues:		
Cafeteria Sales	235,520	
Transfers from Restricted Funds for Research and Education	92,000	
Rental Income	14,680	
Purchase Discounts	23,169	
Total Other Operating Revenues		365,369
Total Operating Revenues		6,030,451
Less Operating Expenses:		
Nursing Services	2,499,194	
Other Professional Services	972,099	
General Services	763,448	
Fiscal Services	355,318	
Administrative Services (including $322,000 of depreciation and $145,820 of interest)	988,296	
Total Operating Expenses		5,578,355
Operating Income		452,096
Add Nonoperating Revenues:		
General Contributions	28,930	
Unrestricted Income from Endowment Fund	41,000	
Interest Income on Unrestricted Fund Investments	14,850	
Total Nonoperating Revenues		84,780
Net Income for the Year		$ 536,876

Figure 15–4 Hartful Hospital Income Statement, Year Ended December 31, 19X1

in Chapter 14, you can see certain indications of the hospital's use of fund accounting.

First, among the revenue deductions, you will notice that the amount of charity service has been reduced by $34,000, which was transferred to the unrestricted fund from a specific purpose fund during 19X1. In other words, the value of charity services provided in 19X1 was $228,920, but the $34,000 received from a specific purpose fund was credited against it to produce the income state-

Impact of Fund Accounting on Income Statement

ment figure of $194,920. Thus, amounts received from a specific purpose fund to finance the hospital's charity work are netted against the charity service figure rather than being shown in the statement as revenues.

Second, the other operating revenues include $92,000 transferred from a specific purpose fund to the unrestricted fund to finance a part of the hospital's research and educational activities. This is the accounting treatment recommended by the AHA *Chart of Accounts for Hospitals* manual for such transfers. It is generally not practical to attempt to credit such transfers to the related research and education expense accounts.

Finally, notice that $41,000 of unrestricted income earned on the investments of the endowment fund is included in the nonoperating revenues classification. If such income were restricted by donors, it would not be reported in the income statement. Instead, it would be recorded as an addition to the fund balance account of either a specific purpose fund or a plant replacement and expansion fund.

Statement of Changes in Fund Balances

A statement of changes in fund balances for the year ended December 31, 19X1, is provided in Figure 15–5. The purpose of this statement is to disclose all of the changes that occurred in the fund balance accounts. It provides essential information that cannot be obtained from an examination of the income statement and balance sheet alone.

Observe that the statement begins with an analysis of the changes in the unrestricted fund balance. In addition to being increased by the year's net income, the fund balance was increased by a $150,000 transfer from the plant replacement and expansion fund to finance the acquisition of plant assets and by the fair market value ($35,000) of medical equipment contributed in kind to the hospital by a donor. You may recall from the preceding discussion that neither of these two items is ever to be recorded as revenue or included in the income statement. Receipts of plant assets in kind or receipts of cash restricted by donors to the acquisition of plant assets are considered contributions to the *permanent capital* of the hospital rather than revenues.

The analysis of changes in the specific purpose fund balance includes the amount ($142,000) of resources received by the hospital during 19X1 that were restricted by donors to specific operating purposes (charity service, research, and education). Such resources, at the time received, are not treated as revenues of the unrestricted fund but, as indicated here, are recorded in the specific purpose

Unrestricted Fund		
Fund Balance, January 1		$4,559,240
Net Income for the Year	*599000*	536,876
Transfers from Plant Replacement and Expansion Fund for Plant Asset Acquisitions	*121*	150,000
Donated Medical Equipment	*40*	35,000
Fund Balance, December 31		$5,281,116

Restricted Funds		
Specific Purpose Fund:		
Fund Balance, January 1		$ 245,612
Donated Resources Received		142,000
Investment Income		18,248
Investment Gains (Net)		7,600
Transfers to Unrestricted Fund for Charity Service	$(34,000)	
Research and Education	(92,000)	(126,000)
Fund Balance, December 31		$ 287,460
Plant Replacement and Expansion Fund:		
Fund Balance, January 1		$1,580,050
Donated Resources Received		196,330
Investment Income		112,477
Investment Gains (Net)		1,472
Transfer to Unrestricted Fund for Plant Asset Acquisitions		(150,000)
Fund Balance, December 31		$1,740,329
Endowment Fund:		
Fund Balance, January 1		$2,800,000
Donated Resources Received		100,000
Investment Gains (Net)		21,400
Fund Balance, December 31		$2,921,400

Figure 15–5 Hartful Hospital Statement of Changes in Fund Balances, Year Ended December 31, 19X1

fund. The balance of the specific purpose fund also was increased during 19X1 by $18,248 of income and $7,600 of net gains on the investments of the fund. The fund balance was decreased by $126,000 of transfers to the unrestricted fund ($34,000 for charity work and $92,000 for research and education costs). As noted earlier, these two items are included in the hospital's income statement.

A similar analysis appears in the statement with respect to the changes in the fund balance accounts of the other two restricted funds. Two points might be emphasized here. First, the $150,000 reduction of the plant replacement and expansion fund balance is

Transfers from Endowment Funds Are Rare

the same item shown as a direct addition to the unrestricted fund balance. Second, notice that investment income is not shown as an element of change in the endowment fund balance. All endowment fund investment income is recorded directly in one of the other funds as previously discussed. Transfers of resources from the endowment fund to other funds (or from other funds to the endowment fund) rarely occur.

Balance Sheet

The December 31, 19X1, balance sheet of Hartful Hospital is presented in Figure 15–6 in accordance with the principles of fund accounting. Notice that the assets, liabilities, and fund balances are segregated by funds. The total assets of each fund equal the total of each fund's liabilities and fund balance. Users of this balance sheet can readily see that $7,960,625 of resources are unrestricted and available for general operating purposes, whereas other resources are restricted by donors or other external authorities to particular purposes. In other words, $299,460 of resources are restricted to specific operating purposes, $1,765,329 of resources are restricted to plant asset acquisitions, and a total of $2,925,400 of resources are restricted for endowment purposes.

Similarly, the liabilities to be paid from the resources of each fund are classified by funds. Note also that the individual fund balance figures as of December 31 are those previously seen in the statement of changes in fund balances (Figure 15–5).

Handling Interfund
Transactions

Among the current assets of the unrestricted fund is an item of $41,000 due from the restricted funds. This is balanced by the ''due to unrestricted fund'' liabilities shown in the restricted funds ($12,000 in the specific purpose fund, $25,000 in the plant replacement and expansion fund, and $4,000 in the endowment fund). Interfund receivables and payables of this sort may arise when interfund transfers are appropriate but resources are not currently available. Such receivables and payables may represent interfund borrowings, however. All such borrowings should be documented and formally approved by the hospital's governing board.

Assets

Unrestricted Fund

Current Assets:			
Cash		$ 192,068	
Temporary Investments		175,000	
Accrued Interest Receivable		8,124	
Receivables—Patients	$1,192,563		
Less Allowance for Uncollectibles	122,056	1,070,507	
Due from Other Funds		41,000	
Inventories		87,000	
Prepaid Expenses		9,260	
Total Current Assets			$1,582,959
Property, Plant, and Equipment:			
Land		175,000	
Buildings		5,000,000	
Equipment		3,505,345	
Total		8,680,345	
Less Accumulated Depreciation		2,302,679	
Net Property, Plant, and Equipment			6,377,666
Total Unrestricted Fund Assets			$7,960,625

Restricted Funds

Specific Purpose Fund:			
Cash		$ 10,300	
Investments		289,160	
Total Specific Purpose Fund Assets			$ 299,460
Plant Replacement and Expansion Fund:			
Cash		$ 9,267	
Pledges Receivable	$ 184,929		
Less Allowance for Uncollectibles	20,450	164,479	
Investments		1,591,583	
Total Plant Replacement and Expansion Fund Assets			$1,765,329
Endowment Fund:			
Cash		$ 1,371	
Investments		2,924,029	
Total Endowment Fund Assets			$2,925,400

Figure 15–6 Hartful Hospital Balance Sheet, December 31, 19X1

Liabilities and Fund Balances

Unrestricted Fund

Current Liabilities:

Notes Payable	$ 125,000	
Accounts Payable	72,384	
Accrued Payroll	31,270	
Payroll Taxes Withheld and Accrued	9,242	
Accrued Interest Payable	40,163	
Deferred Rental Income	1,450	
Total Current Liabilities		$ 279,509
Bonds Payable		2,400,000
Total Liabilities		2,679,509
Unrestricted Fund Balance		5,281,116
Total Unrestricted Fund Liabilities and Fund Balance		$7,960,625

Restricted Funds

Specific Purpose Fund:		
Due to Unrestricted Fund	$ 12,000	
Fund Balance	287,460	
Total Specific Purpose Fund Liabilities and Fund Balance		$ 299,460
Plant Replacement and Expansion Fund:		
Due to Unrestricted Fund	$ 25,000	
Fund Balance	1,740,329	
Total Plant Replacement and Expansion Fund		
Liabilities and Fund Balance		$1,765,329
Endowment Fund:		
Due to Unrestricted Fund	$ 4,000	
Fund Balance	2,921,400	
Total Endowment Fund Liabilities and Fund Balance		$2,925,400

Figure 15–6 Hartful Hospital Balance Sheet, December 31, 19X1 (*continued*)

Questions   Q15–1. Distinguish between unrestricted and restricted resources.

Q15–2. Define fund accounting. Why is fund accounting a useful system of accounting for many hospitals?

Q15–3. What is a "board-designated fund"? Explain why the resources of funds of this kind are not classified as restricted resources.

Q15–4. Offside Hospital received donations of (a) an item of medical equipment having a fair market value of $100,000 and (b) $100,000 cash restricted by the donor to the purchase of medical equipment. How should each of these donations be accounted for when received? Explain why the treatment differs.

Q15–5. Only Hospital received a $300,000 cash donation that is restricted by the donor. In what fund do you think this $300,000 should be recorded?

Q15–6. Only Hospital received a $300,000 cash donation that was not restricted by the donor in any manner. The governing board of the hospital, however, voted to restrict this $300,000 to the purchase of plant assets. In what fund should this donation be recorded? Explain the reason.

Q15–7. When should resources be transferred from the specific purpose funds to the unrestricted fund?

Q15–8. When should resources be transferred from the plant replacement and expansion funds to the unrestricted fund of the hospital?

Q15–9. When, if ever, should resources be transferred from the unrestricted fund to the plant replacement and expansion funds? When, if ever, should resources be transferred from the endowment funds to the unrestricted fund?

Q15–10. If investments held in a restricted fund are sold at a gain, in what fund should the gain be recorded?

Q15–11. In what fund should unrestricted investment income earned on endowment fund investments be recorded?

Q15–12. In the context of "fund accounting," what does the word *fund* mean?

Q15–13. List, and describe briefly, each of the four types of funds used in hospital accounting.

Q15–14. During 19X1, Open Hospital's unrestricted fund received $18,000 cash from its specific purpose funds. Of this total, $13,000 was for charity service and $5,000 for research activities. How should the $18,000 be recorded in the accounts of the unrestricted fund?

P15–1. OK Hospital employs an unrestricted fund, a specific purpose fund, a plant replacement and expansion fund, and an

Problems

endowment fund. Certain of the transactions completed by the hospital during 19X1 are indicated here:

1. The hospital received a $150,000 cash donation not restricted by donors in any manner.
2. The hospital received, as a donation, laboratory equipment having a fair market value of $40,000.
3. The hospital received a $40,000 cash donation restricted by donor to the purchase of new laboratory equipment. The equipment was subsequently purchased at a cost of $45,000.
4. The hospital received a $30,000 cash donation restricted by the donor to the financing of charity service by the hospital. The specified charity service was subsequently provided by the hospital.
5. The hospital received a $14,000 cash donation restricted by the donor to the financing of certain research activities by the hospital. The specified research activity was later completed by the hospital.
6. The hospital received pledges in the amount of $90,000 from donors who wished to contribute to future purchases of plant assets. It is estimated that 85 percent of these pledges will prove to be collectible.
7. The hospital received a $500,000 cash donation that was donor-restricted as a permanent endowment of the hospital. Subsequently:
   a. The $500,000 was invested in corporate securities.
   b. The $500,000 of investments earned $35,000 of dividends and interest during 19X1. According to the provisions of the endowment, 60 percent of the investment income is restricted to the purchase of plant assets and the remaining 40 percent is unrestricted.
8. The unrestricted fund borrowed $75,000 from a specific purpose fund. The loan was subsequently repaid in full along with interest of $3,000.

Required: Prepare, in general journal form, the necessary entries to record all of the above transactions. Specify the particular fund in which each entry should be made.

P15–2. Oldtown Hospital provides you with the following account balances at March 31, 19X1:

Cash—Endowment $ 18,000
Inventories   27,000

Deferred Revenue (Current)	6,000
Accumulated Depreciation	242,000
Investments—Board-Designated	47,000
Notes Payable to Banks	11,000
Receivables—Patients	57,000
Investments—Specific Purpose Fund	92,000
Bonds Payable	80,000
Prepaid Expenses (Current)	5,000
Investments—Unrestricted Fund (Current)	14,000
Accrued Expenses Payable	13,000
Cash—Board-Designated	5,000
Investments—Endowment Fund	303,000
Accounts Payable	41,000
Land	8,000
Allowance for Uncollectible Accounts	15,000
Mortgage Payable (Noncurrent)	135,000
Equipment	260,000
Cash—Plant Replacement and Expansion Fund	17,000
Cash—Unrestricted Fund (Current)	14,000
Building	320,000
Current Portion of Long-Term Debt	10,000
Investments—Plant Replacement and Expansion Fund	174,000
Cash—Specific Purpose Fund	3,000

Required: Prepare, in good form, an all-funds balance sheet for Oldtown Hospital as of March 31, 19X1.

P15–3. Orwell Hospital provides you with the following information taken from its accounting records as of September 30, 19X2, the end of its fiscal year:

Interest expense		$ 11,000
Transfer received from specific purpose fund for:		
Charity service	$14,000	
Education	9,000	23,000
Transfer received from plant replacement and expansion fund for purchase of plant assets		52,000
Nursing service expense		134,000
Deductions from revenues		99,000
Income from board-designated investments		7,000

General services expense	108,000
Depreciation expense	12,000
Unrestricted gifts and bequests	36,000
Gross patient service revenues	422,000
Fiscal services expense	29,000
Unrestricted income from endowment fund	21,000
Other professional services expense	101,000
Other operating revenues	31,000
Administrative services expense	22,000
Unrestricted fund balance, October 1, 19X1	325,000

Required: (1) Prepare an income statement for the year ended September 30, 19X2. (2) Prepare a statement of changes in the unrestricted fund balance for the year ended September 30, 19X2.

P15–4. Oddly Hospital provides you with the following information that relates to the year ended June 30, 19X2:

Cafeteria sales	$ 240,000
Transfer to unrestricted fund from plant replacement and expansion fund for plant asset acquisitions	120,000
Cash—unrestricted fund (current)	190,000
Cash—endowment fund	1,000
Accrued salaries and wages payable	32,000
Nursing services expense	2,500,000
Gross revenues—nursing services	3,600,000
General contributions (unrestricted)	29,000
Donated medical equipment	40,000
Donated resources received— endowment fund	90,000
Land	166,000
Cash—plant replacement and expansion fund	9,300
Unrestricted fund balance, June 30, 19X1	?
Deductions from revenues—bad debts	54,000

General services expense		770,000
Deferred rental income (current)		2,000
Due to unrestricted fund from:		
Specific purpose fund	$15,000	
Plant replacement and expansion fund	34,000	
Endowment fund	6,000	55,000
Revenues—other professional services		2,800,000
Unrestricted income from endowment fund		28,000
Investment income—specific purpose fund		17,000
Endowment fund balance, June 30, 19X1		?
Investment income—plant replacement and expansion fund		108,000
Temporary investments—unrestricted fund (current)		108,000
Equipment		3,500,000
Notes payable		80,000
Bonds payable		2,500,000
Cash—specific purpose fund		12,000
Accrued interest receivable		9,000
Accumulated depreciation		2,400,000
Deductions from revenue—charity service		201,000
Other professional services expense		987,000
Prepaid expenses (current)		8,000
Investments—endowment fund		3,000,000
Accounts payable		75,000
Specific purpose fund balance, June 30, 19X1		?
Buildings		5,500,000
Inventories		110,000
Rental income		15,000
Fiscal services expense		354,000
Purchase discounts		26,000

Deductions from revenue— contractual adjustments		403,000
Payroll taxes withheld and accrued		7,000
Plant replacement and expansion fund balance, June 30, 19X1		?
Accrued interest payable		41,000
Donated resources received— specific purpose fund		124,000
Investment gains:		
Specific purpose fund	$ 8,000	
Plant replacement and expansion fund	3,000	
Endowment fund	14,000	25,000
Administrative services expense		1,004,000
Donated resources received—plant replacement and expansion fund		230,000
Transfers from specific purpose fund to unrestricted fund for:		
Charity service	$29,000	
Research	40,000	
Education	52,000	121,000
Receivables—patients		1,300,000
Investments—specific purpose fund		290,000
Allowance for uncollectible accounts		140,000
Investments—plant replacement and expansion fund		1,600,000
Income on unrestricted fund investments		13,000
Plant asset pledges receivable (net)		206,000

Required: Prepare in good form (1) an income statement for the year ended June 30, 19X2, (2) a statement of changes in fund balances for the year ended June 30, 19X2, and (3) a balance sheet at June 30, 19X2.

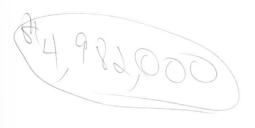

Quick Assets

The *quick assets* of a hospital consist of cash and those other assets (temporary investments and receivables) that can be quickly and directly converted into cash. This chapter discusses certain of the accounting problems and procedures related to such assets. Although cash, marketable securities, and receivables may appear in any fund, most of the materials of this chapter relate to the quick assets of the unrestricted fund. You should understand, however, that the accounting methods and practices described here are generally applicable to the quick assets found in the restricted funds.

Cash

Cash may be defined as consisting of actual money and other immediately available resources or credit instruments generally accepted as media of exchange and used as money equivalents. This includes coin and paper currency, demand deposits in banks, checks, and money orders. Postage stamps, however, are supplies, not cash. Postdated checks and IOUs from employees are properly treated as receivables. The very essence of cash is its availability as a medium of exchange.

Considerable attention is given to cash accounting because of its rather obvious value as the means of financing hospital activities. Cash also is the asset likely to be most susceptible to fraudulent misappropriation by employees and others. Finally, it should be recognized that, because of the large volume of cash transactions hospitals complete, the incidence of honest errors can be quite high unless appropriate accounting procedures and internal controls are observed.

Bank Reconciliations

The bank reconciliation (illustrated in Figure 16–1) should be regarded as one of the more important accounting and internal

	Books		Bank	
	Dr.	Cr.	Dr.	Cr.
Balances, 11/30	$182,062			$168,934

Deposits in transit, 11/30:

Date	Amount				
11/29	21,604				
11/30	18,217				
Total					39,821

Checks outstanding, 11/30:

Date	Number	Amount				
10/19	4529	1,361				
10/27	4326	412				
11/10	4533	89				
.	.	.				
.	.	.				
11/30	4517	145				
Total					$19,655	
Bank service charges for November			$ 37		

NSF checks returned by bank:

		Books Dr.	Books Cr.	Bank Dr.	Bank Cr.
Robert M. Patient check dated 11/14; deposited 11/17			519		
William L. Patient check dated 11/20; deposited 11/21			909		
Collection of treasury bills by bank		25,000			
Bank errors:					
Deposit of 11/27 omitted from bank statement					16,400
Check of Othercity Hospital erroneously charged against Homecity account					187
Book errors:					
Check #4649 for $234, dated 11/15, erroneously journalized as $324		90			
Totals		207,152	1,465	19,655	225,342
Offsets		1,465			19,655
Adjusted balances, 11/30		205,687			205,687

Figure 16–1 Homecity Hospital Bank Reconciliation—General Checking Account, November 30, 19X1

control procedures. It aids in the prevention and detection of fraud, the discovery of errors in accounting records, and the determination of the accuracy of the bank statement. Bank statements, of course, should be delivered unopened to the person who is to perform the reconciliation, and they should remain in that person's control until the reconciliation is completed. Reconciliations should be supervised by the hospital controller and should be performed by someone who does not handle cash or cash records.

A bank reconciliation is primarily a matter of adjusting two incorrect cash balances (the ledger balance and the bank statement balance) to a correct amount representing the actual amount of cash over which the hospital has control, that is, the cash balance to be reported in the balance sheet. Ordinarily, the book balance will be incorrect, for two reasons:

Reasons for Errors in the Book Balance

1. Items may have been properly subtracted from the bank statement balance, but not from the book balance (for example, bank service charges and patients' checks deposited by the hospital that prove to be uncollectible), and
2. Items may have been properly added to the bank statement balance, but not to the book balance (for example, collections of items by the bank on behalf of the hospital).

To reconcile, the Type 1 items are deducted from the book balance, and the Type 2 items are added to the book balance.

On the other hand, the bank statement balance normally will not be correct because

Reasons for Errors in the Bank Statement

1. Items may have been properly added to the book balance, but not to the bank balance (for example, hospital deposits in transit at the bank statement date).
2. Items may have been properly subtracted from the book balance, but not from the bank balance (for example, checks issued and outstanding at the bank statement date).

To reconcile, the Type 1 items are added to the bank statement balance, and the Type 2 items are deducted from the bank statement balance.

In addition, both the book and bank statement balances may not be correct because of errors made by the hospital and the bank. Banks do make errors!

To illustrate the bank reconciliation procedure, assume that the general checking account of Homecity Hospital has a November 30, 19X1, general ledger balance of $182,062. A few days following the end of the month, the hospital receives the November bank statement that reports a November 30, 19X1, balance of only $168,934! Neither of these figures should be reported as the cash balance in the hospital's month-end balance sheet. The two figures must be reconciled to an adjusted (correct) balance. This is accomplished through a reconciliation of the book and bank balances in the manner shown in Figure 16–1.

The reconciliation begins with the entry of the November 30 balances in the respective book and bank columns. The $182,062 book balance is obtained from the general ledger account (1011.0); the $168,934 bank balance is found on the November bank statement. Typically, it is to be hoped, the book balance is a debit balance while the bank balance normally is a credit balance (from the bank's point of view, the hospital's balance is a liability of the bank). If the account is overdrawn, of course, the book balance will be a credit, and the bank balance will be a debit.

The next step is to list the deposits in transit at November 30. A deposit in transit is a deposit made by the hospital (usually on the last day or so of the month) that does not appear on the bank statement for that month. At some banks there may be a lag or delay of a day or so in recording customer's deposits, particularly where the customer makes deposits after banking hours through 24-hour banking stations and night depository systems. Deposits in transit may be identified by a comparison of deposits as shown on the bank statement with entries in the cash receipts journal.

Deposits as Debits to Hospital and Credits on Bank Statements

If the hospital deposits all receipts daily and intact (as it should), daily debits to cash in the journal will be the same amounts as the daily bank deposits. If a deposit was listed as in transit on the prior month's reconciliation, the person making the reconciliation also should ascertain that the deposit appears on the current month's bank statement. (Note that deposits are debits on the hospital's books but appear as credits on the bank statement because, from the bank's point of view, the hospital's cash balance is a liability.)

Note in the figure that Homecity Hospital has two deposits in transit on November 30 that total $39,821. This amount has been included in the hospital's November receipts per books but does not appear as deposits on the November bank statement. To reconcile, therefore, the $39,821 is credited (added) to the bank balance in the reconciliation. As a part of the December 31, 19X1, reconciliation process, the person preparing it should make sure that this $39,821 appears as deposits on the December bank statement.

Checks Compared to Last Month's Reconciliation and Journals

Next, the checks outstanding at November 30 are listed by date, number, and amount on the reconciliation. When the November bank statement is received, the checks included with the statement are arranged in numerical order and are compared (1) with the listing of checks outstanding on the prior month's (October) reconciliation and (2) with the hospital's cash disbursements journal and payroll journal entries of the current month. An investigation should be made of checks that remain outstanding from the prior month's reconciliation to determine whether payment should be stopped on such checks. And, perhaps on a sample basis, the endorsements on canceled checks might be examined for possible irregularities.

As of November 30, Homecity Hospital had a total of $19,655 of outstanding checks. These are checks that were written and included in the hospital's disbursements but that had not yet been presented to the hospital's bank for payment. The bank has no knowledge of this "float" and consequently did not reduce the hospital's checking account balance for those checks. This situation arises because payees sometimes hold the hospital's checks for a few days before cashing them, because delays occur in the postal system, and because time is required for checks to clear the banking system. In any event, the outstanding checks are debited to (deducted from) the bank balance in the reconciliation because the hospital no longer has control of the amount of money represented by such items. The person who prepares the December 31 reconciliation should determine whether these $19,655 of outstanding checks clear the bank in December.

The November bank statement includes a number of debit and credit memos that specify certain special items that have been charged or credited by the bank to the hospital's account. One of the debit memos indicates that the bank service charge for November was $37. This has been deducted by the bank in arriving at the hospital's November 30 balance, but the $37 has not yet been recorded in the hospital's November disbursements. The bank service charges are credited to the books column of the reconciliation.

Debit Memos

Two other debit memos are for *NSF (not sufficient funds)* checks that were received from patients, recorded as cash receipts, and deposited by the hospital during November. Unfortunately, those patients did not have sufficient funds in their checking accounts to cover these checks. These checks appeared as deposits (November 17 and 21) on the bank statement but, when their NSF status was determined, the bank subsequently charged them back against the hospital's account. So, to reconcile, the $1,428 total of bad checks must be credited to the book balance in the reconciliation. These defaulting patients should immediately be contacted to work out a plan to make these checks good. The writing of bad checks is a serious matter, and steps should be taken by the hospital to recover those amounts.

The November bank statement also includes a credit memo representing the collection by the bank of $25,000 of treasury bills for the hospital. These bills, which are issued by the U.S. Treasury Department, were being held as temporary investments by the hospital. They matured late in November and were turned over to

Credit Memos

the bank for collection from the government. (A part of the November service charge includes the fee charged by the bank for this collection service.) The $25,000 appearing on the bank statement as a deposit must be debited to the books column of the reconciliation.

Comparisons made of the bank statement with the hospital's cash records uncovered certain errors made by the bank during November as well as an error made by the hospital's accounting personnel during the month. One of the bank errors was an omission from the bank statement of a $16,400 deposit that was made by the hospital on November 27. Apparently, the bank credited this deposit in error to another customer's account. In order to reconcile, the omitted deposit must be credited to the bank columns of the reconciliation. The bank also made an error in charging one of Othercity Hospital's checks for $187 against Homecity Hospital's account. This is reconciled by a credit to the bank columns.

The error made by Homecity Hospital was in journalizing check number 4649, written for $234 in payment of an account payable, in the incorrect amount of $324. This caused an understatement of $90 ($324 − $234) in the month-end ledger cash balance. To reconcile, the $90 must be added back to the book balance.

Totaling the Columns

After all necessary adjustments have been determined, each of the columns of the reconciliation is totaled. Then, the "books" credit column total is offset against the "books" debit column total, and the bank debit column total is offset against the bank credit column total. This provides the adjusted (correct) cash balance at November 30, or $205,687. This is the cash balance that should be reported in Homecity Hospital's balance sheet at November 30, 19X1. But, because the general ledger account has a $182,062 balance, an adjusting entry is required in the hospital's general journal:

Cash—General Checking Account	$23,625	
Accounts Receivable—Patients	1,428	
Fiscal Services—Supplies and Expense	37	
Temporary Investments		$25,000
Accounts Payable		90
Adjustment of accounts per November 30, 19X1, bank reconciliation.		

The debit of $23,625 increases the general ledger cash balance to $205,687, the debit of $1,428 charges the bad checks back to the patients' accounts, and the $37 debit records the bank service charges as November expenses. The credit of $25,000 eliminates the treasury bills from the temporary investments account, and the credit of $90 corrects the error in accounts payable (when check number 4649 was entered in the cash disbursements journal, $90 too much was debited to the accounts payable account). Notice that no entry is necessary for deposits in transit, outstanding checks, or bank errors. The deposits in transit and the outstanding checks have already been recorded in the hospital's accounts; the bank errors will be called to the bank's attention so that they may be corrected by the bank in its December statement.

The bank reconciliation is an important document; it should not be destroyed. All reconciliations should be retained in appropriate files for review by the hospital's internal and external auditors.

Sometimes bank reconciliations are accomplished by adjusting the bank balance into agreement with the ledger balance (previously adjusted to a correct figure). Although this method will produce a reconciliation and is employed by some auditors, the procedure illustrated in Figure 16–1 is described here for pedagogical reasons and because it always produces the proper balance sheet figure for cash and organizes all the necessary adjustments in one place, and that is in the "books" debit and credit columns. Other reconciliation methods may not necessarily provide these two advantages.

As noted in Chapter 14, the use of a special payroll checking account greatly facilitates the bank reconciliation process. The special payroll account allows the large volume of payroll checks to be removed from the general checking account reconciliation. The payroll checking account ordinarily will require no reconciliation, because it tends to reconcile itself to a zero or imprest balance. This is true because the deposit of the net payroll amount in the account is exactly offset by the total of the individual payroll checks clearing the account. To encourage employees to deposit their payroll checks promptly, payroll checks may be printed to read "void if not presented for payment within 30 days." Other special checking accounts may be established, if useful, for other frequently recurring disbursements such as payroll taxes, equipment purchases, and interest payments on the hospital's long-term debt (bonds payable, for example).

A hospital should not keep unnecessary cash on hand. All cash receipts should be deposited daily and intact; disbursements should

Retention of Bank Reconciliations

Imprest Cash Funds

never be made directly from cash receipts. As a general rule, disbursements should be made only by checks, properly authorized and supported by appropriate vouchers. Any violations of these basic control principles are open invitations to confusion, error, and fraud.

As a practical matter, however, provision usually must be made for the keeping of cash funds in limited amounts from which cash disbursements can be made for items for which the writing of checks is not feasible. For this reason, hospitals often must maintain several so-called petty cash funds, change funds, and check cashing funds. The need for such funds should be evaluated regularly so that their number and size will be neither excessive nor inadequate. All such funds should be accounted for on an imprest basis; that is, each fund should be established in a fixed amount that is replenished periodically when that amount has been exhausted. Responsibility for each imprest (fixed amount) fund should be assigned to a specific employee who, as the fund custodian, has sole control over it.

Petty Cash Funds.   To illustrate the accounting procedures for petty cash funds, assume that Homecity Hospital decides to establish such a fund in the imprest amount of $750. Accordingly, a check for this amount is drawn payable to the appointed petty cash custodian who cashes the check and places the money for safekeeping in a locked petty cash drawer or box. The entries are as follows:

Voucher Register		
Petty Cash Fund	$750	
Accounts Payable		$750
Voucher to establish petty cash fund of $750.		
Cash Disbursements Journal		
Accounts Payable	$750	
Cash—General Checking Account		$750
Check issued to establish an imprest petty cash fund of $750.		

Petty Cash Documentation

Disbursements from the fund are made only by the petty cash custodian, and then only in return for signed receipts, petty cash slips or vouchers, and other supporting documents. A typical petty cash disbursement form is illustrated in Figure 16–2. As cash is paid out of the fund, these forms are completed and retained in the petty cash drawer or box.

```
┌─────────────────────────────────────────────────────────────────────┐
│                                                                       │
│                  PETTY CASH DISBURSEMENT                              │
│                                                                       │
│   No._____      Date_____ 19_____        │
│                                                                       │
│                                       $ _____             │
│                                                                       │
│   TO_____         │
│                                                                       │
│   Amount_____ DOLLARS         │
│                                                                       │
│   For _____                │
│                                                                       │
│   _____                │
│                                                                       │
│   Account Number _____                │
│                                                                       │
│   Approved                     Received                               │
│   By_____  Payment _____                │
│                                                                       │
└─────────────────────────────────────────────────────────────────────┘
```

Figure 16–2 Petty Cash Disbursement Slip

When the fund is found to be nearly exhausted, and routinely at the end of each month, a reimbursement check may be drawn to replenish the fund to its imprest amount. Assume that the contents of the petty cash box at month end are as follows:

Coin and currency	$ 87
Petty cash disbursement slips	635
IOU from employee	25
Total	$747

The coin and currency in the box, of course, were determined by actual count. The disbursement slips are removed from the box, totaled, and summarized according to the accounts to be debited for the expenditures. This summary analysis can be entered on the back of specially printed petty cash disbursements envelopes such as the one shown in Figure 16–3. When the summary is completed, the cash disbursement slips are placed in the envelope and become a part of the voucher package for the check to be drawn to replenish the petty cash fund.

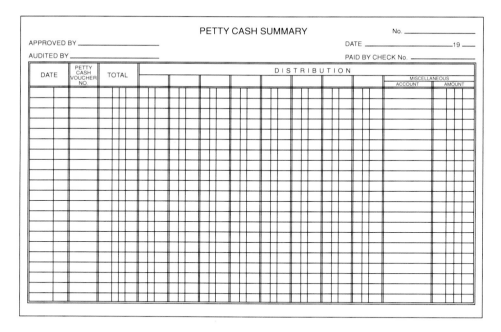

Figure 16–3 Petty Cash Disbursements Summary

For simplicity, let us assume that the petty cash disbursements of $635 are chargeable only to the accounting department ($415) and the laboratory department ($220). The necessary entries to replenish the fund are as follows:

Voucher Register

Accounting—Supplies and Expense	$415	
Laboratory—Supplies and Expense	220	
Accounts Receivable—Employees	25	
Cash Over and Short	3	
Accounts Payable		$663
Voucher for check to replenish the petty cash fund to the imprest amount.		

Cash Disbursements Journal

Accounts Payable	$663	
Cash—General Checking Account		$663
Check issued to replenish the petty cash fund to the imprest amount.		

Notice that the employee's $25 IOU is debited to Accounts Receivable—Employees. This represents an improper use of the petty cash fund, and the custodian should be instructed not to allow employees to borrow from the fund. Note also that the $3 shortage in the fund is debited to a special cash over and short account that is treated as either a miscellaneous expense or miscellaneous income account, depending on its balance at the end of the reporting period.

The $663 check is drawn payable to the petty cash custodian who cashes it and places the money in the petty cash box. This $663 plus the $87, which was remaining in the fund at the time of reimbursement, brings the petty cash drawer up to a total of $750 again. These replenishments are made as often as the fund is depleted, or at least at the end of each monthly reporting period.

It should be recognized that nowhere in the reimbursement process is the petty cash account debited or credited. This is done only when the imprest amount of the fund is increased or decreased. If reimbursements are required often enough to be bothersome, the imprest amount of the fund might be considered inadequate. Assume, for example, that it is decided to increase the above fund to $1,000. A check therefore is drawn for $250 and is debited to the petty cash account. On the other hand, if reimbursements are infrequent, this may be an indication that the imprest amount is excessive. Suppose, for example, that a decision is made to reduce the $750 fund to an imprest amount of $400. In this case, one would remove $350 of currency from the petty cash box and deposit it in the hospital's general checking account, crediting the petty cash account.

Debits and Credits to Petty Cash

Other Imprest Funds. Hospitals often establish change funds in nominal amounts at cash receiving locations for the purpose of providing change to patients, employees, and visitors. These funds should be balanced daily to the total of recorded cash receipts plus the imprest amount of the change fund. In depositing cash receipts, over and short variations are considered to be in the day's receipts and not in the change fund that is retained in its imprest amount.

Funds for Making Change

Although hospital policy ordinarily should be that of not cashing any personal or payroll checks for anyone, check-cashing funds often are established as a convenience to employees. Where such check-cashing funds are necessary, they should be maintained on an imprest basis. The custodian of such funds should be independent of all payroll functions.

Internal cash controls are essential in the hospital's business offices and at all other locations where cash is received or disbursed. These

Internal Cash Controls

safeguards must be built into the accounting system if hospital cash resources are to be accurately recorded and adequately protected from error and misappropriation. A description of many of these controls and the related accounting procedures for the processing of cash receipts and disbursements has been provided in previous chapters, particularly in Chapters 12 and 14. It would now be useful to provide a listing of some of the basic principles typically incorporated into internal cash control systems:

- All hospital employees who handle or have access to cash should be adequately bonded.
- Petty cash and change funds should be limited in number and should be established in minimum imprest amounts.
- Bank accounts should be reconciled regularly by persons other than those who handle cash receipts, sign checks, or maintain the cash journals and records.
- There must be a distinct segregation of duties between cash handling and cash accounting (for example, persons who handle incoming cash should not have control of the accounts receivable records).
- All cash record forms—checks, bank deposit tickets, cash receipt slips, and petty cash vouchers—should be prenumbered and accounted for by numerical sequence whenever this is feasible.
- Definite responsibility for cash-handling functions and for custody of cash funds should be assigned to specific employees.
- The fewest possible employees should be given access to cash.
- The work of business office personnel should be made complementary so that an error made by one automatically will be discovered by another.
- Physical protection should be provided through the use of vaults, bank facilities, cashiers' cages, locked cash drawers, and similar devices.
- Definite procedures should be established in writing for the handling of all cash transactions.
- Office procedures should be so arranged that misappropriations are unlikely to go undetected with the collusion of two or more employees.
- Internal audits and surprise cash counts should be made by a responsible employee at irregular intervals.

Although this listing is not by any means complete, it is indicative of some of the procedures to be observed in a sound internal control system.

Temporarily excessive cash balances should always be invested by the hospital in bank savings accounts, certificates of deposit, U.S. treasury bills, or in some other type of income-producing asset. The investment objectives should be safety, marketability, and a reasonable rate of return. These temporary or short-term investments may appear in the hospital's restricted funds as well as in its unrestricted fund, although long-term investments are more commonly found in the endowment funds and in the plant expansion and replacement funds.

To illustrate the accounting procedures for temporary investments in bonds (sometimes referred to as *marketable debt securities*), assume that Homecity Hospital's cash budget indicates that $40,000 of cash should be available for investment for about four months. Accordingly, on October 1, 19X1, the hospital purchases $40,000 of corporate bonds at face value.

These 6 percent bonds pay interest semiannually on November 1 and May 1 (3 percent each interest payment date). Assuming this is an investment of the hospital's unrestricted fund, the entries for 19X1 are shown in Figure 16–4.

The voucher register entry records the investment at cost, which is the quoted price paid for the securities plus brokerage fees and all other acquisition costs. It is assumed here that the quoted price was 100 percent of face, or par, value and that acquisition costs totaled $65. For accounting purposes, then, the cost of this investment was $40,065. Had these securities been quoted at, say, 98, the price paid for them would have been $39,200 (98 percent of $40,000), and the cost of the investment would have been recorded as $39,265 ($39,200 + $65).

Because these bonds were acquired between interest payment dates, the seller must be paid the accrued interest on the bonds since the last interest payment date—that is, from May 1 to October 1 (five months' accrued interest). This $1,000 is not charged to expense but to accrued interest receivable because it will be recovered by the hospital on November 1, when the bond issuer pays six months' interest to bondholders. Accrued interest settlements always are made in this manner between investors who trade in bonds. It would not be feasible for the bond issuer to attempt to make these adjustments. Instead, the issuer always pays six months' interest on each interest payment date regardless of the length of time the investor has held the bonds.

On October 31, and at the end of each subsequent monthly reporting period so long as Homecity Hospital holds these bonds, a

Temporary Investments

Example of Accounting Procedures for Temporary Investments

Voucher Register

10/1	Temporary Investments		$40,065	
	Accrued Interest Receivable		1,000	
	Accounts Payable			$41,065

Purchase of temporary investments as follows:

Purchase price (face value)	$40,000
Acquisition costs	65
Total cost	40,065
Accrued interest: $40,000 \times 0.06 \times 5/12$	1,000
Total disbursement	$41,065

Cash Disbursements Journal

10/1	Accounts Payable	$41,065	
	Cash—General Checking Account		$41,065
	Check issued for purchase of temporary investments.		

General Journal

| 10/31 | Accrued Interest Receivable | $ 200 | |
| | Interest Income | | $ 200 |

Accrual of interest income earned on temporary investments in
October: $40,000 \times 0.06 \times 1/12$.

Cash Receipts Journal

| 11/1 | Cash—General Checking Account | $ 1,200 | |
| | Accrued Interest Receivable | | $ 1,200 |

Receipt of semiannual interest on temporary investments:
$40,000 \times 0.06 \times 6/12$.

General Journal

| 11/30 | Accrued Interest Receivable | $ 200 | |
| | Interest Income | | $ 200 |

Accrual of interest income earned on temporary investments in
November.

General Journal

| 12/31 | Accrued Interest Receivable | $ 200 | |
| | Interest Income | | $ 200 |

Accrual of interest income earned on temporary investments in
December.

Figure 16–4 Entries for Temporary Investments

general journal adjusting entry is required to record the accrued
interest income on the investment. The amount of this entry is an
approximation of interest for one month; precise computations to
exact days or cents can be made but are not necessary in recording
most accruals of this type. Note that the October 31 entry increases

the balance of the accrued interest receivable account to $1,200, that is, the amount of the semiannual interest received the following day (November 1).

On December 31, the interest income account has a balance of $600, which is reported in Homecity Hospital's 19X1 income statement as nonoperating revenue. The $400 of accrued interest receivable will be reported in the hospital's year-end balance sheet as a current asset. The December 31, 19X1, balance sheet also will report the investment at its cost of $40,065.

Suppose, however, that the December 31 quoted market price of these bonds has risen to 102 ($40,800), or has fallen to 97 ($38,800). Should the carrying value of the investment be adjusted (written up or down) to current market value? Under current generally accepted accounting principles, temporary investments in bonds usually are carried in the accounts and in the balance sheet at their *original acquisition cost* with *market value indicated parenthetically or by footnote.* Some accountants argue, however, that such investments should be valued at the lower of cost or market value; others believe that such investments should be reported at market value, whether this is higher or lower than cost. We shall use the cost valuation.

To complete this illustration, let us assume that these investments are sold by the hospital at 102.5 and accrued interest on January 1, 19X2, with brokerage fees and other expenses of sale amounting to $76. The cash receipts journal entry is as follows:

Cash—General Checking Account	$41,324	
Accrued Interest Receivable		$ 400
Temporary Investments		40,065
Gain on Sale of Temporary		
Investments		859
Sale of temporary investments as		
follows:		
Sale price ($40,000 × 102.5)	$41,000	
Less brokerage and other		
expenses of sale	76	
Net proceeds from sale	$40,924	
Add accrued interest:		
$40,000 × 0.06 × 2/12	400	
Total cash received	$41,324	

The credit to Accrued Interest Receivable is necessary to eliminate the balance of that account as established by the income accruals at the end of November and December 19X1. A gain of $859 is realized on the sale; it is computed as the difference between the net proceeds ($40,924) and the cost of the investment ($40,065). This gain will be reported in the 19X2 income statement of the hospital among the nonoperating revenues.

Similar procedures are followed in accounting for temporary investments in bonds by the hospital's restricted funds. The accounting procedures for long-term investments in bonds, however, are somewhat different. This matter is pursued at length in Chapter 19.

Short-term investments in corporate stocks usually are reported at the lower of aggregate cost or market. This matter is beyond the scope of this book, but is covered in *Hospital Financial Accounting: Theory and Practice* (Chicago: HFMA, 1987).

Receivables

The term *receivables,* as employed in hospital accounting, refers to the realizable cash value of the hospital's legal claim against its patients, third-party payers, and others. Such receivables arise primarily from the provision of healthcare services to patients on a credit basis. In effect, the hospital exchanges its services, including goods and supplies, for the patient's and/or the third party's promise to pay for such services in the future. It is an economic exchange measured in terms of the hospital's full established rates regardless of expectations about future collectibility.

The resulting revenues and related receivables are recorded on the accrual basis in the time period in which the associated healthcare services are provided. Because there is usually a considerable time lag between the provision of services and the receipt of payment for those services, this practice gives rise to substantial amounts of accounts and notes receivable in the balance sheet.

Receivables may also exist in relatively small amounts from transactions that are only indirectly related to the provision of services to patients. Included in this category are accruals for various miscellaneous items such as interest and rental income earned but not miscellaneous items such as interest and rental income earned but not yet received in cash, advances to employees, tuition charges receivable from students, and donors' pledges receivable. Full and separate disclosure should be made in the hospital balance sheet of all material amounts of these miscellaneous receivables.

Much of the accounting procedure relating to receivables was dealt with in earlier chapters. Here, the discussion is confined to the balance sheet valuation of receivables, accounting for notes receivable, and internal controls for receivables.

Receivables should be reported in the hospital balance sheet at their net realizable value. In other words, the gross amount of receivables recorded at established service rates in the accounts should be reduced to the net amount that can be reasonably estimated to be actually collectible in cash. Appropriate estimates, as described later, should be made of the amounts uncollectible due to bad debts, contractual adjustments, charity service, and other factors. Such estimates are treated as reductions of gross receivables in the balance sheet by the use of the allowance for uncollectibles account. These amounts should also be included as "revenue deductions" in the income statement of the period in which the receivables arose. This procedure is required to secure a proper balance sheet valuation of the receivables as well as to properly match revenues and revenue deductions on an accrual basis.

Bad Debts. It is reasonable to expect that a certain amount of receivables arising from services provided to self-responsible patients will prove to be uncollectible. Uncollectible amounts also may arise from the uninsured portion of the accounts of patients covered by Blue Cross or other third-party payers. At the time of admission, or as soon thereafter as practicable, the financial status of each patient should be determined so that uncollectible amounts can be properly classified and distinguished as arising from bad debts, contractual adjustments, or charity service. After adequate collection efforts have been expended to the point at which additional expenditures cannot be justified on the basis of prospective benefits, amounts still remaining uncollected should be treated as bad debts.

At the end of each reporting period, an estimate must be made of the amount of receivables that ultimately will prove to be bad debts. This is necessary to prevent an overstatement of assets (receivables) in the balance sheet and to provide for a proper matching of revenues and revenue deductions in the income statement of the period in which the receivables originated. It is a procedure required under the accrual basis of accounting.

To illustrate, let us assume that 19X1 is the initial year of operations for Homecity Hospital. During this year, the hospital provided $3.6 million of services to patients and collected $3 million of this amount. At the end of the year, then, accounts receivable total $600,000. Also assume that operating expenses for the year are $3.5 million and that there were no charity patients or contractual adjustments. If nothing is done to consider the possibility of bad debts, the

Valuation of Receivables

Receivables Reported at Net Realizable Value

Estimating Bad Debts

hospital's year-end balance sheet will include $600,000 of accounts receivable among the assets, and the 19X1 income statement will report a net income of $100,000 ($3.6 million–$3.5 million).

In the first several months of 19X2, $564,000 of the 19X1 accounts receivable are collected. The remaining sum of $36,000 (after diligent efforts to collect it) is deemed to be uncollectible, or bad debts. An entry is made to write off these receivables and charge the $36,000 to the 19X2 revenue deductions (Bad Debts) account. Observe, however, that the receivables and the related revenues were recorded in 19X1.

This procedure obviously places the bad debts in the wrong year! The $36,000 of bad debts should have been given accounting recognition as a deduction from revenue in 19X1—the year in which the related revenue was recorded. This means that the net income for 19X1 was overstated by $36,000. In addition, there was a $36,000 overstatement of assets (accounts receivable) in the December 31, 19X1, balance sheet. The receivables should have been stated in that balance sheet at net realizable cash value, or $564,000 ($600,000 − $36,000).

The Three Methods of Estimating Bad Debts

The difficulty, of course, is that it is impossible to predict precisely which individual accounts will prove to be bad debts. It also is impossible to determine precisely the total dollar amount of accounts that will prove to be uncollectible in the future; no one has perfect foresight. Nevertheless, a reasonable estimate can, and should, be made so that the degree of misstatement in the financial statements will be minimized. There are three methods by which bad debts may be estimated for accrual basis accounting purposes:

Method 1: Application of a percentage, based on past experience, to the balance of accounts receivable at the end of the reporting period

Method 2: Application of a percentage, based on past experience, to the total of charges to patients' accounts during the reporting period

Method 3: Determination through an analysis of individual accounts in the patients' ledger, taking into account the length of time each account has remained unpaid ("aging the accounts receivable")

As a matter of actual practice, hospitals often employ all three methods, comparing the results of each so as to arrive at the most accurate estimate of probable bad debts.

The percentage used in these methods often is an average percentage based on several prior years' experience and tempered by expectations of conditions that might exist in the future collection period. Computations of these percentages, of course, are based only on the self-responsible portions of patients' accounts receivable, because billings to third parties are generally collectible in full. In the following example, we assume that an average of about 60 percent of the hospital's charges are billed to third-party payers, leaving 40 percent payable by patients themselves.

Let us return to the end of 19X1 and attempt to estimate the amount of bad debts likely to arise in 19X2 from the $600,000 of accounts receivable. If we use the first method noted and assume that the estimated bad debts percentage is 12 percent, bad debts will be estimated at $28,800:

Using Method 1

Accounts receivable, 12/31/X1	$600,000
Less third-party portion (60%)	360,000
Self-responsible portion	240,000
Percentage of bad debts	12%
Estimated bad debts	$ 28,800

However, if we use the second method and assume that the estimated bad percentage is 2.4 percent of revenues, bad debts will be estimated at $34,560:

Using Method 2

Charges to patients—19X1	$3,600,000
Less third-party portion (60%)	2,160,000
Self-responsible portion	1,440,000
Percentage of bad debts	2.4%
Estimated bad debts	$ 34,560

You should not assume from this example that Method 2 will always provide a larger estimate than Method 1 or that it will produce the most accurate estimate. It can be argued that Method 2 may be statistically superior to Method 1 because of the larger base (charges rather than receivables) used. Under either method, the critical factor is the soundness of assumptions and judgments underlying the determination of the bad debts percentage.

The aging procedure (Method 3) is likely to provide the most accurate estimate of bad debts. It also is the most managerially useful

Using Method 3

| Patient Name | Account Balance | Third-Party Portion | Total | Inhouse | Self Responsible Portion — Elapsed Days Since Discharge | | | | | | Remarks |
					1-30	31-60	61-90	91-180	Over 180	DLP	
Able, Marcus C.	1,420	690	730	730							
Active, James R.	2,466	1,314	1,152		1,152						
Adams, Mary P.	608		608						608		
Agar, Thomas J.	1,190		1,190				1,190				
Akron, Louise M.	782		782			782					
Allen, Richard Q.	532		532					532			
Ammons, Peter C.	808	355	453	453							
Etc.											
Totals	600,000	360,000	240,000	90,000	50,000	40,000	30,000	20,000	10,000		
Bad debt percentages				.05	.08	.12	.20	.40	.90		
Estimated bad debts			6,300	4,500	4,000	4,800	6,000	8,000	9,000		

Figure 16-5 Accounts Receivable Aging Schedule, December 31, 19X1

method in that it requires a detailed, account-by-account examination of patients' receivables. The procedure involves the classification of account balances into "age" groups, depending on the number of days that have elapsed since the date of discharge, as illustrated in Figure 16–5. (In some cases, the aging may be made on the basis of time elapsed since the date of the last payment received on the account. Our illustration merely provides a DLP—date of last payment—column to indicate this information when it is desired.)

As you can see in the aging schedule, a total is obtained for each age group. For example, $90,000 of receivables are inhouse accounts, $50,000 of receivables are 1–30 days "old"; $40,000 are 31–60 days "old"; $30,000 are 61–90 days "old"; and so on. Appropriate percentages based on past experience are then applied to these totals to obtain an estimate of total probable bad debts. As you might expect, the percentage used increases with the age of the accounts. The older the account, the less likely it is to be collected.

Using the bad debt estimate provided by the aging schedule, the required adjusting entry at the end of 19X1 is as follows:

Revenue Deductions—Bad Debts	$ 36,300	
Allowance for Uncollectible		
Accounts—Bad Debts		$ 36,300
Required provision for bad debts per accounts receivable aging schedule.		

Thus, the 19X1 income statement will include the $36,300 of estimated bad debts as a deduction from the patient service revenues of the year. And the balance sheet at December 31, 19X1, will present the receivables as follows:

Accounts Receivable	$600,000	
Less Allowance for Uncollectible		
Accounts—Bad Debts	36,300	$563,700

In this way, the accounts receivable are reduced to net realizable value for balance sheet presentation purposes.

Let us now assume that, during 19X2, $564,000 of these accounts are collected by the hospital. The hospital credit manager concludes that the remaining $36,000 of accounts are definitely uncollectible. The summary entries are the following:

Cash Receipts Journal

Cash—General Checking Account	$564,000	
Accounts Receivable		$564,000
Collections on 19X1 accounts receivable during 19X2.		

General Journal

Allowance for Uncollectible Accounts— Bad Debts	$ 36,000	
Accounts Receivable		$ 36,000
Writeoff of accounts receivable deemed to be bad debts.		

The specific 19X1 accounts written off during 19X2 are removed or otherwise eliminated from the active section of the patients' subsidiary ledger. The ledger cards and related records are placed in an inactive file and are retained under the control of a responsible employee who does not have any access to incoming cash receipts. This is designed to prevent the theft of subsequent cash collections on previously written-off accounts. Where such recoveries are made, the credit should be made to the allowance account or to a special account titled "recoveries of accounts written off."

To complete this illustration, assume that Homecity Hospital's accounts receivable at the end of 19X2 total $685,000. Bad debts are estimated at $41,000, determined in the manner previously described for the end of 19X1. The required adjusting entry for bad debts at December 31, 19X2, is as follows:

General Journal

Revenue Deductions—Bad Debts	$40,700	
Allowance for Uncollectible Accounts—Bad Debts		$40,700
Required provision for bad debts:		
Required allowance account balance (credit)	$41,000	
Present allowance account balance (credit)	300	
Required adjustment	$40,700	

Recall that bad debts were estimated in the amount of $36,300 at the end of 19X1, but actual writeoffs during 19X2 were only $36,000. This means that the allowance account is left with a $300 credit balance at December 31, 19X2. Because a credit balance of $41,000 is required (based on an aging schedule) at the end of 19X2, the adjustment is made for only $40,700. On the other hand, if 19X2 writeoffs had been $38,000, the allowance account would have had a December 31, 19X2, debit balance of $1,700. In that case, the above entry would have been made for $42,700 ($41,000 + $1,700) to obtain the desired $41,000 credit balance in the allowance account.

The same procedure is followed when bad debts are estimated as a percentage of year-end receivables (Method 1). When bad debts are estimated as a percentage of charges (Method 2), however, the estimated amount of bad debts is simply debited to revenue deductions and credited to the allowance for uncollectible accounts. In other words, when Method 1 or Method 3 is employed, the result is the required balance in the allowance for uncollectibles account at the end of the reporting period. The allowance account is adjusted to that balance. When Method 2 is used, however, the result is the amount to be debited to revenue deductions and credited to the allowance account.

Contractual Adjustments.   Under contractual agreements with third-party payers, hospitals often receive less than their full rates and are sometimes prohibited from collecting the difference from patients that are covered by the contract. In such cases, the amount of these differences—called *contractual adjustments*—included in end-of-period receivables must be determined. This may be done by a direct analysis of individual accounts or on a percentage basis developed either from a sample of the accounts or from past experience. The procedure is similar to that for estimating bad debts.

To illustrate, recall (from Figure 16–5) that the third-party portion of Homecity Hospital's December 31, 19X1, receivables was $360,000, measured in terms of the hospital's full service rates. Earlier, it was assumed that the third-party payers paid 100 percent of such rates; now let us assume that the hospital is reimbursed on the average at only 95 percent of such rates. If this 5 percent difference is not billable to the patients involved, the following adjusting entry is required at December 31, 19X1:

Estimating Contractual Adjustments

General Journal

| Revenue Deductions—Contractual Adjustments | $ 18,000 | |
| Allowance for Uncollectible Accounts—Contractual Adjustments | | $ 18,000 |

Required provision for estimated contractual adjustments included in year-end receivables: $360,000 × 5% = $18,000.

Including the previously determined estimate of bad debts, the December 31, 19X2, balance sheet presentation of receivables is the following:

| Accounts Receivable | $600,000 | |
| Less Allowance for Uncollectible Accounts (Estimated Bad Debts, $36,300, and Contractual Adjustments, $18,000) | 54,300 | $545,700 |

The 19X1 income statement, of course, will include the $18,000 of estimated contractual adjustments as a deduction from the patient service revenues of the year. Where the precise amounts of contractual adjustments can be determined, they may be credited directly to accounts receivable rather than to the allowance account.

Assume now that payments received on these accounts from third-party payers in 19X2 amount to $341,000. The necessary entries are summarized below in a single cash receipts journal entry:

Cash Receipts Journal

Cash—General Checking Account	$341,000	
Revenue Deductions—Contractual Adjustments	19,000	
Accounts Receivable		$360,000

Receipt of payments for third-party portion of 12/31/X1 receivables.

Notice that the $19,000 debit is made here to revenue deductions and not to the allowance account because of the assumed design of the cash receipts journal (see the cash receipts journal illustrated in Figure 11–4).

So, at the end of 19X2, the allowance for uncollectible accounts for contractual adjustments remains with the $18,000 credit balance established at the end of 19X1. If the amount of contractual adjustments at December 31, 19X2, is estimated at $19,500, the required adjusting entry is as follows:

General Journal

Revenue Deductions—		
Contractual Adjustments	$1,500	
Allowance for Uncollectible		
Accounts—Contractual		
Adjustments		$1,500
Required provision for		
contractual adjustments at		
12/31/X2:		
Required allowance	$19,500	
Present balance of		
allowance account	18,000	
Required adjustment	$ 1,500	

On the other hand, if the $19,000 were debited to the allowance account in this cash receipts journal entry, the December 31, 19X2, adjustment would be made in the amount of $20,500 ($19,500 plus the debit balance of $1,000 in the allowance account). Either procedure is acceptable.

The preceding illustrations for bad debts and contractual adjustments were presented in annual terms for ease of exposition. You must understand, however, that these adjustments are made monthly in actual practice. This is necessary to make the monthly financial statements more accurate and useful for internal management purposes.

Charity Service.   As indicated in previous chapters (see particularly Chapter 7), uncollectible receivables arising from the provision of charity service to patients may be accounted for using an allowance account in the manner described here for contractual adjustments. This method may be used where the amount of charity service in receivables is determined by estimate rather than by specific identification. In many cases, however, such amounts are readily determinable, and the use of the allowance account method is not necessary. Instead, charity service is recorded by direct credits to the receivables account.

Accounting for Notes Receivable

It is not uncommon for hospitals to accept interest-bearing promissory notes from patients who, faced with a substantial hospital bill, require an extended period of time to accumulate the resources with which to pay their accounts. To illustrate the accounting procedures, assume that a patient gives Homecity Hospital an 8 percent, 90-day promissory note on March 1, 19X1, in settlement of a $9,000 account with the hospital. The total interest on this note is $180 ($9,000 × 0.08 × [90 ÷ 360]), or $2 per day. It should be recognized as earned income by the hospital through monthly accruals, as shown in Figure 16-6. Elapsed days between any two dates are computed by counting the first day or the last day, but not both; in other words, the number of days between March 1 and March 31 is 30.

It is assumed here that the note in question is a *term note receivable,* that is, that the face amount of the note and all interest is payable in a single sum on the maturity date of the note (May 30,

Figure 16-6 Accounting for Notes Receivable

General Journal		
3/1 Notes Receivable	$9,000	
Accounts Receivable		$9,000
Receipt of 8%, 90–day note receivable in settlement of patient's account.		
3/31 Accrued Interest Receivable	$ 60	
Interest Income		$ 60
Interest income earned in March: $9,000 × 0.08 × 1/12 = $60.		
4/30 Accrued Interest Receivable	$ 60	
Interest Income		$ 60
Interest income earned in April: $9,000 × 0.08 × 1/12 = $60.		
Cash Receipts Journal		
5/30 Cash—General Checking Account	$9,180	
Interest Income		$ 60
Accrued Interest Receivable		120
Notes Receivable		9,000
Collection of note receivable and accrued interest.		

19X1). Accounting for installment notes receivable, where the principal amount and interest is payable in periodic installments, is discussed fully in the author's *Hospital Financial Accounting: Theory and Practice* (HFMA, 1987).

Should the patient fail to pay the note at maturity, the debit of $9,180 is made to dishonored notes receivable rather than to cash. The failure of the patient to honor the note, however, in no way changes the fact that interest income of $180 was earned. If further collection efforts are unsuccessful, the $9,180 is written off as a bad debt.

To illustrate how patients' notes receivable may be used as a source of funds by the hospital, let us backtrack to March 31. Assume that the first two entries in Figure 16–6 have already been made, and that the hospital discounts the note receivable at a local bank. Assuming that the bank discount rate is 12 percent, the entry to record the discounting of the note is as follows:

Notes Receivable Used as a Source of Funds

	Cash Receipts Journal		
3/31	Cash—General Checking Account	$8,996	
	Interest Expense	64	
	Accrued Interest Receivable		$ 60
	Notes Receivable Discounted		9,000
	Discounting of a $9,000 note		
	receivable at 12% at local bank.		

The maturity value of this note is $9,180, and there are 60 days remaining before that maturity date. The discount charged by the bank (rounded to the nearest dollar) therefore is $184 [$9,180 × 0.12 × (60 ÷ 360)]. The proceeds of the note to the hospital are $8,996 ($9,180 − $184); that is, on March 31 the bank gives the hospital $8,996 for the patient's note. The hospital gives up the right to receive the $9,180 maturity value of the note. The maturity value will be collected by the bank.

Notice here the credit to notes receivable discounted. This is a contingent liability account. So, assuming that the note was discounted "with recourse" (as is usual), the hospital is obligated to pay the bank $9,180 at the maturity date of the note if the patient does not. This account is presented in the hospital's balance sheet as a direct deduction from notes receivable in the asset section.

No other entries related to this note are made by the hospital until the May 30 maturity date. Following are the two sets of entries to be made on May 30 by the hospital, assuming (1) that the patient pays the bank and (2) that the patient does not pay the bank:

---

(1)	General Journal		
	Notes Receivable Discounted	$9,000	
	Notes Receivable		$9,000
	Payment by patient of discounted note receivable.		
(2)	Voucher Register		
	Notes Receivable Discounted	$9,000	
	Notes Receivable Dishonored	9,195	
	Notes Receivable		$9,000
	Accounts Payable		9,195
	Voucher for payment of discounted note receivable dishonored by patient.		
	Cash Disbursements Journal		
	Accounts Payable	$9,195	
	Cash—General Checking Account		$9,195
	Check issued to pay bank for dishonored note receivable discounted.		

Protest Fee for Dishonored Discounted Notes

When a discounted note is dishonored, the bank generally makes a charge often called a "protest fee." In this case, the fee was $15, making the total payment to the bank $9,195 ($9,000 + $180 + $15). Notice that the face amount of the note, the interest, and the protest fee is charged back to the patient by the debit to notes receivable dishonored. If collection efforts are not fruitful, the $9,195 is written off as a bad debt.

Internal Control

Various internal control principles and procedures have been discussed in earlier chapters, particularly in Chapter 12 where you observed that the control of receivables and the control of revenues are closely linked. Thus, let us limit this discussion to a few general observations about the internal control of hospital receivables.

Initiating Receivables Control in the Admitting Process

Receivables control begins in the admitting process, where complete and accurate information must be secured so that an initial determination can be made of each patient's financial status and unnecessary delays may be avoided in subsequent billing and collection efforts. Once patients are admitted, the system should be such as to provide a high degree of assurance that all billable services rendered are promptly and accurately charged to patients' accounts. Unrecorded revenues are unlikely to be charged; if not charged, they will not be billed; and, if not billed, they will not be collected. Having complete and accurate charges to patients' accounts, the objective becomes that of maximum collection of such charges at the earliest practicable time.

The billing function usually should be performed by someone other than those who maintain the patients' subsidiary ledger records or the cashiers. Sound procedures should be followed (as described in Chapter 12) as collections are received to ensure that patients' accounts are promptly and accurately credited. Noncash credits made to accounts receivable deserve particular attention, as such credits may be used to hide errors and defalcations.

Separating Billing and Collections Responsibilities

Finally, the regular reconciliation of subsidiary ledgers with receivables control accounts must be recognized as an essential internal control practice.

Reconciling Ledgers with Control Accounts

Questions

Q16–1. What are *quick assets*?

Q16–2. Define *cash*. Are postage stamps, postdated checks, and employee IOUs properly includable in "cash"? If not, how should such items be classified in the balance sheet?

Q16–3. For what reasons are bank reconciliations prepared? By whom should bank reconciliations be prepared?

Q16–4. Explain how you would determine the appropriate imprest amount with which to establish a petty cash fund.

Q16–5. Under what circumstances is the petty cash account debited or credited?

Q16–6. List 10 of the most important basic principles typically incorporated into internal cash control systems.

Q16–7. Name three methods by which bad debts may be estimated for accrual basis accounting purposes. Which method is best?

Q16–8. Describe briefly some of the procedures that should be observed to maintain effective internal control over receivables.

Q16–9. Identify and explain the nature of three deductions that may be made to arrive at a balance sheet valuation for accounts receivable.

Q16–10. Define the term *temporary investments*. List some common types of temporary investments available to hospitals.

Q16–11. Purr Hospital's general ledger cash in bank account has a balance of $213,597 as of November 30. The November bank statement, however, shows a balance of $244,129 at the same date. List four types of factors that may cause such a difference and give an example of each.

Q16–12. Briefly describe the imprest system for operating a petty cash fund and state the principal advantages of the imprest system from the standpoint of internal control.

Exercises

E16–1. Pike Hospital's bank statement shows a March 31 balance of $4,200. An analysis discloses that $1,500 of checks are outstanding and that there is a deposit in transit of $900 at March 31. Bank service charges for March were $25 and an "NSF" check of $175 was charged against the hospital's account by the bank on March 28.

The hospital had deposited this patient's check on March 19. The hospital made a deposit of $400 on March 21 that does not appear on the March bank statement, and the bank admitted its error when contacted about it. On March 25, one of the hospital's bookkeepers journalized a properly drawn $50 check (issued in payment of a supplier's invoice) as $500.

Required: What amount should the hospital report as cash in bank in its March 31 balance sheet? What adjusting entry should the hospital make on March 31?

E16–2. Pack Hospital maintains a petty cash fund in the imprest amount of $275. The fund is reimbursed at a time when the contents of the petty cash box are as follows:

Petty cash vouchers	$131
Employee's personal check made payable to Pack Hospital	25
IOU from another employee	10
Coin and currency	106

Here petty cash vouchers include a voucher for a $50 purchase of postage stamps. Unused stamps having a face value of $19 remain in the petty cash box.

Required: In the entry to record the reimbursement of the petty cash fund, what amount should be credited to the petty cash account?

E16-3. Pick Hospital provides you with the following 19X1 information:

Accounts receivable, 1/1	$ 45,000
Charges to patients' accounts	639,200
Cash collections on patients' accounts	634,200
Accounts written off as bad debts	4,690
Collection of accounts previously written off as bad debts	350
Allowance for bad debts, 1/1	5,400

The hospital's aging schedule indicates that $6,000 of the 12/31/X1 accounts receivable will prove uncollectible.

Required: What amount should the hospital's 19X1 income statement report as revenue deductions (bad debts)?

E16-4. Pink Hospital maintains an allowance for bad debts as a contraaccount to receivables from patients. On 12/31/X1, the allowance account had a credit balance of $2,000. Each month, the hospital accrues bad debts equal to 1 percent of charges to patients' accounts. Charges to patients' accounts during 19X2 amounted to $500,000. During 19X2, accounts receivable totaling $8,000 were written off as bad debts. An aging of receivables at 12/31/X2 indicates that $10,000 of 12/31/X2 receivables are likely to prove to be bad debts.

Required: By what amount should revenue deductions (bad debts) previously accrued during 19X2 be increased on 12/31/X2?

E16-5. Poke Hospital provides you with the following data relating to October activity in its checking account with a local bank:

	Per Books	Per Bank
Balances, 9/30	$11,863	$12,310
October receipts	51,422	50,827
October disbursements	48,705	49,107
Balance, 10/31	14,580	14,030
Deposits in transit:		
9/30	$139	
10/31	?	
Checks outstanding:		
9/30	$586	
10/31	?	

Bank service charges for October, $14.

NSF check of patient returned with October bank statement, $108.

In reconciling the account, you discover two errors: (1) one of the hospital's accountants journalized a $620 check, issued in payment of an account payable, as $260, and (2) the bank charged the hospital for a $150 check drawn by another of the bank's depositors.

Required: What amount should be reported as cash in bank in the hospital's October 31 balance sheet?

Problems

P16–1. On June 1, Pixie Hospital established a petty cash fund in the imprest amount of $500. On June 14, the contents of the petty cash fund were as follows when the fund was reimbursed:

Coin and currency	$221
Petty cash expense vouchers	216
IOU from employee	10
Check of another employee made payable to Pixie Hospital	50

On June 16 the imprest amount of the petty cash fund was reduced to $300.

Required: (1) Prepare the necessary entries in general journal form at June 1, 14, and 16. (2) Why do you think the imprest amount of the petty cash fund was reduced on June 16?

P16–2. Plato Hospital decided to establish a petty cash fund on May 1 in the imprest amount of $750. The following transactions relating to the fund took place during May:

1. The fund was established on May 1.
2. The fund was replenished on May 15 at a time when the contents of the fund were as follows:

Currency and coin	$42
Expense vouchers	$681
Employee IOU	25

3. On May 16, it was decided to increase the imprest amount of the fund to $1,000.
4. The fund was replenished on May 31 at a time when the contents of the fund were as follows:

Currency and coin	$173
Expense vouchers	837

Required: (1) Prepare general journal entries to record all the petty cash transactions for May. (2) Assuming that the petty cash fund was not reimbursed on May 31, prepare the necessary May 31 adjusting entry.

P16–3. Painless Hospital's general ledger cash in bank account reports a balance of $346,920 as of October 31. An examination of the October bank statement in comparison with the cash records of the hospital, however, discloses the following information:

1. The October 31 balance per bank statement was $465,900.
2. A deposit in transit at October 31 was for $12,800.
3. Checks outstanding at October 31 totaled $89,300.
4. A patient's NSF $5,100 check was returned by the bank with the October statement.
5. Bank service charges for October were $120.
6. The bank inadvertently credited another of its depositors for the Painless Hospital's October 26 bank deposit of $10,600.
7. Matured temporary investments of $50,000, plus interest of $2,000, were collected and credited by the bank to the hospital's checking account on October 29.
8. A hospital employee journalized a properly drawn check for $700 as $7,000 on October 11 in settlement of an account payable.

Required: Prepare (1) a bank reconciliation at October 31 for Painless Hospital and (2) the necessary adjusting entry at October 31.

P16–4. Parkway Hospital's comparison of its cash records with its March bank statement provides the following information:

	Per Books	Per Bank
1. Balances, February 28	$14,755	$15,862
Receipts	15,431	17,495
Disbursements	13,744	16,087
Balances, March 31	16,442	17,270

2. Deposits in transit totaled $1,375 at February 28 and $946 at March 31. Checks outstanding were $2,482 at February 28 and $1,949 at March 31.
3. Bank service charges on the March bank statement were $16.
4. An NSF $479 check of a Parkway Hospital patient was returned by the bank with the March statement.

5. On March 30, the bank collected a Parkway Hospital patient's note to the hospital of $2,000 plus $40 interest. The bank credited the hospital for collection of the note and debited the hospital $7 for the service provided.

6. A hospital bookkeeper on March 12 journalized a $487 deposit as $847. This was a collection on a patient's account.

7. On March 22, the bank charged the hospital's account with a $300 check of another of the bank's depositors. The bank has stated that this mistake would be corrected on the April bank statement.

8. On March 27, one of the hospital's bookkeepers journalized a $10 check as $100. This check was issued in settlement of an account payable.

9. On March 29, the bank failed to give the hospital credit for a $1,055 deposit of that date. When notified of the error on April 4, the bank made a correction, to appear on the April bank statement.

Required: (1) Prepare a bank reconciliation at February 28. (2) Prepare a bank reconciliation at March 31. (3) Prepare the required March 31 adjusting entry.

P16-5. According to its books, Peerless Hospital has a cash balance of $438,104 at June 30. The June bank statement, however, reports a June 30 balance of $486,681. An investigation produces the following information:

1. The bank credited, in error, Peerless Hospital for a deposit of $28,417 made by Peerless Hospital on June 22.

2. Bank service charges for June amounted to $27.

3. Outstanding checks at June 30 were $107,092.

4. A deposit of $39,865 was in transit at June 30.

5. The June bank statement shows a credit of $10,600 (including $600 interest) representing the proceeds of a patient's note collected for the hospital by the bank.

6. The bank returned patients' checks marked "not sufficient funds" in the amount of $2,606.

7. Check number 1791 issued in payment of an account payable of $200 was recorded in error by a hospital bookkeeper as $2,000 even though the check was drawn in the correct $200 amount.

Required: (1) Prepare a bank reconciliation at June 30. (2) Prepare the necessary adjusting journal entry at June 30.

P16–6. Parson Hospital purchased $60,000 of U.S. government bonds at face value and accrued interest on September 1, 19X1. These 8 percent bonds pay interest semiannually on April 1 and October 1. Brokerage and other acquisition costs totaled $94. The bonds mature on April 1, 19X6, but the hospital intends to hold these securities as a short-term investment in its unrestricted fund. On January 1, 19X2, the bonds are sold by the hospital at 103 and accrued interest, with brokerage fees and other expenses of sale amounting to $105. The hospital closes its books annually on December 31.

Required: (1) Prepare, in general journal form, all necessary entries for 19X1 in connection with this investment. (2) Indicate how all matters relating to this investment should be presented in the hospital's 19X1 financial statements. (3) Prepare the necessary entry, in general journal form, to record the sale of the bonds on January 1, 19X2.

P16–7. Potter Hospital purchased $75,000 of corporate bonds at face value and accrued interest on August 1, 19X1, with brokerage and other acquisition costs amounting to $88. These 6 percent bonds pay interest semiannually on June 1 and December 1, and mature on June 1, 19X5. The hospital intends to hold these bonds as a temporary investment of its unrestricted fund. On January 1, 19X2, the bonds are sold by the hospital at 98 and accrued interest, with brokerage fees and other expenses of sale amounting to $73. Potter Hospital closes its books annually on December 31.

Required: (1) Prepare, in general journal form, all necessary entries for 19X1 with respect to this investment. (2) Indicate how all matters relating to this investment should be presented in the hospital's 19X1 financial statements. (3) Prepare the necessary entry, in general journal form to record the sale of the bonds on January 1, 19X2.

P16–8. A patient gave Peppy Hospital a 9 percent, 90-day promissory note on November 1, 19X1, in settlement of a $12,000 account with the hospital. The hospital closes its books annually on December 31.

Required: (1) Prepare, in general journal form, all necessary entries with respect to this note for 19X1 and 19X2. (2) Indicate how all matters relating to this note should be presented in the hospital's 19X1 financial statements.

P16–9. A patient gave Popover Hospital a 6 percent, 180-day promissory note on October 1, 19X1, in settlement of an $8,000 account with the hospital. The hospital discounted this note on November 1, 19X1, at a local bank whose discount rate is 9 percent. The hospital closes its books annually on December 31.

Required: (1) Prepare, in general journal form, all necessary entries with respect to this note for 19X1 and 19X2. (2) Indicate how all matters relating to this note should be presented in the hospital's 19X1 financial statements. (3) Prepare, in general journal form, the necessary entry at the maturity date of the note, assuming that the note is dishonored by the patient and the bank makes a protest fee charge of $22.

P16–10. Packer Hospital has $760,000 of accounts receivable as of December 31, 19X1. An aging schedule is prepared that indicates that bad debts should be estimated in the amount of $58,000. Before adjustment, however, the allowance for bad debts account has a December 31, 19X1, credit balance of $3,700. During 19X2, $64,800 of the 19X1 accounts receivable are written off as bad debts; the remainder of the accounts are collected. On December 31, 19X2, Packer Hospital has $827,000 of accounts receivable, and an aging schedule is prepared that indicates that bad debts should be estimated in the amount of $71,000.

Required: (1) Make the necessary entry at December 31, 19X1, to record the required provision for bad debts. (2) Make the necessary summary entry to record the writeoff of uncollectible accounts in 19X2. (3) Make the necessary entry as of December 31, 19X2, to record the required provision for bad debts. (4) Indicate the presentation of receivables in the hospital's December 31, 19X2, balance sheet.

P16–11. During 19X1, Pirate Hospital charged patients' accounts for a total of $3,500,000. Its general ledger at December 31, 19X1 (the end of the fiscal year), shows the following balances:

Patients' accounts receivable	$425,000 Dr.
Allowance for uncollectible accounts—bad debts	4,300 Cr.

Required: Prepare the necessary adjusting entries for estimated bad debts under each of the following assumptions:

(1) Bad debts are estimated at 1 percent of charges,
(2) Bad debts are estimated at 6 percent of receivables, and
(3) Bad debts, based on an aging of the receivables, are estimated at $31,900.

P16–12. Parker Hospital's adjusted trial balance at December 31, 19X1, included the following accounts:

Accounts receivable—patients	$500,000 Dr.
Allowance for uncollectible accounts:	
Bad debts	40,000 Cr.
Contractual adjustments	50,000 Cr.
Charity service	20,000 Cr.

In 19X2, with respect to the 19X1 accounts receivable, writeoffs were made as follows: bad debts $37,400, contractual adjustments $51,700, and charity service of $19,200. The remainder of the 19X1 receivables were collected.

Parker Hospital's accounts receivable at December 31, 19X2, were $600,000. Estimated uncollectibles at that date were bad debts 9 percent, contractual adjustments 11 percent, and charity service 1 percent.

Required: Prepare the receivables section of the hospital's balance sheet as of December 31, 19X2. Present all necessary computations of the amounts included in the presentation.

Inventories and Current Liabilities

17

The first part of this chapter is concerned with accounting procedures pertaining to the acquisition, usage, and valuation of hospital inventories. In a hospital, inventories include, besides drugs and pharmaceuticals shelved in the pharmacy, the foodstuffs located in dietary storerooms and numerous other items ranging from the cleaning supplies used in housekeeping to laboratory chemicals and radiological film. Although the inventory of the hospital may not be of substantial size relative to other assets, the annual usage of supplies is a significant cost element. As much as 15 percent of total operating expense may be represented by the cost of supplies. And, like cash, much of the inventory is highly susceptible to theft. It also should be recognized that the cost of maintaining an inventory—purchasing, receiving, storing, issuing, and insuring—is substantial. Finally, it is necessary for accounting purposes that proper determinations be made of the costs of supplies used and of the costs of supplies remaining unused in the hospital inventory. Therefore, the accountant should not underestimate the importance of adequate accounting and internal control procedures with respect to inventories.

The second part of this chapter pulls together some of the previously discussed materials dealing with current liabilities. Certain other related matters not covered before are also introduced from the context of a balance sheet. The balance sheet classification of current liabilities, as you know, includes a wide variety of debts representing goods and services purchased on account, borrowings from banks, accruals for payrolls, payroll-related obligations, interest, and various other obligations. In fact, *all* cash disbursements made by the hospital ordinarily must pass through current liability accounts of one kind or another. These accounts consequently deserve a considerable amount of accounting and managerial attention.

Inventories

The operations of a hospital enterprise require the purchase and use (or sale) of a variety of goods and supplies. The purchasing and receiving functions were discussed in Chapter 14, and now we turn to the problems of determining (1) the costs of supplies used (the debits to supplies expense accounts) and (2) the costs of supplies unused and on hand (the valuation of the inventory) for balance sheet purposes. These determinations require an inventory accounting system and the adoption of an inventory valuation method.

Inventory Accounting Systems

Most hospitals employ two different inventory accounting systems concurrently. Certain types of supplies are accounted for by the periodic inventory system; others are concurrently maintained on a perpetual inventory basis. To illustrate the two systems, assume that we have the following information for a particular supply item that we shall refer to as Item X:

	Units		Unit Cost
Inventory, April 1	100	x	$6
Purchase, April 15	400		$6
Usage, April 20	350		$6

The month begins with $600 (that is, 100 units @ $6) in the inventory account. What entry is made on April 15 when 400 additional units are purchased? What entry should be made on April 20 to record the usage of 350 units? By what procedure is the inventory at April 30 determined? The last two questions would be much more difficult to answer if the April 15 purchase were made at a unit cost other than $6, but we defer this complication to a later point.

Periodic Inventory System.   Under the periodic inventory system, no day-to-day record of supplies in inventory is maintained in the accounting records. As supplies are purchased, they may be charged either to inventory (the asset account) or directly to expense. Assuming the latter, this is the April 15 entry:

Supplies Expense	$2,400	
Accounts Payable		$2,400
Purchase of supplies:		
400 units @ $6 per unit = $2,400.		

Generally, the debit is made to a supplies expense account only if the department that will use the supplies is known. Otherwise, the debit is made to an inventory account.

Whether the above debit is made to supplies expense or to inventory, no entry is made on April 20 when 350 units of these supplies are used in departmental activities. At the end of April, then, the accounts would appear as follows:

Debit to Expense at Time of Purchase, Not Use

Inventory	Supplies Expense
600	2,400

The inventory account shows the inventory balance at April 1, not April 30. The supplies expense account indicates the cost of supplies purchased, not the cost of supplies used. Both account balances are incorrect.

So, at April 30, either a physical inventory (actual count) must be taken or an estimate must be made of the number of units in the month-end inventory. In the absence of error or theft, this quantity will be found to be 150 units (100 + 400 − 350). Cost prices then are assigned to these units, and the account balances are adjusted accordingly:

Adjusting the Periodic Inventory Accounts

Inventory	$300	
Supplies Expense		$300
Increase in inventory and corresponding		
reduction in supplies expense.		

This entry adjusts the inventory to the proper April 30 balance of $900 (150 units @ $6) and reduces the supplies expense account balance to $2,100 (the 350 units used that cost $6 each).

If we assume that the April 15 purchase of 400 units was debited to inventory rather than to supplies expense, the necessary April 30 adjusting entry is the following:

Supplies Expense	$2,100	
Inventory		$2,100
Cost of supplies used during April:		
350 units $\times$ $6 = $2,100.		

So, regardless of the debit made in the April 15 entry, we end April with $900 in inventory and $2,100 in supplies expense.

Advantages and Disadvantages of Periodic Inventory System

The periodic inventory system has the advantage of simplicity; it is clerically inexpensive. Because monthly physical inventory counts usually are not practical (and accurate monthly inventory estimates may not be available), however, the account balances may be somewhat distorted until actual counts and appropriate adjustments can be made. The degree of misstatement usually is not serious for interim reporting purposes, but physical inventories must be taken at least once each year, generally at the end of the fiscal period. The major disadvantage of the periodic inventory system is that the accounting records do not provide a means for control. The physical inventory indicates what the inventory is, of course, but the accounting records do not indicate what the inventory *should* be. Significant shortages therefore may go undetected.

Perpetual Inventory System.   Under the perpetual inventory system, records are maintained to provide a continuous record of supplies purchased, used, and on hand. Supplies accounted for on this basis are always charged to inventory accounts when purchased. The necessary April 15 entry is as follows:

Inventory	$2,400	
Accounts Payable		$2,400
Purchase of 400 units of supplies at $6		
per unit.		

An entry is also made in subsidiary inventory ledger records to reflect this inventory acquisition, increasing the inventory balance to 500 units having a total cost of $3,000 (the April 1 inventory of 100 units at $6 each plus the April 15 purchase of 400 units at $6

LOCATION _____ ITEM _____						STOCK NO. _____						

Figure 17–1 Perpetual Inventory Ledger Card

each). Perpetual inventory ledger cards such as the one illustrated in Figure 17–1 may be used, or inventory subsidiary records may be maintained by computer. Whatever the means employed, a continuous record is maintained of the units (with unit costs) received, issued, and remaining on hand.

As the supplies are required by departments for use in day-to-day activities, stores requisition forms (see Figure 17–2) are executed. The forms provide a record of the quantities and costs of supplies used by the various departments of the hospital. Copies of these forms are routed to the accounting department, where they serve as the basis for entries debiting the supplies expense accounts and crediting the inventory accounts. The April 20 entry, for example, is as follows:

Perpetual Inventory System Forms

Supplies Expense	$2,100	
Inventory		$2,100

Requisition from inventory of 350 units of supplies that cost $6 per unit.

| STORES REQUISITION | REQUISITION NO. _____ |

DEPARTMENT_____ DATE_____ 19____

FLOOR OR DIVISION _____ DATE REQUIRED _____ 19____

QUANTITY		DESCRIPTION OF SUPPLIES NEEDED	TO BE USED IF PERPETUAL INVENTORIES ARE KEPT			
WANTED	DELIVERED		PRICE	PER	AMOUNT	ACCT. NO.

REQUESTED BY _____   APPROVED BY _____

SEND ORIGINAL TO STORE ROOM CLERK. DUPLICATE IS RETAINED BY DEPARTMENT HEAD.

Figure 17–2 Stores (Inventory) Requisition Form

An entry also is made in the subsidiary ledger records to reflect a reduction of 350 units in the inventory, thus lowering the inventory balance to 150 units of this supply item. These subsidiary ledger records may be kept in terms of quantities only, unit costs only, or in both quantities and costs as illustrated in Figure 17–1.

Adjusting the Perpetual Inventory Accounts

At least once each year, a physical inventory is taken and the perpetual records are adjusted, if necessary, to reflect the actual count. The main point is that the perpetual inventory ledger, in the absence of accounting errors, indicates precisely what the inventory *should* be at any time.

Advantages and Disadvantages of Perpetual Inventory System

The choice of inventory system depends mainly on the characteristics of particular supply items. If the dollar value of annual usage is substantial, if the supplies have a high unit cost and are susceptible to theft, or if the supplies are directly billable to patients, the perpetual inventory system is often desirable. The perpetual system provides continuous control over the inventory, because information is immediately available as to inventory levels. Purchasing is facilitated, the adequacy of supplies on hand is more likely, and shortages are readily identified. Perpetual records also are useful for maintaining adequate insurance coverage and for documentation of losses. Because it is a costly system to administer, however, careful studies should be made to determine whether the benefits derived from perpetual records exceed the costs of installing and maintaining them.

The preceding example assumed a single unit cost of supplies. In actual practice, however, supplies typically are purchased during a given time period at different unit costs. A problem therefore arises in determining which unit costs relate to the supply items that have been used during the period and which apply to the units remaining in inventory at the end of the period. These determinations are important because of their direct effect on the hospital's reported operating expenses and net income as well as on the balance sheet valuation of the end-of-period inventory.

    As a basis for subsequent illustrations, let us assume the following data concerning a particular supply item:

Inventory Valuation Methods

19X1 Date		Units	Cost Unit	Cost Total
May 1	Inventory	200	$2.00	$ 400
5	Purchase	400	2.50	1,000
10	Usage	300		
15	Purchase	500	3.00	1,500
20	Usage	600		
25	Purchase	100	3.50	350
				$3,250

The month begins with an inventory of 200 units that cost $2 each. During the month of May, a total of 1,000 more units were purchased at steadily increasing prices; and, because 900 units were used during the month, the May 31 inventory consists of 300 units. In this illustration, the total cost of the opening inventory and purchases is $3,250. What part of this total cost is the cost of supplies used during the month? What part should be assigned to the 300 units remaining in the month-end inventory? There are

INVENTORY

Date_____19____   Sheet No._____

DEPARTMENT_____ Location_____

Called by_____ Entered by_____ Priced by_____ Extended by_____ Verified by_____

DESCRIPTION	✔	QUANTITY	PRICE	UNIT	EXTENSION

Figure 17–3 Physical Inventory Record

several different possible answers to these questions, depending on the inventory valuation method that is adopted by the hospital.

Specific Identification. It may be feasible to make a specific identification of unit purchase costs with individual items of inventory. Where the inventory items are packaged or are in containers of some kind, the packages or cartons may be crayon-marked or tagged in some manner to show actual unit costs. Then, as items are issued from inventory to departments, the stores requisition forms can be completed to indicate the specifically identified unit costs. When the annual physical inventory is taken, the marked containers will provide the necessary unit figures for the costing of the units in the inventory. Figure 17–3 illustrates the type of form sometimes used to take the physical inventory and to assign costs to the units counted.

The specific identification method, however, is generally impractical, if not impossible, to apply. This is because of the multiplicity of products in hospital inventories and because the marking of unit costs on each item either is not feasible or is too labor-costly. It therefore is necessary to turn to some assumed flow of inventory units or costs. Some generally accepted assumptions are (1) average; (2) first-in, first-out; and (3) last-in, first-out. Different assumptions may be made for different classifications of inventory; the same assumption need not be applied to all supply items in the inventory.

Weighted-Average Costing. Weighted-average costing assumes that the units issued from inventory are drawn more or less *equally* from each acquisition of supplies. It is not necessary, however, that the actual physical flow of the units in inventory correspond with this assumption.

If the periodic inventory system is employed, a weighted-average cost for the month of May would be computed as indicated in Figure 17–4. This computation, which is made at the end of the month, indicates that the weighted-average cost per unit was $2.71 (rounded to the nearest cent). The May 31 inventory is therefore valued at $813 (300 units @ $2.71). This leaves $2,437 ($3,250 − $813) as the cost of supplies used during the month. Computing the Weighted-Average Cost

The necessary May 31 journal entry, assuming that the month's purchases were debited to the inventory account, is as follows:

Supplies Expense	$2,437	
Inventory		$2,437
Cost of supplies used during May, under		
the weighted-average cost method		
(periodic inventory system).		

The credit in this entry reduces the inventory account balance from $3,250 ($400 + $1,000 + $1,500 + $350) to $813. Had purchases been debited to supplies expense, the month-end adjustment would have been a debit to inventory and a credit to supplies expense for $413.

If the perpetual inventory system is employed but the cost of units issued is recorded only at the end of each month or other Computing the Moving Weighted-Average Cost

Figure 17–4 Computation of
Weighted-Average Cost Periodic
Inventory System

May 1	Inventory	200	units @ $2.00	=	$ 400
5	Purchase	400	units @ $2.50	=	1,000
15	Purchase	500	units @ $3.00	=	1,500
25	Purchase	100	units @ $3.50	=	350
	Totals	1,200			$3,250
	Weighted-average cost ($3,250 ÷ 1,200)			=	$ 2.71

convenient period, the computation of the weighted-average cost
can be the same as shown in Figure 17–4. On the other hand, it
may be desirable to compute and record costs as supplies are issued
from the inventory. This requires the computation of a new
weighted-average cost after each purchase of supplies at a unit cost
different from the current average cost of the inventory. In other
words, a "moving" weighted-average cost is computed. Figure
17–5 shows how this computation might appear on an inventory
ledger card.

Thus, a new weighted-average cost is determined after each
additional purchase. After the purchase of May 5, for instance, the
recomputed average cost is $2.33, determined by a division of
$1,400 by 600 units. As a result, the cost of supplies used is
computed to be $2,350 (compared to $2,437 under the periodic
inventory system), and the ending inventory is $900 (compared to
$813 under the periodic inventory system).

First-In, First-Out (FIFO) Costing. The first-in, first-
out (FIFO) costing method assumes that the supplies issued from
inventory are pulled from the oldest stock. This means that the
remaining units in inventory are valued in terms of the most
recently incurred costs (last-in, still-here, or LISH, if you wish).
The assumption appears logical in that some effort usually is made
to issue the oldest stock first. Nevertheless, the actual physical flow
of the units need not conform with the underlying FIFO assumption for this method to be acceptable.

If the periodic inventory system is used, the 300-unit inventory at May 31 would be valued as follows:

100	units @ $3.50	=	$350	(most recent purchase)
200	units @ $3.00	=	600	(from next most recent pur-chase)
300	units		$950	May 31 inventory valuation

Date	Purchases			Issues			Balance		
	Units	Cost Unit	Total	Units	Cost Unit	Total	Units	Cost Unit	Total
May 1							200	$2.00	$ 400
5	400	$2.50	$1,000				600	2.33	1,400
10				300	$2.33	$ 700	300	2.33	700
15	500	3.00	1,500				800	2.75	2,200
20				600	2.75	1,650	200	2.75	550
25	100	3.50	350				300	3.00	900
				Cost of supplies used		$2,350			

Figure 17–5 Computation of Weighted-Average Cost Perpetual Inventory System

Because the ending inventory is composed of the most recently incurred costs, the cost assigned to supplies used during the month is $2,300 ($3,250 − $950), the "oldest" costs.

If the perpetual inventory system is used in conjunction with FIFO costing, the same results as noted above are obtained. The procedure is illustrated in Figure 17–6 as it might appear on a subsidiary inventory ledger card. This allows the cost of supplies used to be determined at the time of issuance from inventory rather than only at the end of the month or year.

Last-In, First-Out (LIFO) Costing. The last-in, first-out (LIFO) method of inventory valuation assumes that the supplies issued from inventory are drawn from the *most recently purchased stock*; the units are charged out of inventory at the most recently incurred costs. This means that the ending inventory will be stated in terms of the earliest (oldest) costs experienced (or, if you wish, FISH: first-in, still-here). It may be somewhat difficult to imagine a hospital supplies situation in which there would actually be a LIFO flow of physical units, but you must remember that the physical flow need not conform to the LIFO assumption for the use of the method to be acceptable. The LIFO procedure is really based on an assumed flow of costs rather than of units.

If the periodic inventory system is used, the physical inventory of 300 units at May 31 would have a cost computed as follows:

Determining Costs at Time of Inventory Issuance

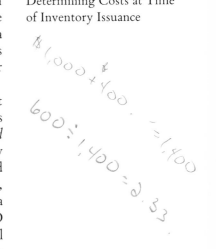

200 units @ $2.00 = $400 (earliest costs; May 1 inventory)
100 units @ $2.50 = 250 (next earliest costs; May 5 purchase)
300         $650 May 31 inventory valuation

Date	Purchases			Issues			Balance		
		Cost			Cost			Cost	
	Units	Unit	Total	Units	Unit	Total	Units	Unit	Total
May 1							200	$2.00	$ 400
5	400	$2.50	$1,000				200	2.00	400
							400	2.50	1,000
10				200	$2.00	$ 400			
				100	2.50	250	300	2.50	750
15	500	3.00	1,500				300	2.50	750
							500	3.00	1,500
20				300	2.50	750			
				300	3.00	900	200	3.00˙	600
25	100	3.50	350				200	3.00	600
							100	3.50	350
				Cost of supplies used		$2,300			

Figure 17–6 Computation of FIFO Cost Perpetual Inventory System

Because the May 31 inventory is composed of the earliest costs incurred, the cost of supplies issued during the month consists of the most recently incurred costs, or $2,600 ($3,250 − $650). Again, although it is unlikely that the oldest physical units compose the inventory at May 31, the LIFO method's validity does not depend on the actual physical flow of the units of inventory.

Results Differ with LIFO under Perpetual and Periodic Systems

If the perpetual inventory system is employed in conjunction with the LIFO method, the required procedure is illustrated in Figure 17–7 as it may appear on a subsidiary inventory ledger card. As indicated, the perpetual LIFO cost of supplies used is $2,500 and the May 31 inventory is $750 ($400 + $350), while the periodic LIFO figures were $2,600 and $650. It should be noted that the periodic and perpetual inventory systems ordinarily do not produce the same results when the LIFO method is employed; they *do* produce the same results, however, when the FIFO method is used.

Conclusions About Costing Methods.   The hospital management has a choice among the inventory costing methods in most instances. Which method should be adopted? The method should, of course, be theoretically sound and clerically feasible. Consideration also should be given to the probable effect of the method on the reported results of operations and financial position. The implications of each method for third-party cost reimbursement contracts also may be important.

Date	Purchases			Issues			Balance		
		Cost			Cost			Cost	
	Units	Unit	Total	Units	Unit	Total	Units	Unit	Total
May 1							200	$2.00	$ 400
5	400	$2.50	$1,000				200	2.00	400
							400	2.50	1,000
10				300	$2.50	$ 750	200	2.00	400
							100	2.50	250
15	500	3.50	1,500				200	2.00	400
							100	2.50	250
							500	3.00	1,500
20				500	3.00	1,500			
				100	2.50	250	200	2.00	400
25	100	3.50	350				200	2.00	400
							100	3.50	350
				Cost of supplies used		$2,500			

Figure 17–7 Computation of LIFO Cost Perpetual Inventory System

	Costing Method		
	FIFO	Average	LIFO
Inventory, May 1	$ 400	$ 400	$ 400
Purchases	2,850	2,850	2,850
Total	3,250	3,250	3,250
Less inventory, May 31	950	900	750
Cost of supplies used in May	$2,300	$2,350	$2,500

Figure 17–8 Summary of Inventory Costing Methods Perpetual Inventory System

Summary of Results When Prices Are Rising

Figure 17–8 summarizes the results obtained by the use of FIFO, LIFO, and weighted-average costing (the three most widely used methods), assuming the perpetual inventory system. This illustration reveals that, in a period of rising prices, the LIFO method produces the highest operating expenses and the lowest inventory valuation. FIFO produces the opposite results. Weighted-average costing will provide results somewhere between those obtained from FIFO and LIFO.

Internal Control

Internal controls over the purchase and receipt of supplies for inventory were discussed in Chapter 14. Once supplies are acquired, the initial internal control objective is largely that of protecting the inventory items from theft, damage, waste, and obsolescence, as they remain in storage and then are consumed in hospital operations. A major requirement is the assignment of responsibility to specific employees for management of inventories at each location in the hospital. The number of such locations should be minimized so that centralized control may be better achieved.

The storage areas should be kept clean, adequately lighted, and locked, with access limited strictly to authorized employees. Supplies should be released from the storerooms only on presentation of properly executed inventory requisition forms. Listings of approved authorization signatures should be issued by administration and reviewed periodically. Maximum-minimum controls should be devised that permit inventories to be maintained in amounts that are neither inadequate nor excessive. Where perpetual inventory records are kept, these records should be reconciled with physical inventories taken at least annually.

Current Liabilities

The traditional working definition of *current liabilities* commonly employed identifies them as obligations that mature and normally will be paid within approximately one year from the balance sheet date. Included in the current liability classification are notes payable, accounts payable, current maturities of long-term debt, accrued liabilities for expenses and other items, and deferred revenues.

Notes Payable

Notes payable are obligations in the form of promissory notes issued to trade creditors for the purchase of goods and services, to banks for loans of a short-term character, and to other organizations. Whereas accounts payable generally fall due within a month, notes may be outstanding for 90, 180, or more days from the balance sheet date. This requires, for interim reporting purposes, the accrual of interest expense on a monthly basis.

To illustrate the accounting procedures involved, assume that a hospital issues its 90-day, 10 percent note for $36,000 to a local bank on August 1, 19X1. The interest on this note is $900 [$36,000 $\times$ 0.10 $\times$ (90 $\div$ 360)]. The maturity date of the note is October 30, 19X1. All necessary entries for the 90-day term of the note are summarized in Figure 17–9.

Prepaid Loan Expenses

In some instances, local banking practices may dictate that interest on loans be deducted in advance from the loan proceeds. This, in effect, means that the hospital is prepaying the interest expense. If that were the case for this loan, the proceeds would be only $35,100 ($36,000 − $900), and the $900 would be accounted

Cash Receipts Journal			
8/1	Cash—General Checking Account	$36,000	
	Note Payable		$36,000
	Issuance of 90-day, 10% note to a local bank for a short-term loan of $36,000.		

General Journal			
8/31	Interest Expense	$ 300	
	Accrued Interest Payable		$ 300
	Accrual of interest expense on note for August: [$36,000 × 0.10 × (30 ÷ 360)].		

General Journal			
9/30	Interest Expense	$ 300	
	Accrued Interest Payable		$ 300
	Accrual of interest expense on note for September.		

Voucher Register			
10/30	Interest Expense	$ 300	
	Accrued Interest Payable	600	
	Notes Payable	36,000	
	Accounts Payable		$36,900
	Issuance of voucher for payment of note and interest to maturity date.		

Cash Disbursements Journal			
10/30	Accounts Payable	$36,900	
	Cash—General Checking Account		$36,900
	Issuance of check in payment of note and interest.		

Figure 17–9 Accounting for Notes Payable Interest Not Prepaid

for as prepaid interest expense as illustrated in Figure 17–10. It should be noted here that the hospital is paying $900 interest for the use of $35,100 for 90 days; so the effective (true) rate of interest is actually higher than the 10 percent rate quoted by the bank.

Accounts Payable

Trade accounts payable originate from the purchase of supplies and services on account. In many such purchases, a cash discount is allowed to the hospital if the related invoices are paid within a specified period of time. It is important, therefore, that the accounting system provide assurance that invoices are paid, whenever possible, within the discount period. It can be a costly omission to fail to take these discounts. (It should be noted that *trade* discounts, which may be obtained from a supplier because of large-volume buying or other reasons, are always considered a reduction in cost. Only the billed price, net of any trade discount, should be recorded in the hospital's accounts.)

Cash Receipts Journal			
8/1	Cash—General Checking Account	$35,100	
	Prepaid Interest Expense	900	
	Notes Payable		$36,000
	Issuance of 90-day, 10% note to a local bank for a short-term loan of		
	$36,000, with interest prepaid.		
General Journal			
8/31	Interest Expense	$ 300	
	Prepaid Interest Expense		$ 300
	Recognition of interest expense on note for August ($900 × 1/3).		
General Journal			
9/30	Interest Expense	$ 300	
	Prepaid Interest Expense		$ 300
	Recognition of interest expense on note for September.		
Voucher Register			
10/30	Interest Expense	$ 300	
	Notes Payable	36,000	
	Prepaid Interest Expense		$ 300
	Accounts Payable		36,000
	Issuance of voucher for payment of note and to recognize interest expense		
	for October.		
Cash Disbursements Journal			
10/30	Accounts Payable	$36,000	
	Cash—General Checking Account		$36,000
	Issuance of check in payment of note.		

Figure 17–10 Accounting for Notes Payable Interest Prepaid

Purchase Discounts

To illustrate, assume that the hospital purchases $5,000 of supplies on account, with terms of 2/10, n/30, on October 31. This means that, if the invoice is paid within 10 days (by November 10), a 2 percent cash discount can be taken by the hospital. The discount would amount to $100 (2 percent of $5,000), and a payment of only $4,900 ($5,000 − $100) would be required. If the hospital does not pay the invoice within 10 days, however, the supplier must be paid the full $5,000 within 30 days. So, if the hospital waits until, say, November 30 to pay the invoice, it is in effect paying an additional $100 (or 2 percent) for delaying its payment for 20 days. Because there are roughly 18 periods of 20 days in a year, missing the discount would be the equivalent of paying 36 percent interest (18 × 2 percent) per year on purchases!

The procedure described in earlier chapters is indicated by the following journal entries for the example:

Voucher Register

10/31	Supplies Expense	$5,000	
	Accounts Payable		$5,000
	Voucher for purchase of supplies on account.		

Cash Disbursements Journal

11/10	Accounts Payable	$5,000	
	Purchase Discounts Earned		$ 100
	Cash—General Checking Account		4,900
	Check issued in payment of voucher.		

Notice here that purchase discounts are recorded only when taken, and they are treated as other operating income. If we can assume that all available discount opportunities will be taken, this procedure has a number of weaknesses. First, the voucher register entry overstates both the cost of the supplies and the amount of the liability. Second, income is not earned by purchasing. Last, if the discount is missed, no recognition is given to the discount lost in the accounting records. That is, the cash disbursements journal entry would be simply a debit to accounts payable and a credit to cash for $5,000.

An alternative procedure designed to overcome the weaknesses of the system is indicated by the following entries:

Recording Supplies at the Amount Hospital Should Pay

Voucher Register

10/31	Supplies Expense	$4,900	
	Accounts Payable		$4,900
	Voucher (net of discount) for purchase of supplies on account.		

Cash Disbursements Journal

11/10	Accounts Payable	$4,900	
	Cash—General Checking Account		$4,900
	Check issued in payment of voucher.		

In this way, the supplies and the related liability are recorded at the amount that the hospital should pay; no discount earned is recorded if the invoice is paid on time. If the discount is missed, however, the payment entry will be as follows:

	Cash Disbursements Journal		
11/10	Accounts Payable	$4,900	
	Purchase Discounts Lost	100	
	Cash—General Checking Account		$5,000
	Check issued in payment of voucher after discount period has elapsed.		

Here, the use of the purchase discounts lost account (which is treated as a financial expense) points up an inefficiency in the hospital's processing of its accounts payable. Thus, management's attention is drawn to a situation that requires corrective action. Management should be more interested in the amount of purchase discounts lost than in the amount of discounts taken.

Current Maturities of Long-Term Liabilities

Mortgages, bonds, and other long-term obligations of the hospital should be reported as current liabilities to the extent that they are to be paid within one year from resources classified as current assets. In many instances, such as with mortgage notes and bonds that mature in annual installments, a portion of the total obligation is presented as a current liability, and the balance of the debt remains in the long-term liability classification. Assume, for example, that a hospital issues $5 million of bonds on January 1, 19X1, and that $500,000 of this bond issue matures each year for 10 years, beginning January 1, 19X2. The December 31, 19X1, balance sheet therefore should report $500,000 among the current liabilities and $4.5 million as long-term debt.

Accrued Liabilities

Accrued liabilities are obligations that arise as a result of past transactions—usually ones involving contractual commitments and tax legislation. Included in this balance sheet classification are accrued salaries and wages payable, payroll withholdings and tax accruals, and various expense items such as interest and rent. Because of their materiality, accrued payroll and payroll-related liabilities typically are reported separately from other accrued liabilities. Accounting procedures for these liabilities were discussed in several earlier chapters, particularly Chapters 5 and 13.

Deferred Revenues

Hospitals sometimes receive cash advances from patients, third-party payers, and others for services that are to be provided in the future. Prepayments of this kind—including patients' admission deposits, advances from third-party reimbursement agencies, and tuition, rent, and interest received in advance—are recorded as liabilities when they are received. If the provision of such future services will involve significant costs to be financed from the hospital's current resources, these advances are properly classified as current liabilities.

Preferred Balance Sheet Listing of Deferred Revenues

It sometimes has been the practice to report all deferred revenues in a balance sheet classification separately located between current liabilities and long-term liabilities. This practice, however, should be avoided. Deferred revenues should be identified as either current or long-term liabilities and be reported in the balance sheet accordingly.

Internal Control

The key to effective internal control over liabilities lies in (1) an appropriate authorization of purchase, borrowing, payroll, or other transactions giving rise to liabilities and (2) an accurate determination of the amounts in which such liabilities are recorded. The voucher system employed should require that authorizations and approvals be fully evidenced in writing before any liabilities are recorded and before disbursements are made to discharge them. Appropriate subsidiary ledger records should be maintained by employees who are independent of the general ledger accounting function. These detailed records should be reconciled with the related general ledger control accounts on a regular basis.

Questions

Q17–1. Indicate some of the major requirements for a good system of internal control over hospital inventories.

Q17–2. Distinguish between the periodic inventory system and the perpetual inventory system. What are the advantages and disadvantages of each system? Which system should be used by hospitals?

Q17–3. Indicate the reasons that a considerable amount of importance should be assigned to inventory accounting and management in a hospital.

Q17–4. Distinguish between the FIFO and LIFO inventory costing methods. In a period of rising prices, which method would tend to result in the recording of the highest costs for supplies used? In a period of rising prices, which method would tend to result in the highest end-of-period inventory?

Q17-5. Quiet Hospital had a 19X1 net income of $164,000. The cost of supplies used during the year totaled $713,000. The hospital's inventory of supplies increased by $27,000, and accounts payable to suppliers increased by $39,400 during the 19X1 year. What was the amount of cash payments to suppliers during 19X1?

Q17-6. Because of an error, Quest Hospital's December 31, 19X1, inventory was understated by $19,000. What is the effect of this error on the hospital's reported net income for 19X1 and its balance sheet at December 31, 19X1? What effect, if any, will this error have on the hospital's 19X2 net income?

Q17-7. Define current liabilities. Give six examples of accounts that are reported in the current liability section of the hospital's balance sheet.

Q17-8. What are the financial consequences of a continued failure to take advantage of cash discount opportunities in the payment of accounts payable?

Q17-9. Quaint Hospital purchased supplies on account and paid the related invoice within the specified discount period. The following entries were made:

Supplies Expense	$3,000	
Accounts Payable		$3,000
Accounts Payable	$3,000	
Purchase Discounts		$ 60
Cash—General Checking		
Account		2,940

From a theoretical and practical point of view, what is "wrong" with these entries? Briefly explain the alternative "discounts lost" procedure.

Q17-10. What are some of the major features of a satisfactory system of internal control over hospital liabilities?

Exercises

E17-1. Quitt Hospital provides you with the following information relating to its activities for January:

Accounts payable to suppliers, 1/1 $ 10,000

Inventory, 1/1 — 14,000
Payments on accounts payable to suppliers — 80,000
Revenues — 335,000
Inventory, 1/31 — 17,000
Accounts payable to suppliers, 1/31 — 15,000
Operating expenses (excluding cost of supplies
used) — 233,000

Required: What amount should the hospital's January income statement report as net income?

E17–2. Quirk Hospital made inventory errors as follows:
• 12/31/X1 inventory overstated by $400.
• 12/31/X2 inventory understated by $100.

Required: By what amount was the hospital's 19X2 net income overstated or understated due to these errors? By what amount was the hospital's equity (fund balance) overstated or understated at 12/31/X2 due to these errors?

E17–3. Quark Hospital issues its 12 percent, 90-day, $100,000 promissory note to a local bank to obtain a short-term loan on April 1. Interest was not prepaid.

Required: Prepare, in general journal form, the necessary entry on June 30 to record payment of the note and interest.

E17–4. Following is a series of multiple-choice questions:
1. The use of a discounts lost account indicates that the recorded cost of a purchased inventory item is its
   a. Invoice price.
   b. Invoice price plus the purchase discount lost.
   c. Invoice price less the discount taken.
   d. Invoice price less the discount allowable, whether or not taken.
2. A hospital has been using the FIFO method of inventory valuation for 15 years. Its inventory at the end of the 15th year was $26,000, but it would have been $15,000 if LIFO had been used. Thus, if LIFO had been used during the 15-year period, the hospital's net income would have been
   a. $11,000 less over the 15-year period.
   b. $11,000 greater over the 15-year period.
   c. $11,000 less for the 15th year.
   d. $11,000 greater for the 15th year.

3. A hospital's inventory valuation in its balance sheet was lower using FIFO than LIFO. Assuming no beginning inventory, in what direction did the unit cost of purchases move during the period?
   a. Up.
   b. Down.
   c. No change.
   d. Cannot be determined from the information given.
4. The September 30 physical inventory of a hospital properly included $13,000 of supplies that were not recorded as purchases until October. What effect will this error have on September 30 assets, liabilities, equity (fund balance), and net income for the year then ended, respectively?
   a. No effect; overstate; understate; understate.
   b. No effect; understate; understate; overstate.
   c. Understate; no effect; overstate; overstate.
   d. No effect; understate; overstate; overstate.

Problems

P17–1. Quick Hospital provides you with the following information for a single supply item purchased and used in its radiology department:

May	1	Inventory	400 units @	$7
	8	Usage	300 units	
	15	Purchase	200 units @	$8
	22	Purchase	200 units @	$9
	27	Usage	200 units	

Required: Compute the cost of supplies used in May, assuming (1) periodic LIFO costing, (2) perpetual LIFO costing, (3) periodic FIFO costing, (4) periodic weighted average costing.

P17–2. Given the following data relating to a single billable supply item purchased and sold by Quack Hospital:

		Cost	
	Units	Per Unit	Total
Inventory, October 1	200	$1.00	$ 200
Purchases:			
October 5	200	2.00	400
October 15	400	3.00	1,200
October 25	200	4.50	900

Sales:

October 10	300
October 20	400

Required: Compute the cost of supplies sold to patients during October and the inventory valuation at October 31, assuming the following:

1. Periodic inventory system.
   a. Weighted average costing.
   b. FIFO costing.
   c. LIFO costing.
2. Perpetual inventory system.
   a. Weighted average costing.
   b. FIFO costing.
   c. LIFO costing.

P17–3. Queen Hospital began operating a new department on April 1. This department purchased and issued a single supply item as follows:

April	1	Purchased 500 units @ $5.
	5	Issued 300 units.
	10	Purchased 200 units @ $6.
	15	Purchased 300 units @ $7.
	25	Issued 400 units.

Required: Assuming that this supply item is billed to patients at $10 per unit, compute the gross profit made by this department during April if the department uses:

1. Perpetual FIFO costing method.
2. Perpetual LIFO costing method.

P17–4. Quip Hospital issues its 90-day, 10 percent note to a local bank for a short-term loan of $48,000 on September 1, 19X1. Interest on the note was not deducted in advance. The hospital's fiscal year ends on September 30.

Required: Prepare, in general journal form, all necessary entries for 19X1 in connection with this note.

P17–5. Quinn Hospital issues its 120-day, 12 percent note to a local bank for a short-term loan of $75,000 on October 1, 19X1. Interest on the note was deducted in advance. The hospital's fiscal year ends on December 31.

Required: Prepare, in general journal form, all necessary entries for 19X1 and 19X2 in connection with this note.

P17–6. Quaker Hospital provides you with the following information about the purchase and usage of one of its billable supply items:

June Date	Units	Unit	Cost Total	
1	Inventory	300	$4.00	$1,200
5	Purchase	500	4.60	2,300
10	Usage	400		
15	Purchase	450	5.20	2,340
20	Usage	550		
27	Purchase	200	5.50	1,100

This supply item is billed to patients at $8.00 per unit.

Required: Assume that Quaker Hospital employs the perpetual LIFO system of accounting for this supply item. (1) Prepare an inventory ledger card for the month of June. (2) Prepare, in general journal form, all necessary entries for the month of June. (3) Assume that the physical inventory at June 30 indicates that 480 units are on hand in the inventory. What adjusting entry, if any, would you suggest?

Plant Assets and Depreciation

18

A hospital's plant assets consist of land, land improvements, buildings, and equipment. Other descriptive terms such as fixed assets, capital assets, and tangible assets also are often used as synonyms for this classification of resources. In any event, these assets are not intended for sale in the normal course of business but are held for use over a period of years in the provision of hospital services. Except for land, plant assets deteriorate with use and the passage of time; they eventually wear out. This "wearing out" process, as you already know, is recognized in accounting through *depreciation,* the rational and systematic allocation of the cost of plant assets to expense over their useful lives.

Previous chapters gave only minimum attention to the problems of accounting for plant assets and depreciation. We should now explore in some detail the accounting concepts and procedures employed by hospitals in recording the acquisition, depreciation, and disposal of plant properties. These are matters of considerable significance, because it is not at all unusual to find 60 percent or more of a hospital's assets invested in land, buildings, and equipment. Developing and maintaining adequate records of these long-lived assets clearly must be one of the imperatives of hospital accounting.

Acquisition of Plant Assets

Hospitals generally acquire plant assets either by purchase or by donation. A purchase of plant assets should result only from a budgetary process and a carefully constructed program of capital expenditures. The amounts that can be spent for this purpose are limited, and the available funds must be allocated in the most effective manner consistent with the long-range objectives of the hospital. This program should also include an ongoing effort to secure plant assets by donation so that donors are encouraged to contribute in a form and manner best suited to the hospital's real needs. All plant asset acquisitions, whether by purchase or by donation, should also require the approval of the governing board of the hospital.

Initiating Accounting Records for Plant Assets

As plant assets are acquired, appropriate accounting records should be established. This requires a proper account classification of the assets and an accurate determination of their "cost." In addition to the general ledger record, a suitable subsidiary ledger record also must be maintained for accounting and internal control purposes.

Classification of Plant Assets

Hospital plant assets, with the related accumulated depreciation accounts, traditionally have been classified in the following manner:

Account Numbers	
1130	Land
1140	Land Improvements
1240	Accumulated Depreciation—Land Improvements
1150	Buildings
1250	Accumulated Depreciation—Buildings
1170	Fixed Equipment
1270	Accumulated Depreciation—Fixed Equipment
1180	Major Movable Equipment
1280	Accumulated Depreciation—Major Movable Equipment
1190	Minor Equipment
1290	Accumulated Depreciation—Minor Equipment

This classification, or some variation of it, probably is employed by a majority of hospitals. Let us briefly examine the nature and content of each of the six primary asset accounts.

Land. The land account includes the cost of earth surface owned by the hospital and used in the ordinary course of hospital operations. It includes all land used for building sites, yards and grounds, and parking areas. Land acquired for future expansion and not currently in use should not be included in the land account but should be reported among the long-term investments in the hospital's balance sheet. Because land does not deteriorate with use or the passage of time, it is not subject to depreciation.

Land Improvements.   Land improvements consist of the cost of on-site water and sewer systems, fencing and walls, sidewalks, shrubbery and trees, and paving of roadways and parking lots. These costs are depreciable and therefore should be separately recorded in the accounts to distinguish them from land costs that are not depreciable.

Buildings.   This account should reflect the cost of all buildings owned by the hospital and used in its normal day-to-day activities. Included in this account are the hospital buildings themselves, personnel residences, garages and storage houses, and utility structures such as an outlying heating and cooling plant. A building that has been donated to the hospital for endowment investment purposes and that is not used in regular hospital activities should be reported among the assets of the endowment fund. All hospital buildings, of course, are depreciable.

Fixed Equipment.   The fixed equipment account includes the cost of equipment that is affixed to, and constitutes a structural component of, the hospital building. Another characteristic of fixed equipment is that it is not subject to transfer or removal from its fixed location. Equipment in this classification includes such items as mechanical and electrical systems, elevators, generators, pumps, boilers, and refrigeration machinery. All of this equipment is depreciable over a relatively long life.

Major Movable Equipment.   The following are general characteristics of equipment included in this category:

- A capability of being readily moved from one location to another in the hospital
- A unit cost sufficiently large to justify the expense incident to control by means of a subsidiary equipment ledger
- A minimum useful life usually of three years or more

Some examples of major movable equipment are desks, chairs, beds, automobiles and trucks, accounting machines, sterilizers, operating tables, and radiology equipment. Major movable equipment items are depreciable over lives generally much shorter than for fixed equipment.

Minor Equipment.   Minor equipment items include wastebaskets, bedpans, glassware, sheets, basins, buckets, silverware, and most surgical instruments. As a matter of expedience, many accounting systems provide that only the cost of the original supply of minor equipment should be charged to this asset account. This original cost generally is depreciated over a short period (perhaps three years), with all additional purchases charged to expense at acquisition. Other hospitals record all minor equipment (both the original supply and replacement purchases) to the asset account and depreciate it over a three-year period. Because it is not feasible to attempt to inventory this equipment annually and the costs involved are relatively immaterial, no other accounting procedures are generally workable.

Determination of Cost

The "cost" of a purchased plant asset includes all expenditures related to the acquisition of the asset, bringing it to the desired location, and making it ready for use in hospital activities. Such costs may include the following:

- The billed price of the asset, net of any trade or cash discounts allowed
- Freight charges
- Sales taxes
- Fees and commissions paid
- Installation costs

Excluding Interest from Cost of Purchased Plant Asset

The cost of a purchased plant asset, however, generally should not include interest. A hospital, for example, may acquire expensive equipment under a conditional sales or other deferred payment plan requiring a series of installment payments that include interest. Such interest charges should be excluded from asset cost, being recorded instead as interest expense. When a hospital constructs a building, however, interest costs incurred during the construction period are capitalized as a part of the cost of the building.

Recording Donated Plant Assets

When plant assets are acquired by gift or donation, the assets should be recorded at their fair market values as of the date of donation. The offsetting credit is made directly to the unrestricted fund balance account, not to a revenue account. All receipts of plant assets by donation are considered contributions to the permanent capital of the hospital. Depreciation should be recorded on donated plant assets as if the assets had been purchased.

Accounting Procedure

To illustrate the accounting procedure for plant asset acquisitions, let us assume that on January 1, 19X1, Hopewell Hospital purchased a new item of radiology equipment for $75,000. This equipment has an estimated useful life of five years and an estimated salvage value of 20 percent, or $15,000. The necessary entries to record the acquisition are the following:

Voucher Register

1/1/X1   Major Movable Equipment $75,000
           Accounts Payable $75,000
           Voucher for purchase of new
           item of radiology equipment.

Cash Disbursements Journal

1/1/X1   Accounts Payable $75,000
           Cash—General Checking
             Account $75,000
           Check issued for purchase of
           new radiology equipment.

The major movable equipment account, as you know, is a general ledger control account whose balance reflects the cost of all hospital equipment items in the major movable equipment classification. Detailed information concerning these individual items of equipment is contained in some form of plant asset subsidiary ledger record.

One form of subsidiary ledger record is illustrated in Figure 18–1. When an item of equipment is acquired, it is entered on one of these cards. This provides a detailed record including a full description of the equipment, its cost, date of acquisition, salvage value, estimated life, depreciation method and amounts, and whatever additional information may be desired. Such records support the periodic depreciation charges, and the balance sheet asset valuations provide the basis for insurance coverage and claims, permit the accurate recording of asset retirements and disposals, and assist in securing effective internal controls over the plant asset investment.

Subsidiary Ledger Records

Notice that the plant ledger card indicates that the x-ray equipment was assigned identification number 7040-8510-67. (As you may recall, 7040 is the expense account number for the radiology department, and 8510 is the account number for depreciation expense. The 67 indicates that this equipment is the sixty-seventh item of equipment in the department. Numbering systems, of course, vary; this is simply an example.) A metal tag showing this number is attached to the equipment to facilitate its identification with the accounting records whenever an inventory is taken of the hospital's equipment.

Description Radiology Equipment (details)   I.D. #7040–8510–67

Cost $75,000	Useful Life 5 years	Method SL
Salvage value 15,000	Depreciation:	
	Annual $12,000	
Depreciable cost $60,000	Monthly 1,000	

| Date | Asset | | | Accumulated Depreciation | | | Book |
	Dr.	Cr.	Balance	Dr.	Cr.	Balance	Value
1 1 X1	$75,000		$75,000				$75,000

Figure 18–1 Plant Asset Subsidiary Ledger Card

Even when electromechanical accounting equipment is employed, however, it may not be feasible to attempt to maintain this type of separate subsidiary record for each individual item of equipment. Instead, similar items of equipment may be grouped on a single card. All beds in a particular nursing unit, for example, might be entered on one card. In other systems, a separate plant asset subsidiary record is maintained for the equipment in each department. When one of these variations is found, depreciation often can be computed on a group or composite basis, such as is described later in this chapter.

Depreciation of Plant Assets

When Hopewell Hospital purchased the equipment, it acquired a "bundle of services" at a cost of $75,000. Each year, as this equipment is used in hospital activities, a portion of its total service capability is expended. After five years of use, it is estimated that this bundle of services will have been exhausted. Clearly, the cost of the services consumed each year should be recognized as an expense to be matched against the revenues produced by those services. As noted before, this consumption of cost, or expense, is depreciation. Depreciation is fully as valid an expense as is the hospital payroll. But how is it measured?

The determination of periodic depreciation charges is dependent on three important factors: (1) depreciable cost, (2) service life, and (3) choice of depreciation method. In past years, hospitals have employed various techniques of depreciation, including the straight-line method and accelerated methods such as the declining balance method and the sum-of-years'-digits method. All of these methods are in conformity with generally accepted accounting principles and are widely used by industrial commercial firms for accounting and income tax purposes. The use of accelerated depreciation methods by hospitals for cost reimbursement purposes, however, may be disallowed by governmental and certain other third-party payers. For this reason, the discussion in this book is limited to the straight-line depreciation method. A complete discussion of accelerated depreciation methods can be found in the author's *Hospital Financial Accounting: Theory and Practice.*

Three Factors in Determining Periodic Depreciation

The depreciable cost, sometimes called the *depreciation base* or *basis,* of a plant asset is its acquisition cost minus its estimated salvage value:

Depreciable Cost

Acquisition cost − Salvage value = Depreciable cost

The residual salvage value of a depreciable plant asset is the estimated amount for which the asset can be sold when it is retired from use in hospital activity. There is no simple formula by which salvage value determinations can be made. It is largely a matter of judgment applied by the individual hospital in view of its plant asset retirement policy and experience, expected future market conditions for used or scrapped equipment, and other factors. Some assistance, however, may be obtained from the hospital's auditors and from equipment manufacturers.

The useful service life of a plant asset ordinarily is expressed in terms of years. In selecting a service life, consideration should be given to both the functional and the physical factors that limit the service life. The functional factors include obsolescence resulting from technological change, growth in the scale of a hospital's activities, and major changes in methods of delivering health care services. The physical factors include wear and tear resulting from use, and deterioration caused by the elements. As was true of salvage value deter-

Service Life

minations, however, the determination of service lives also is largely a matter of judgment and depends heavily on the individual hospital's plant asset retirement policy and experience. Although a plant asset remains in very sound condition, its economical service life may be at an end from the standpoint of a particular hospital. Various guides are published by hospital associations and governmental agencies that offer assistance in establishing useful service lives.

Basic Straight-Line Depreciation Method

The straight-line (SL) method of depreciation assigns an equal amount of depreciation to each year of useful life. The following formula is used to calculate annual depreciation:

$$\frac{\text{Cost} - \text{Salvage value}}{\text{Estimated useful life}} = \text{Annual depreciation expense}$$

Application of the formula to the data assumed in this example for the new item of equipment produces annual depreciation expense of $12,000, as follows:

$$\frac{\$75,000 - \$15,000}{5} = \underline{\$12,000}$$

Thus, each year of the 19X1–19X5 period would be charged with $12,000 of depreciation expense for this item of equipment.

Because monthly financial statements should reflect all expenses, including depreciation, the following adjusting entry is required at the end of each monthly reporting period:

General Journal

Depreciation Expense	$1,000	
Accumulated Depreciation—Major		
Movable Equipment		$1,000
Monthly straight-line depreciation		
expense on radiology equipment		
($12,000 × 1/12).		

Although the entry is posted to the general ledger accounts, monthly postings generally are not made to the plant asset subsidiary ledger cards. The plant asset subsidiary ledger cards ordinarily are posted only on an annual basis, as shown in Figure 18–2. The information in the subsidiary ledger is reconciled with the balances of the general ledger control accounts (for plant assets, depreciation

Description Radiology Equipment (details)   I.D. #7040–8510–67

Cost	$75,000			Useful Life	5 years	Method	SL
Salvage value	15,000			Depreciation:			
				Annual	$12,000		
Depreciable cost	$60,000			Monthly	1,000		

Date	Asset			Accumulated Depreciation			Book Value
	Dr.	Cr.	Balance	Dr.	Cr.	Balance	
1 1 X1	$75,000		$75,000				$75,000
12 31 X1					$12,000	$12,000	63,000

Figure 18–2 Depreciation Posting to Plant Ledger Card

expense, and accumulated depreciation) at the end of each fiscal year.

A special policy may be followed in recording depreciation on plant assets acquired during the course of a fiscal year. Because depreciation expense is, after all, merely an estimate, it is acceptable to adopt a policy of a half-year's depreciation on all plant asset additions in the year acquired, regardless of the month of acquisition. Once this policy is adopted, however, it should be consistently followed.

Recording a Half-Year's Depreciation on Plant Asset Additions

The procedure described so far has assumed *unit depreciation*— that is, the straight-line method was applied to a single unit or item of equipment. Because the computation of depreciation on an item-by-item basis involves considerable clerical effort, hospitals often find it more efficient to compute depreciation by groups of related plant assets. The procedure (known as *group depreciation* or *composite depreciation*) involves the application of a single depreciation rate to the total cost of a combined group of assets.

Figure 18–3 Computation of
Composite Depreciation Rate

Asset	Acquisition Cost	Salvage Value	Depreciable Cost	Useful Life (Years)	Annual Depreciation
A	$ 4,000	$ 400	$ 3,600	4	$ 900
B	22,000	2,000	20,000	20	1,000
C	9,000	-0-	9,000	5	1,800
D	20,000	4,000	16,000	8	2,000
E	6,000	1,200	4,800	6	800
F	19,000	1,000	18,000	12	1,500
	$80,000	$8,600	$71,400		$8,000

Composite depreciation rate = $8,000 ÷ $71,400 = 11.2%

Group Rates. Under the group depreciation method, a number of similar plant assets are depreciated as a single unit. All the beds in a particular nursing unit, for example, might be grouped on a single subsidiary ledger record. Depreciation is then computed as if these beds were a single plant asset. If these beds have a total depreciable cost of $45,000 and an average service life of 15 years, the annual depreciation expense is $3,000 ($45,000 ÷ 15).

Composite Rates. Under the composite depreciation method, a number of dissimilar assets may be depreciated as a single unit. To illustrate, assume that six different equipment items are acquired on January 1, 19X1, for a particular department of a hospital. Each equipment item has a different cost, salvage value, and useful life. When acquired, these items are entered on a single subsidiary ledger record, and a composite rate of depreciation is determined, as shown in Figure 18–3. The composite rate of depreciation for this departmental group of assets is 11.2 percent ($8,000 ÷ $71,400); the composite life is 8.925 years ($71,400 ÷ $8,000). Thus, $8,000 of depreciation expense is recorded each year so that, at the end of 8.925 years, accumulated depreciation will amount to $71,400.

Funding of Depreciation

The funding of depreciation refers to the process by which cash resources are set aside periodically and accumulated for the purpose of financing the renewal or replacement of plant assets. To illustrate the procedure, assume that Hopewell Hospital's depreciation expense for a particular year is $185,000:

Depreciation Expense	$185,000	
Accumulated Depreciation		$185,000
Depreciation expense for the year.		

Now assume that the funding of depreciation by the hospital is a voluntary action prescribed by the governing board. This is the appropriate entry, assuming 100 percent funding:

Board-Designated Assets—Cash	$185,000	
Cash—General Checking		
Account		$185,000
Funding of depreciation expense		
for the year.		

Thus, $185,000 is transferred from the hospital's general checking account and set aside in a special board-designated cash account within the unrestricted fund. Although these resources are earmarked for a specific purpose, the future use of this money remains entirely under the control of the board. It would be improper to transfer the $185,000 to the plant replacement and expansion fund as if it were donor-restricted.

The hospital, of course, may fund more or less than the amount recorded as depreciation expense. The amount actually funded, however, has no bearing whatever on the amount of depreciation expense to be recorded. Naturally, the cash set aside in this way should be invested until such time as new plant assets are required. Income earned on such investments is accounted for as unrestricted resources and must be reported as nonoperating revenues in the hospital's income statement. This income, however, may be designated by the board for the purchase of new plant assets and added to board-designated assets.

Amount Funded Is Distinct from Depreciation Expense

It should be pointed out that the funding of depreciation is the only means through which the value of plant assets is maintained and converted into cash during the assets' useful lives. The alternative is to do nothing, allowing the plant asset values to decline over time; this, in reality, gradually depletes and impairs the hospital's permanent capital.

Disposal of Plant Assets

It is important to make an accurate accounting of disposals of plant assets through normal retirement, sale, or exchange. Each of these possibilities is examined in this discussion. As a basis for the illustrations, we again assume that radiology equipment was acquired for $75,000 on January 1, 19X1. The equipment, which has an estimated useful life of five years and a $15,000 salvage value, is depreciated by the straight-line method.

Normal Retirement

If the equipment's useful service life ends on December 31, 19X5, as was estimated, and its expected salvage value is realized, the entry to record the retirement of the equipment is as follows:

Cash Receipts Journal

12/31/X5	Cash—General Checking Account	$15,000	
	Accumulated Depreciation—Major Movable Equipment	60,000	
	Major Movable Equipment		$75,000
	Retirement of equipment.		

In addition to the general ledger postings arising from this entry, suitable notations are made on the plant ledger card, as indicated in Figure 18–4. At this time, the card is removed to an inactive file and retained for the period of time required by the hospital's record retention policies.

Should the actual salvage value prove to be more or less than $15,000, the entry just shown would include an account for the recognition of a gain or loss on retirement of the asset. If the salvage proceeds proved to be $16,500, for example, the entry would include a credit to a "gain on retirement of plant assets" account for $1,500. This gain would be reported among the nonoperating revenues in the hospital's 19X5 income statement.

Handling Fully Depreciated Assets Remaining in Use

In cases where fully depreciated assets remain in service, the usual practice is to take no further depreciation and to make no adjustment of previously recorded depreciation. The cost of such assets and the related accumulated depreciation remain on the books until the assets are eventually retired from service.

Sale of Plant Assets

A plant asset may be sold prior to the end of its scheduled useful service life for reasons not anticipated when it was acquired.

Assume, for example, that the equipment is sold for $49,400 on May 1, 19X3:

Cash Receipts Journal

5/1/X3	Cash—General Checking Account	$49,400	
	Accumulated Depreciation— Major Movable Equipment	28,000	
	Major Movable Equipment		$75,000
	Gain on Sale of Plant Assets		2,400

Sale of item of equipment:

Cost	$75,000
Accumulated depreciation:	
19X1 (12 months)	12,000
19X2 (12 months)	12,000
19X3 (4 months)	4,000
Total	28,000
Book value	47,000
Sale proceeds	49,400
Gain	$ 2,400

Description Radiology Equipment (details)   I.D. #7040–8510–67

Cost	$75,000	Useful Life	5 years	Method	SL
Salvage value	15,000	Depreciation:			
		Annual	$12,000		
Depreciable cost	$60,000	Monthly	1,000		

Date	Asset Dr.	Asset Cr.	Asset Balance	Accum. Dep. Dr.	Accum. Dep. Cr.	Accum. Dep. Balance	Book Value
1 1 X1	$75,000		$75,000				$75,000
12 31 X1					$12,000	$12,000	63,000
12 31 X2					12,000	24,000	51,000
12 31 X3					12,000	36,000	39,000
12 31 X4					12,000	48,000	27,000
12 31 X5					12,000	60,000	15,000
12 31 X5		$75,000	–0–	$60,000			–0–

Retired 12/31/X5; salvage value was $15,000.

Figure 18–4 Retirement Recorded on Plant Ledger Card

If this equipment had been sold on this date for an amount less than its $47,000 book value, the transaction would have produced a "loss on sale of plant assets." Such losses usually are treated as reductions of nonoperating revenues in the income statement.

Exchanges (Trades) of Plant Assets

In certain instances, an old plant asset may be given up (along with cash) in exchange for a new plant asset. To illustrate, assume that the radiology equipment along with $33,800 cash is given in exchange for a new item of radiology equipment. The necessary accounting entry, assuming that the exchange occurs on May 1, 19X3, is as follows:

Cash Receipts Journal

5/1/X3	Major Movable Equipment		$80,800	
	Accumulated Depreciation—			
	Major Movable Equipment		28,000	
	Major Movable Equip-			
	ment			$75,000
	Cash—General			
	Checking Account			33,800
	Acquisition of new			
	equipment in exchange			
	for old equipment and			
	cash as follows:			
	Book value of old			
	equipment	$47,000		
	Cash paid	33,800		
	Cost of new equipment	$80,800		

The general accounting rule is that the "cost" of an asset received in an exchange is the fair market value of the assets given up, or the fair market value of the asset received, whichever is more clearly evident. Any gain or loss is recognized. An exception to that general principle is made when, as in this case, the noncash assets exchanged are similar in nature and use. In such cases, the "cost" of the asset received is the book value of the noncash asset given up, plus cash paid, and no gain or loss is recognized. There are other exceptions, but a discussion of them is beyond the scope of this book. These matters are covered, however, in the author's *Hospital Financial Accounting: Theory and Practice.*

Q18-1. Distinguish between land and land improvements.

Questions

Q18-2. Distinguish between fixed equipment and major movable equipment. Give examples of the types of equipment that are includable in each of these classifications.

Q18-3. Describe briefly the proper accounting procedure for minor equipment.

Q18-4. List five items that generally should be included in the cost of purchased equipment. Should interest be included in the cost of equipment purchased on an installment or deferred payment plan?

Q18-5. Rex Hospital obtained an item of equipment by dona- tion. At the date received, the equipment had a fair mar- ket value of $25,000. This equipment has an estimated useful life of 8 years and a 20 percent salvage value.
   a. Make the entry to record the acquisition of the equipment.
   b. Compute the annual depreciation to be recorded on this equipment.

Q18-6. What are the advantages of maintaining a detailed subsid- iary ledger for plant assets?

Q18-7. How is each of the following determined?
   a. Depreciable cost
   b. Useful life
   c. Salvage value

Q18-8. "Depreciation expense is a measure of the decline in the value of plant assets during an accounting period." Do you agree? Explain.

Q18-9. Distinguish briefly between the group depreciation method and the composite rate depreciation method.

Q18-10. What is meant by the "funding" of depreciation? What entry is made to record the funding of, say, $79,000 of depreciation?

Q18-11. Righton Hospital purchased an item of equipment for $40,000 on January 1, 19X1. This equipment has an estimated useful life of eight years and a 10 percent sal- vage value. On June 30, 19X4, the equipment is sold for $23,100. Assuming the straight-line depreciation method, prepare the necessary entry to record the sale of the equipment.

New Equip 72,000
Dep 22,800
Old equip 60,000
Cash 26,000
Loss 8,800

Q18–12. Ragtag Hospital purchased an item of equipment for $60,000 on January 1, 19X1. This equipment has an estimated useful life of 10 years and a 20 percent salvage value. On October 1, 19X5, this equipment is traded, along with $26,000 cash, for similar equipment having a list price of $72,000. Assuming the straight-line depreciation method, prepare the necessary entry to record the trade.

Rule is cost of assets received in an exchange is the fair market value of the assets given up plus cash.

Q18–13. Summarize briefly the accounting procedure to be followed when an existing item of equipment having a book value of $40,000 and a fair market value of $45,000 is traded, along with $13,000 cash, for a new item of equipment having a list price of $60,000. *Cost*

$18,000 \div 3 \text{ yrs} = \$6,000$
$6,000 \times 12 = \$72,000$
$72,000 \div 90\% = \$80,000$

Q18–14. Ritter Hospital purchased an item of equipment on April 1, 19X1. This equipment has an estimated useful life of 12 years and a 10 percent salvage value. The accumulated depreciation on this equipment on March 31, 19X4, was $18,000. Assuming straight-line depreciation has been recorded, what was the acquisition cost of the equipment?

Exercises

Cash 535
AccDep 150
Loss 115
Equip 800
$(800-80) \div 8 = 90 \times 2 (1\frac{1}{2}) = 150$

E18–1. Right Hospital purchased a new item of equipment for $800 on 5/1/X1. The equipment has an estimated useful life of eight years and an estimated salvage value of $80. This equipment was sold for $535 on 7/1/X2. The equipment is depreciated by the straight-line method.

Required: What was the loss on the sale of the equipment?

Cost ÷ Dep per yr

$22\% \quad 12.5\% \quad \frac{2200}{2750}$

E18–2. Ready Hospital provides you with the following list of depreciable assets acquired at the beginning of the current year:

Asset	Cost	Estimated Salvage Value	Estimated Useful Life (Years)	
A	$4,000	$400 *3600*	3	*1200*
B	1,500	300 *1200*	4	*300*
C	7,000	750 *6250*	5	*1250*

Required: What is the composite depreciation rate on cost? *2750*

New Equip 950
AccDep 270
Old equip 800
Cash 420
$(800-80) \div 8 = 90 \times 3 = 270$

E18–3. Realgood Hospital purchased a new item of equipment for $800 on 1/1/X1. The equipment has an estimated salvage value of $80 and an estimated useful life of eight years. The equipment, which was depreciated by the straight-line method, was traded on 1/1/X4 for a similar item of equipment. Cash "boot" of $420 was paid to effect the trade. The old equipment had a fair value of $530; the new equipment had a fair value of $950.

Required: What is the cost of the new equipment?

E18–4. Realfine Hospital provides you with the following information about one of its depreciable assets at 12/31/X3:

Year of acquisition	19X1
Estimated useful life	Five years
Cost	$70,000
Estimated salvage value	14,000
Accumulated depreciation	33,600

The hospital takes a full year's depreciation in the year of a depreciable asset's acquisition, and no depreciation in the year of a depreciable asset's disposition. On 6/30/X4, this depreciable asset was sold for $28,000.

Required: What is the gain (loss) on the sale?

P18–1. On January 1, 19X1, Rainy Hospital acquired five items of equipment, as follows:

Problems

Asset	Acquisition Cost	Salvage Value	Useful Life (Years)
#1	$10,000	$2,000	8
#2	45,000	5,000	10
#3	24,000	4,000	5
#4	30,000	6,000	12
#5	19,000	1,000	6

Required: Prepare a depreciation table, similar to the one illustrated in Figure 18–3, showing a computation of the composite rate of depreciation and the composite life of these five items of equipment.

P18–2. On January 1, 19X1, Restful Hospital acquired an item of equipment for $90,000. This equipment has an estimated useful life of five years and a 20 percent salvage value. On March 1, 19X4, this equipment is sold for $44,000.

Required: Assume that Restful Hospital's fiscal year ends on December 31 and that adjustments for depreciation are made only at the end of each year. (1) Prepare all necessary journal entries from January 1, 19X1, through March 1,

19X4. (2) Draw up and complete a plant ledger card for this item.

P18–3. Redhot Hospital purchased an item of laboratory equipment on October 1, 19X1, at a billed price of $20,000. In addition, the hospital paid $200 for freight and $800 for the construction of a wooden base and for making the proper electrical connections. The estimated useful life of the equipment is six years with no salvage value. The hospital's fiscal year ends September 30.

Required: Prepare journal entries to record (1) the purchase of the equipment, (2) depreciation expense for the first year, (3) the write-off of the fully depreciated equipment after six years, and (4) the funding of depreciation at the end of the first year.

P18–4. Roadway Hospital's preadjusted trial balance at December 31, 19X3 (the end of the hospital's fiscal year) includes the following accounts:

	Dr.	Cr.
Land	$ 13,000	
Land Improvements	18,000	
Accumulated Depreciation—Land Improvements		$ 2,000
Buildings	900,000	
Accumulated Depreciation—Buildings		28,800
Fixed Equipment	300,000	
Accumulated Depreciation—Fixed Equipment		20,000
Major Movable Equipment	440,000	
Accumulated Depreciation—Major Movable Equipment		60,000
Minor Equipment	24,000	
Accumulated Depreciation—Minor Equipment		16,000

The following additional information is available:

1. Roadway Hospital began operations on January 1, 19X1, when (with the exception noted below) all of its plant assets were acquired. The correct amounts of depreciation have been recorded for 19X1 and 19X2, but no depreciation entries have as yet been made for 19X3.

2. The land improvements are being depreciated over an 18-year life with no expected salvage value.
3. The building has an estimated useful life of 50 years and an estimated salvage value of 20 percent.
4. The fixed equipment has an estimated useful life of 25 years and an estimated salvage value of $50,000.
5. An analysis of the major movable equipment account is as follows:

1/1/X1	Equipment purchased having an estimated useful life of 12 years and a 10% salvage value	$400,000
3/1/X3	Equipment purchased having an estimated useful life of eight years and a 20% salvage value	60,000
9/1/X3	Proceeds from sale of equipment purchased on 1/1/X1 for $20,000	(15,000)

6. Minor equipment is being depreciated over a three-year period with no salvage value expected.

Required: (1) Prepare the necessary journal entries at December 31, 19X3. (2) Prepare a presentation of the plant assets section of the hospital's December 31, 19X3, balance sheet.

Long-Term Investments

19

Temporary, or short-term, investments in stocks and bonds are those that are readily marketable and that management intends to hold for only a short period (generally not in excess of one year). The proceeds from their disposition ordinarily are used to meet current obligations. Investments not meeting these criteria are separately classified in the balance sheet as long-term investments. Short-term investments were discussed in Chapter 16; this chapter is concerned with long-term investments.

Long-term investments may appear in any fund, but often they are found as assets of the endowment fund or of the plant replacement and expansion fund. The funding of depreciation by action of the hospital's governing board may result in long-term investments that are properly reported as board-designated assets in the unrestricted fund. In any case, these investments typically consist of government bonds, corporate bonds, and corporate stocks.

When securities of a long-term investment nature are acquired by gift or by endowment, they are recorded in the appropriate fund at their fair market value when received. The cost of bonds and stocks purchased, on the other hand, will include the quoted purchase price, brokerage fees, and other expenditures that are necessary to the acquisition. Income from long-term investments, usually consisting of interest and dividends, should be recognized on the accrual basis and in the appropriate fund. All income on unrestricted fund investments and all unrestricted income on investments of the restricted funds must be reported as nonoperating revenues of the unrestricted fund. Donor-restricted investment income generally is recorded in either the specific purpose fund or the plant replacement and expansion fund. Gains and losses on the disposition of long-term investments usually are recorded in the fund in which the investments were carried as assets.

Long-term investments in debt securities, regardless of the fund in which they are recorded, are usually recorded in the accounts at cost, plus or minus unamortized premium or discount. Departures from the cost basis are not currently acceptable, unless there is clear evidence of a material and apparently permanent decline in the market value of those investments. The "write-downs" to the lower market values are reported as losses of the period in which the decline in value occurs. In no event is it presently in accord with generally accepted accounting principles to adjust the carrying value of long-term investments upward to reflect market values higher than cost.

Valuing Long-Term Investments Under Cost Principle

Certain authorities, however, are challenging this position. The AHA *Chart of Accounts for Hospitals* (in both the 1976 and the 1966 editions), for example, expresses a preference for the valuation of long-term security investments at market value, whether it be higher or lower than historical cost. Nevertheless, in spite of its supposed merit, this practice is not yet a generally accepted accounting principle. So, in this book we assume that long-term investments in debt securities are to be valued under the cost principle, with appropriate supplemental disclosures of market values. The valuation of long-term investments in stocks is discussed later in this chapter.

Investments in Bonds

A major part of the hospital investment portfolio is likely to consist of investments in government and corporate bonds because of the emphasis usually put on safety of principal and stability of income. Both government and corporate bonds are available in varying types and denominations, although bonds of $1,000 face, or maturity, value are most common. Bond interest is quoted at annual percentage rates of face value but often is paid to bondholders semiannually on specified dates six months apart.

Acquisition of Bonds

To illustrate the accounting procedures for long-term investments in bonds, assume that Goodcare Hospital purchases 60 of the $1,000, 8 percent, 10-year bonds of National Company on September 1, 19X1. The bonds have a May 1, 19X8, maturity date and pay interest semiannually on May 1 and November 1. Although bonds may be purchased at face value at times, it is more likely that the acquisition price will be either more or less than face value; that is, the bonds will be purchased either at a premium or at a discount. This occurs largely because the current market rate of interest (which changes frequently) is higher or lower than the fixed nominal or coupon rate of interest paid on the bonds.

Discount Acquisition. If the current market rate of interest is in excess of 8 percent, the National Company bonds may be quoted at a price that is less than face value. Assume, for example, that the bonds are quoted at 92 (at 92 percent of face value), or $55,200 (92 percent of $60,000). Let us also assume that brokerage fees and other acquisition costs total $400. The entries for the acquisition of the bonds therefore are as follows:

Voucher Register

9/1/X1	Investments—Bonds		$55,600	
	Accrued Interest Receivable		1,600	
	Accounts Payable			$57,200
	Voucher for purchase of			
	National Company bonds			
	at a discount:			
	Quoted price (92% of			
	$60,000)	$55,200		
	Acquisition costs	400		
	Cost of bonds	55,600		
	Accrued interest:			
	($60,000 × 0.08 × 4/12)	1,600		
	Disbursement	$57,200		

Cash Disbursements Journal

9/1/X1	Accounts Payable	$57,200	
	Cash—General		
	Checking Account		$57,200
	Check issued for purchase of		
	National Company bonds.		

Notice that the brokerage fees and other acquisition expenditures are treated as a part of the cost of the bonds. Note also that because these bonds were purchased between interest payment dates, the hospital must pay the seller the amount of interest accrued since the last interest payment date (May 1, 19X1). This, however, will be recovered by the hospital on November 1, 19X1, as National Company will always pay a full six months' interest on each interest payment date regardless of the number of months the bonds have been held by the investor. (This was explained earlier in

Handling Brokerage Fees and Acquisition Expenditures

Chapter 16.) If these bonds had been purchased on an interest payment date (May 1 or November 1 in this example), no accrued interest would have been involved in the acquisition.

Premium Acquisition.   In instances where the nominal or coupon rate of interest is higher than the current market rate of interest, bonds tend to sell at a *premium,* a price greater than the face value. Assume, for example, that Goodcare Hospital purchased the above National Company bonds at 105 and that acquisition costs were $600. The following shows the necessary entries:

Voucher Register

9/1/X1	Investments—Bonds	$63,600	
	Accrued Interest Receivable	1,600	
	Accounts Payable		$65,200
	Voucher for purchase of National		
	Company bonds at a premium:		

Quoted price (105% of $60,000)	$63,000	
Acquisition costs	+ 600	
Cost of bonds	63,600	
Accrued interest ($60,000 × 0.08 × 4/12)	1,600	
Disbursement	$65,200	

Cash Disbursements Journal

9/1/X1	Accounts Payable	$65,200	
	Cash—General Checking Account		$65,200
	Check issued for purchase of National Company bonds.		

Observe that Goodcare Hospital will receive annual interest of $4,800 (8 percent of $60,000). Because $63,600 was paid for the bonds, however, the effective (actual) rate of return on this investment to the hospital will be somewhat less than 8 percent. In the previous example, which assumed that the bonds were acquired at a cost of $55,600, the effective yield will be greater than 8 percent.

Bond Interest Income   The amount of bond interest to be recorded as investment income by Goodcare Hospital depends on whether the bonds were purchased at a discount or premium. This is because the amount of discount or premium must be amortized over the number of months between the date of acquisition and the maturity date of the bonds. Let us examine the amortization process through the following illustrations.

Amortization of Discount. Again assume the purchase of the National Company bonds (details provided earlier) at a discount on September 1, 19X1. At the end of September (and at the end of each ensuing month), the hospital will make an adjusting entry to record bond interest income for the month. Assuming that the bond discount is amortized by the straight-line method, the following is the necessary entry:

General Journal

9/30/X1	Accrued Interest Receivable	$400	
	Investments—Bonds	55	
	Bond Interest Income		$455
	Accrual of interest and amortization of		
	bond discount:		

Nominal interest
($60,000 × 0.08 × 1/12) $ 400

Discount amortization:

Maturity value of bonds	−60,000	
Cost of bonds	−55,600	
Discount	−4,400	
Divide by months to maturity	80	
Discount amortization	55	
Monthly interest income	$ 455	

Note that the discount ($4,400) will be taken into the accounts as bond interest income over the 80 months from the acquisition date to the maturity date of the bonds at the rate of $55 per month. The resulting $455 credit to income is a rough approximation of the effective amount of interest earned each month on the investment.

Notice also that the preceding entry debits the monthly amortization to the investment account, thereby increasing its carrying value by $55 each month. By the maturity date (May 1, 19X8), the investment account will have a balance of exactly $60,000, that is, $55,600 + ($55 × 80 months). So, when the face amount of the bonds is paid to the hospital on the maturity date by National Company, the following entry is made:

Debiting the Monthly Amortization

Cash Receipts Journal

5/1/X8   Cash—General Checking
            Account $60,000
                Investments—Bonds $60,000
            Receipt of face value of
            matured National
            Company bonds.

If the discount were not amortized over the 80-month period, the entire $4,400 discount would have to be recorded as 19X8 income in the above entry. It seems quite clear, however, that the discount is earned by the hospital ratably over the 80-month period rather than just in the year of maturity alone. Thus, long-term investments in bonds purchased at a discount are carried in the accounts at acquisition cost plus discount amortization to date.

On November 1, 19X1, the hospital will receive six months' interest on its investment in National Company bonds:

Cash Receipts Journal

11/1/X1   Cash—General Checking
            Account $2,400
                Accrued Interest
                    Receivable $2,400
            Receipt of semiannual
            interest on investment in
            National Company bonds
            ($60,000 × 0.08 × 6/12).

Remember that the accrued interest receivable account was debited for $1,600 on September 1, when the bonds were acquired, for $400 on September 30, in an adjusting entry, and for $400 again on October 31, in an adjusting entry. The resulting $2,400 debit balance is then cleared from the accounts by the credit in the cash receipts journal entry on November 1. The adjusting entry required at the end of each month to record the nominal monthly interest income also includes the monthly discount amortization.

To help you understand this process, Figure 19–1 shows the postings of all 19X1 entries relating to Goodcare Hospital's investment in the National Company bonds. The hospital's 19X1 income statement will report bond interest income of $1,820. Its December 31, 19X1, balance sheet will include $800 of accrued interest receivable and will report the long-term investment at $55,820 (acquisition cost plus discount amortization to date).

Amortization of Premium.   Earlier, this section described the purchase of the National Company bonds on September 1, 19X1, at a cost of $63,600. At the end of each month, an adjusting entry will be required to record bond interest income and amortization of bond premium for the month. Assuming that the premium is amortized by the straight-line method, the entry at September 30, 19X1, is as follows:

General Journal			
9/30/X1	Accrued Interest Receivable	$400	
	Investments—Bonds		$45
	Bond Interest Income		355
	Accrual of interest and		
	amortization of bond premium:		

Nominal interest:		
($60,000 × 0.08 × 1/12)	$ 400	
Premium amortization:		
Cost of bonds	63,600	
Maturity value of bonds	60,000	
Premium	3,600	
Divide by months to maturity	80	
Premium amortization	45	
Monthly interest income	$ 355	

Exactly the same adjusting entry is made at the end of each month until the maturity date of the bonds. Notice that the amortization of bond premium has the effect of reducing bond interest income. The resulting $355 is roughly the effective amount of monthly bond interest income.

Notice that the adjusting entry credits the monthly amortization of premium to the investment account, thereby decreasing its carrying value by $45 monthly. By the maturity date of the bonds, the investment account will have a balance of precisely $60,000, that is, $63,600 − ($45 × 80 months). Thus, long-term investments in bonds purchased at a premium are carried in the accounts at acquisition cost minus premium amortization to date.

Monthly Premium Amortization Credited to the Investment Account

Figure 19-1 Accounting for Bonds Purchased at a Discount

Cash—General Checking Account			Accrued Interest Receivable			Investments—Bonds		
(5) 2,400	(2) 57,200	(1) 1,600	(5) 2,400		(1) 55,600			
		(3) 400			(3) 55			
		(4) 400			(4) 55			
		(6) 400			(6) 55			
		(7) 400			(7) 55			
		Bal. 800			Bal. 55,820			

Accounts Payable		Bond Interest Income	
(2) 57,200	(1) 57,200		(3) 455
			(4) 455
			(6) 455
			(7) 455
			Bal. 1,820

Posting references:
(1) 9/1/X1 acquisition of bonds—voucher register.
(2) 9/1/X1 acquisition of bonds—cash disbursements journal.
(3) 9/30/X1 adjusting entry—general journal.
(4) 10/31/X1 adjusting entry—general journal.
(5) 11/1/X1 receipt of interest—cash receipts journal.
(6) 11/30/X1 adjusting entry—general journal.
(7) 12/31/X1 adjusting entry—general journal.

Figure 19-2 Accounting for Bonds Purchased at a Premium

Cash—General Checking Account			Accrued Interest Receivable			Investments—Bonds		
(5) 2,400	(2) 65,200	(1) 1,600	(5) 2,400		(1) 63,600	(3) 45		
		(3) 400				(4) 45		
		(4) 400				(6) 45		
		(6) 400				(7) 45		
		(7) 400			Bal. 63,420			
		Bal. 800						

Accounts Payable		Bond Interest Income	
(2) 65,200	(1) 65,200		(3) 355
			(4) 355
			(6) 355
			(7) 355
			Bal. 1,420

Posting references:
(1) 9/1/X1 acquisition of bonds—voucher register.
(2) 9/1/X1 acquisition of bonds—cash disbursements journal.
(3) 9/30/X1 adjusting entry—general journal.
(4) 10/31/X1 adjusting entry—general journal.
(5) 11/1/X1 receipt of interest—cash receipts journal.
(6) 11/30/X1 adjusting entry—general journal.
(7) 12/31/X1 adjusting entry—general journal.

Figure 19–2 presents the postings of all 19X1 entries for Goodcare Hospital's investment (at a premium) in the National Company bonds. You should study this illustration in comparison with Figure 19–1.

The entry to be made when bond investments are held to maturity has been illustrated earlier. Suppose, however, that bonds held as long-term investments are sold prior to their maturity. Refer to the facts given earlier in this section relating to the purchase of the National Company bonds for $55,600 on September 1, 19X1, and now assume that the bonds are sold on April 1, 19X3, at 102 and accrued interest. The required entry is as follows:

	Cash Receipts Journal		
4/1/X3	Cash—General Checking Account	$62,725	
	Accrued Interest Receivable		$ 2,000
	Investments—Bonds		56,645
	Gain on Sale of Investments		4,080
	Sale of investment in National Company bonds:		
	Sales price ($60,000 @ 102)	$61,200	
	Less brokerage fees	475	
	Net sales proceeds	60,725	
	Accrued interest:		
	($60,000 × 0.08 × 5/12)	2,000	
	Cash received	$62,725	
	Net sales proceeds (above)	$60,725	
	Book value of bonds:		
	Acquisition cost	55,600	
	Add amortized discount:		
	($55 × 19 months)	1,045	
	Book value of bonds	56,645	
	Gain on sale	$ 4,080	

As can be seen, the cash account is debited for the quoted price at which the bonds were sold (net of brokerage fees) plus the five months of bond interest accrued since the last interest payment date (November 1, 19X2). This accrued interest, of course, had previously been established in the accounts by the month-end adjusting entries. At the date of the sale, the bond investment account had a balance of $56,645, having been written up to that amount because of the amortization of discount at the rate of $55 per month for the 19 months since the date of acquisition. Then, the difference between this carrying amount and the net sales proceeds is recorded as the gain on the sale. Make special note of the fact that the accrued interest at the date of sale has no bearing on the amount of gain or loss on the sale.

Instead of selling all the bonds, let us now assume that only 40 percent (face value of $24,000) of the bonds are sold on April 1, 19X3, at 102 and accrued interest, with brokerage fees amounting to $200. The necessary entry is as follows:

Cash Receipts Journal

4/1/X3	Cash—General Checking Account	$25,080	
	Accrued Interest Receivable		$ 800
	Investments—Bonds		22,658
	Gain on Sale of Investments		1,622
	Sale of 40% of the investment in		
	National Company bonds:		

— Sales price ($24,000 @ 102)	$24,480	
Less brokerage fees —	200	
Net sales proceeds	24,280	
Accrued interest:		
($24,000 × 0.08 × 5/12)	800	
Cash received	$25,080	
Net sales proceeds (above)	$24,280	
Book value of bonds sold:		
(40% × $56,645)	22,658	
Gain on sale	$ 1,622	

Interest and discount amortization, of course, will continue on the remaining $36,000 face value of the National Company bond investment until these bonds are either sold or reach maturity. The monthly interest and discount amortization, however, will be only 60 percent of the amounts illustrated earlier. In other words, the monthly amortization will be $33 (60 percent of $55) and the monthly credit to bond interest income $273 (60 percent of $455), starting April 30, 19X3.

The procedures described here are also applicable to bonds acquired by the hospital as a gift or an endowment. In these cases, the fair market value of the bonds at the date of donation is regarded to be their cost. If the fair market value is less than maturity value, accounting procedures are those described for bonds acquired at a discount. If the fair market value is greater than maturity value, the accounting procedure is that described for bonds acquired at a premium.

The investment of hospital resources in corporate stocks involves some degree of risk with regard to price declines, but such investments may offer large rewards in the form of dividends and appreciation in value if they are managed intelligently. Investments may be made in either preferred or common stocks. Preferred stock has certain preferences over common stock, as the name implies. Dividends, for example, must be paid to a company's preferred stockholders before any dividends may be paid to its common stockholders. Accounting procedures for investments in capital stocks, however, are not much affected by the particular type of stock involved.

Investments in Stocks

Assume that Goodcare Hospital purchases 400 shares of Bluchip Company's common stock for $22,000 (including brokerage fees and other acquisition costs) on January 2, 19X1:

Acquisition of Stocks

	Voucher Register		
1/2/X1	Investments—Stocks	$22,000	
	Accounts Payable		$22,000
	Purchase of 400 shares of Bluchip Company's common stock.		
	Cash Disbursements Journal		
1/2/X1	Accounts Payable	$22,000	
	Cash—General Checking Account		$22,000
	Check issued for purchase of Bluchip Company stock.		

For investments in both bonds and stocks, a subsidiary ledger record should be maintained to provide the details of each investment and to support the general ledger investment control accounts. These subsidiary records sometimes are kept in the form illustrated in Figure 19–3.

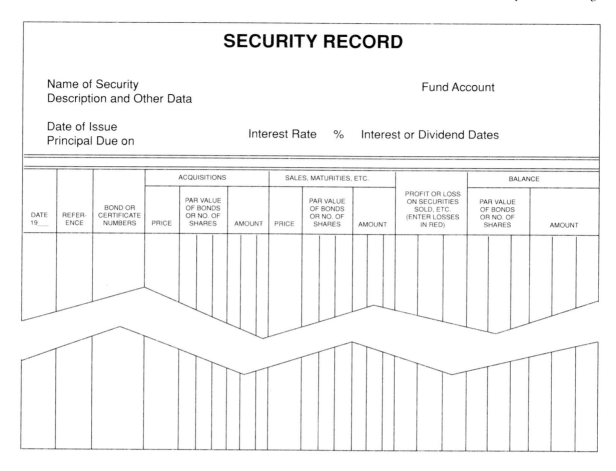

Figure 19–3 Subsidiary Ledger Record for Investments

Receipt of Dividends   Hospitals having capital stocks in their investment portfolios may receive cash dividends and perhaps stock dividends. We will illustrate the receipt of both types of dividends below with respect to Goodcare Hospital's investment in Bluchip Company stock.

Cash Dividends.   There are three important dates with respect to dividends. A typical cash dividend announcement reads somewhat as follows:

> On April 20, 19X1, the board of directors of Bluchip Company declared a cash dividend of $1.50 per share payable on May 19, 19X1, to common stockholders of record at May 5, 19X1.

You can find dividend announcements of this sort in the financial pages of newspapers, in business journals, and even in certain popular magazines. These announcements always provide three dates:

1. The declaration date (here, April 20), that is, the date on which the board of directors voted dividend payment approval.

2. The payment date (May 19 in this case), that is, the date on which the company will mail out the dividend checks.

3. The record date (May 5 here), that is, the date on which a determination is made of the names of the stockholders entitled to the dividend on the basis of the company's records.

Once a dividend has been declared, it must be paid. It also should be noted that all stockholders listed as such in the company's records on the record date will receive the dividend although they may sell their stock prior to the payment date. If the stock is purchased or sold between the declaration date and the record date, the quoted price per share includes the declared dividend. If the stock is purchased or sold after the record date, the per share price does not include the dividend.

An entry for cash dividends should be made at the declaration date by the investor because the dividend has been earned at that time and because the payment of the declared dividend by the corporation is legally required. Goodcare Hospital's entry follows:

Entry for Cash Dividends at Declaration Date

General Journal

4/20/X1 Dividends Receivable	$600	
Dividend Income		$600
Dividend income on Bluchip Company stock (400 shares × $1.50).		

Assuming that the hospital continues to hold the 400 shares of Bluchip stock, no entry will be necessary at the record date. But when the dividend check is received on May 19, the following entry is made:

Cash Receipts Journal

5/19/X1 Cash—General Checking Account	$600	
Dividends Receivable		$600
Receipt of cash dividends on Bluchip Company stock.		

Carefully note that the stock's dividend income was recorded in April (the month in which the dividend was earned) whereas the cash receipt was recorded in May. This, you see, is accrual basis accounting; income is recorded in the time period in which it is earned rather than in the time period in which the income is received in cash.

Stock Dividends.   In addition to paying cash dividends, corporations sometimes will distribute *stock dividends,* that is, their stockholders are given additional shares of stock without charge. As is true of cash dividends, there are three important dates in recording the distribution: the declaration date, the record date, and the stock distribution date. Announcements similar to those for cash dividends are made.

Journal Entry Not Required for Stock Dividends

To illustrate, assume that on June 2, 19X1, Bluchip Company's board of directors declared a 10 percent common stock dividend to be distributed on July 10, 19X1, to common stockholders of record at June 26, 19X1. As a result, Goodcare Hospital receives 40 (10 percent × 400 shares) additional common shares without cost. No formal entry of any kind, however, is necessary because stock dividends do not give rise to income, regardless of the market value of the shares received. Stock dividends simply increase the number of shares outstanding without any change in the issuing corporation's net assets. Subsequent to a stock dividend, each shareholder has the same percentage ownership interest as before.

The effect of a stock dividend on the stockholder is simply to reduce the cost per share of stock. Goodcare Hospital, for example, had 400 shares of stock that had cost $22,000, or $55 per share. On receipt of the 40–share stock dividend, the hospital has 440 shares that cost $22,000, or $50 per share. Thus, the effect of the stock dividend in this example is simply an increase in the number of shares held and a decrease in the cost per share. Naturally, the subsidiary ledger investment records would be adjusted accordingly, but no journal entry is required.

Disposition of Stocks

When stock is sold, the difference between the proceeds of sale (net of any brokerage fees and other expenses of sale) and the cost of the stock (as it may be adjusted for stock dividends, if any) is recorded as a gain or loss of the fund in which the stock was carried as an investment. Assume, for example, that Goodcare Hospital sells 100 shares of the Bluchip Company common stock for $6,425 on September 4, 19X1. Assuming brokerage fees of $92, the entry to record the sale is as follows:

Cash Receipts Journal

9/4/X1	Cash—General Checking Account	$6,333	
	Investments—Stocks		$5,000
	Gain on Sale of Investments		1,333
	Sale of 100 shares of Bluchip		
	Company stock:		

Sales price	$6,425	
Less brokerage fees	92	
Net sales proceeds	6,333	
Less cost of stock:		
(100 shares × $50)	5,000	
Gain on sale	$1,333	

The subsidiary ledger records should be properly adjusted for the shares sold. It should be clear that 340 (440 − 100) shares of stock remain in the investment account at a cost of $17,000 (340 shares × $50).

Suppose, however, that the Bluchip stock had been acquired at different times and at different costs per share. In such cases, to determine the cost of shares subsequently sold, it may be necessary to assume first-in, first-out (FIFO) or other costing methods (see Chapter 17) in much the same manner as is done for inventories of supplies. Of course, if the subsidiary record of investments provides a record of cost per share according to stock certificate numbers, a specific identification can be made to determine the cost of shares sold.

Entries for Sale of Shares Purchased at Various Prices

Depending on the circumstances, investments in equity securities may be accounted for at cost, at the lower of aggregate cost or market value, or at an amount resulting from the use of the equity method. We assume the use of the cost method in this book. The other methods are treated at length in the author's *Hospital Financial Accounting: Theory and Practice*.

Valuation of Equity Investments

Suitable internal controls should be maintained to safeguard the hospital's investments in stocks and bonds, as well as the related interest and dividend income, against loss through fraud, error, or mismanagement. It is important that all purchases and sales of investment securities be authorized by the hospital's governing

Internal Controls

board or its investment committee. Once acquired, stock and bond certificates should be kept in a safe place, preferably in a bank safe-deposit box with access requiring two hospital executives. Employees who can access the accounting records or cash should not, of course, have access to investment securities. Finally, regular reports of investments should be submitted to management and to the hospital's governing board.

Questions

Q19-1. Distinguish between temporary investments and long-term investments.

Q19-2. When securities of a long-term investment nature are acquired by donation, at what amount are such assets initially recorded in the hospital's accounts?

Q19-3. When securities are purchased for long-term investment purposes by the hospital, what is their "cost"?

Q19-4. In what fund should the hospital record income earned on long-term investments? In what fund should gains and losses on sales of long-term investments be recorded?

Q19-5. Explain what is meant by the declaration date, the record date, and the payment date with respect to corporate dividend distributions resulting from hospital investments in corporate stocks.

Q19-6. What are some of the major features of a satisfactory system of internal control over hospital investments in securities?

Q19-7. Sara Hospital holds an investment in the capital stock of an industrial corporation. The hospital receives 50 shares of the corporation's common stock as a dividend at a time when the stock is quoted on the market at $40 per share. Should Sara Hospital record $2,000 of dividend income? Explain.

Q19-8. Saint Hospital owns investment securities that cost $100,000 but have a current market value of $140,000. At what amount should these securities be presented in the hospital's balance sheet? Explain.

Q19-9. A hospital owns 300 shares of stock that were acquired as follows:

1/1/X1   100 shares purchased for $4,000.
1/1/X2   100 shares purchased for $5,000.
1/1/X3   100 shares purchased for $6,000.

On 2/1/X3, 150 of these shares are sold for $9,750. What is the amount of the gain on the sale?

Q19-10. When corporate bonds are purchased between interest payment dates, the hospital purchaser must pay accrued interest since the last interest payment date. Why?

Q19-11. When corporate bonds are purchased at a price higher or lower than face value, the premium or discount must be amortized by the purchaser. What is the purpose of amortizing bond premium or discount?

Q19-12. In what sections of the hospital balance sheet does one find the following accounts?
  a. Temporary investments
  b. Long-term investments—bonds
  c. Accrued interest receivable
  d. Long-term investments—stocks
  e. Dividends receivable

Exercises

E19-1. Samson Hospital purchased $1,200 (face value) of the 5 percent bonds of XYZ Company at 92 on 7/1/X1. Brokerage and other acquisition costs were $32. Interest is payable semiannually on 5/1 and 11/1. The maturity date of the bonds is 11/1/X6. On 9/1/X1, $480 (face value) of the bonds are sold at 95 and accrued interest; brokerage costs were $12.

Required: What was the gain (loss) on the sale?

E19-2. Sitdown Hospital purchased $900 (face value) of the 8 percent bonds of Robin Company at 109 on 10/1/X1. Brokerage costs were $31. Interest is payable semiannually on 6/1 and 12/1. The maturity date of the bonds is 6/1/X6. On 1/1/X3, $450 (face value) of the bonds are sold at 114 and accrued interest; brokerage costs were $13.

Required: What was the gain (loss) on the sale?

E19-3. On 11/1/X1, Sheraton Hospital purchased Maybell Company 10-year, 7 percent bonds with a face value of $50,000 for $49,167. Interest is payable semiannually on 1/1 and 7/1. The bonds mature on 7/1/X8.

Required: What is the hospital's 19X1 interest income?

E19-4. On 1/1/X1, Sideway Hospital purchased 200 shares of Pickard Company stock for $5,760 plus brokerage costs of $240. An additional 200 shares were purchased on 5/1/X1 for $6,912 plus brokerage costs of $288. On 8/1/X1, Pickard declared and distributed a 20 percent stock dividend. On 10/1/X1, Sideway sold 100 shares of the Pickard stock at 32³/₈ less brokerage costs of $129.50.

Required: Assuming FIFO, what was the gain on the sale?

E19–5. On 10/1/X1, Safeway Hospital purchased 100 shares of Paul Company stock at $45 per share; brokerage costs were $26. A $3 per share cash dividend had been declared on 9/25/X1 to be paid on 10/18/X1 to stockholders of record at 10/8/X1.

Required: At what amount should the investment in Paul stock be reported in Safeway's 10/31/X1 balance sheet?

Problems

P19–1. Sample Hospital purchased 90 of the $1,000, 8 percent, 10-year bonds of ABC Company on August 1, 19X1, at 91 and accrued interest. Brokerage and other acquisition costs were $560. These bonds mature in 116 months and pay interest semiannually on April 1 and October 1. The hospital's fiscal year ends on December 31. Although the hospital intended to hold these bonds as long-term investments, the bonds were sold on January 1, 19X2, at 98 and accrued interest. Brokerage and other expenses of sale amounted to $610.

Required: Prepare a chart, such as the one illustrated in Figure 19–1 of the text, showing all necessary entries from August 1, 19X1, through January 1, 19X2.

P19–2. Simple Hospital purchased 90 of the $1,000, 8 percent, 10-year bonds of ABC Company on August 1, 19X1, at 108 and accrued interest. Brokerage and other acquisition costs were $572. These bonds mature in 116 months and pay interest semiannually on April 1 and October 1. The hospital's fiscal year ends on December 31. Although the hospital intended to hold these bonds as long-term investments, the bonds were sold on January 1, 19X2, at 102 and accrued interest. Brokerage and other expenses of sale amounted to $520.

Required: Prepare a chart, such as the one illustrated in Figure 19–2 of the text, showing all necessary entries from August 1, 19X1, through January 1, 19X2.

P19–3. Supple Hospital purchased $100,000 face value of XYZ Company bonds at 96 on May 1, 19X1. These bonds pay 6 percent interest per year, payable semiannually on April 1 and October 1. These bonds mature in 107 months. Brokerage fees and various other acquisition costs totaling $255 were paid. It was management's intent to hold these securities as long-term investments, but on January 1, 19X2, 60 percent of the bonds were sold at 94 and accrued interest, less brokerage fees and other expenses of sale amounting to $210.

Required: Prepare all necessary entries relating to this investment from May 1, 19X1, through January 1, 19X2.

P19–4. Setsail Hospital purchased $100,000 face value of XYZ Company bonds at 104 on May 1, 19X1. Brokerage and other acquisition costs were $280. These bonds pay 7.5 percent interest per year, payable semiannually on April 1 and October 1. The maturity date of the bonds is April 1, 19X6. It was management's intent to hold these securities as long-term investments, but on January 1, 19X2, 40 percent of the bonds were sold at 106 and accrued interest, less brokerage fees of $310.

Required: Prepare all necessary entries relating to this investment from May 1, 19X1, through January 1, 19X2.

P19–5. Signoff Hospital purchased 200 shares of the $10 par value common stock of Mohawk Company on May 15, 19X1, for $12,700. Brokerage fees amounted to $60. On June 1, the board of directors of Mohawk declared a cash dividend of $2.50 per share payable June 18 to stockholders of record at June 10. On August 4, the board of directors of Mohawk declared a 10 percent stock dividend payable August 30 to stockholders of record at August 15. As of August 4, Mohawk stock was selling on the market at $80 per share. On September 19, the hospital sold 120 shares of the Mohawk stock for $10,000, with brokerage fees amounting to $140.

Required: Prepare entries to record all matters relating to the investment in Mohawk Company stock for 19X1.

P19–6. Situp Hospital purchased Eastcoast Company common stock, as shown here:

Date	Shares	Price Per Share	Brokerage	Total Cost
1/1/X1	20	$11.00	$20.00	$240.00
1/1/X2	20	14.50	30.00	320.00

On April 1, 19X2, Eastcoast Company declared a cash dividend of $1.50 per share payable May 1, 19X2, to stockholders of record as of April 20, 19X2. On July 2, 19X2, Eastcoast Company declared a 25 percent stock dividend distributable August 15, 19X2, to stockholders of record on July 21, 19X2. On October 3, 19X2, Situp Hospital sold 10 shares of the Eastcoast Company stock for $160, less brokerage costs of $25.

Required: Prepare entries to record all matters relating to the investment in Eastcoast Company stock for 19X1 and 19X2.

Long-Term Liabilities

20

In addition to the current liabilities described in Chapter 17, a hospital has economic obligations that will not be discharged with resources classified in the balance sheet as current assets. These obligations are variously referred to as *long-term, noncurrent,* or *fixed liabilities.* Whereas current liabilities generally arise from informal contractual arrangements, long-term liabilities are ordinarily based on a written contract such as a mortgage document, bond indenture, or lease agreement. A proper distinction between current and noncurrent liabilities in the balance sheet is of considerable importance in evaluating the financial position of a hospital as well as in managing its financial affairs.

Long-term liabilities typically consist of mortgages and bonds payable, long-term contracts and capital lease obligations, employee pension and retirement plan liabilities, and the noncurrent portion of deferred revenues. The discussion in this chapter will be limited, however, to accounting procedures relating to hospital bond issues.

Because most hospitals can no longer expect to obtain significant amounts of new long-term funds from philanthropy, public subscription, government grants, and other traditional sources, the only recourse is for the hospital to borrow through bond issues and then to repay with internally generated cash. The rapid increase in debt financing by hospitals in recent years provides sufficient documentation on this matter. This practice, encouraged by various state laws that enable hospitals to issue tax-free revenue bonds, naturally places a premium on superior financial management and its accounting prerequisites. It is largely for these reasons that we devote this chapter entirely to the subject of accounting for bonds payable. Accounting procedures relating to long-term leases, pension plans, and other noncurrent liabilities are described at length in the author's *Hospital Financial Accounting: Theory and Practice.*

Nature of Bonds Payable

The power of a hospital corporation to issue bonds arises in the corporation laws of the state and is exercised by authorization of the governing board. For state and municipal hospitals, bonded indebtedness also may require the approval of a majority of citizens. Many states have created statutory authority for issuing tax-exempt bonds to finance not-for-profit hospitals' long-term capital needs.

The Bond Indenture

Bonds ordinarily are issued in $1,000 denominations referred to as *face* (or *maturity*) *value*. The terms of a bond issue are spelled out in a contract known as a bond indenture. It details the rights and obligations of the bondholders and the hospital, names the agency that is to act as trustee to protect the rights and enforce the covenants and obligations of both parties, and describes the bonds as to security, interest rate, maturity date, and other matters. Although bonds may be sold directly to the general public, they more often are underwritten by investment bankers or a syndicate of brokerage firms who market the bonds on a commission basis.

Types of Bonds

Several different types of bonds may be issued by hospitals. *Registered bonds* are those on which interest is paid only to "bondholders of record" (that is, those whose holdings are recorded by the issuing hospital or its registrar agent). No record is kept of the owners of coupon bonds; rather, interest on coupon bonds is paid to all bondholders who present the periodic interest coupons that accompany the bond certificates. *Serial bonds* mature in installments over a period of years, whereas a *term bond* issue matures on a single fixed maturity date. Some bonds, at the option of the hospital, may be callable at specified times on payment of a "call price" that usually is higher than the face value of the bonds.

In addition, bonds may be either secured or unsecured. *Secured bonds, often known as mortgage bonds,* involve pledging specific plant assets under liens as security to bondholders. Hospital bond issues may also be secured in the sense that payment of principal and/or interest may be guaranteed by a governmental authority or some parent organization. The security for a hospital bond issue may also arise from the accumulation of a bond *sinking fund* (a pool of resources earmarked for the payment of interest charges and for the retirement of the bonds). In many instances, hospitals have issued revenue bonds on which interest is paid from specified revenue sources. Finally, hospitals having extremely high credit ratings may sometimes issue *general obligation bonds* that are secured only by the hospital's reputation and general financial resources. Unsecured bonds of this type are called *debentures*.

The decision to issue bonds is a critical matter. All relevant factors must be carefully considered and evaluated. It should be evident that the bond issue is the most desirable means of obtaining the necessary long-term funds at reasonable cost and on acceptable terms. There must be assurances that the debt burden, periodic interest charges, and principal retirement will not lead to financial embarrassment and endanger the hospital's ability to meet its obligations to the community it serves. In all cases, the assistance of reputable professional firms specializing in hospital financing should be obtained.

Issuance of Bonds

When the hospital corporation issues bonds, it contracts to pay (1) the face value of the bonds at a specified maturity date and (2) interest (expressed as a percentage of face value) at periodic intervals, usually every six months. This nominal, or coupon, interest rate is predetermined on the basis of expectations concerning the rate of interest investors will demand at the time the bonds are actually issued. The market rate of interest varies according to the degree of credit risk, the term of the bonds, the supply-and-demand situation for long-term money, and the taxability of the bond interest to investors, among other factors.

Premium and Discount Prices

If the nominal interest rate should equal the market rate, the hospital's bonds will sell at face value. There often is a difference, however, between the nominal and market rates of interest. Bonds sell at a premium (a price greater than face value) if the nominal interest rate is higher than the market rate; they sell at a discount (a price lower than face value) if they pay interest at a rate less than the market rate. Thus, differences between the contractual and market rates of interest are reflected in the prices investors are willing to pay for the bonds, thereby eliminating the need to amend the bond contract. Because issuing bonds at a discount or a premium is most common, we will discuss only those two possibilities.

Issuance at a Discount

To illustrate the accounting procedures for bonds issued at a discount, let us assume that Supercare Hospital issues $400,000 (face value) of 6 percent, 20-year bonds at $92^5/8$ (92.625 percent of face value, or $370,500) on August 1, 19X1. (Hospital bond issues generally are much larger amounts, but $400,000 is a convenient amount for purposes of illustration.) These bonds pay interest semiannually on April 1 and October 1. Semiannual interest payments are \$12,000 (\$400,000 $\times$ 0.06 $\times$ 6/12). The bonds are dated April 1, 19X1, so the maturity date is 20 years later. Also assume that bond issue costs amount to \$17,700, which include sales commissions paid to investment bankers, legal and accounting fees, registration and filing fees, appraisal costs, and printing expenses.

As noted earlier, the bond certificates are dated April 1, 19X1, but the hospital postponed the actual sale of the bonds until August 1, 19X1, in order to take advantage of an expected decline in the market rate of interest. Assuming that all of the bonds are sold on August 1, 19X1, then, the following entries are made in the unrestricted fund accounts of the hospital:

Cash Receipts Journal

8/1/X1	Cash—General Checking Account	\$378,500	
	Unamortized Bond Discount	29,500	
	Accrued Interest Payable		\$ 8,000
	Bonds Payable		400,000
	Issue of \$400,000 of 6%, 20-year bonds:		
	Face value	\$400,000	
	Proceeds:		
	($400,000 @ 92.625)	370,500	
	Discount	\$ 29,500	
	Proceeds (above)	\$370,500	
	Accrued interest:		
	($400,000 $\times$ 0.06 $\times$ 4/12)	8,000	
	Total cash received	\$378,500	

Voucher Register

8/1/X1	Unamortized Bond Issue Costs	\$ 17,700	
	Accounts Payable		\$ 17,700
	Voucher issued for payment of bond issue costs.		

Cash Disbursements Journal

8/1/X1	Accounts Payable	\$ 17,700	
	Cash—General Checking Account		\$ 17,700
	Check issued in payment of bond issue costs.		

When bonds are issued (sold) between interest payment dates, as these bonds were, the issuing hospital collects accrued interest from the purchasers as a part of the transaction. This procedure enables the hospital to pay a full six months' interest at each semiannual interest payment date, regardless of how long individual bondholders may have held their bonds. It would be impractical for the hospital to try to compute the amount of interest actually due each bondholder at each interest payment date. Accrued interest settlements are made between sellers and buyers of bonds at the trading date as an adjustment of the price to be paid by the buyers.

If a balance sheet were prepared immediately after the bond issue, it would present the bonds as a long-term liability of Supercare Hospital's unrestricted fund in the following manner:

6% Bonds Payable	$400,000	
Less Unamortized Bond Discount	29,500	$370,500

Thus, the unamortized bond discount is deducted from the face amount of the outstanding bonds in the long-term liability section of the balance sheet. The unamortized bond issue costs of $17,700, on the other hand, should be included in the noncurrent assets of the unrestricted fund in a "deferred charges" or "other assets" category. Only the unamortized bond discount should be shown in the contraliability position. It is never correct to classify the bond discount as an asset. Finally, the balance sheet also would present the $8,000 of accrued interest payable among the current liabilities of the hospital.

When the nominal interest rate is higher than the market rate of interest, bonds will be issued at a premium. Assume, for example, that Supercare Hospital issues $400,000 (face value) of 9 percent, 20-year bonds at 108.85 (108.85 percent of $400,000, or $435,400) on August 1, 19X1. These bonds pay interest semiannually on April 1 and October 1, and are dated April 1, 19X1. Also assume that bond issue costs amounted to $23,600. If all of the bonds are sold on August 1, 19X1, the following entries are made in the unrestricted fund accounts:

Issuing Bonds Between
Interest Payment Dates

Reporting Discounts and
Issue Costs in the Balance
Sheet

Issuance at a Premium

Cash Receipts Journal

8/1/X1	Cash—General Checking		
	Account	$447,400	
	Unamortized Bond Premium		$ 35,400
	Accrued Interest Payable		12,000
	Bonds Payable		400,000
	Issuance of $400,000 of 9% bonds:		

Proceeds:

$400,000 @ 108.85	$435,400	
Face value	400,000	
Premium	$ 35,400	
Proceeds (above)	$435,400	
Accrued interest:		
($400,000 × 0.09 × 4/12)	12,000	
Total cash received	$447,400	

Voucher Register

8/1/X1	Unamortized Bond Issue Costs	$ 23,600	
	Accounts Payable		$ 23,600
	Voucher issued for payment of bond issue costs.		

Cash Disbursements Journal

8/1/X1	Accounts Payable	$ 23,600	
	Cash—General Checking Account		$ 23,600
	Check issued in payment of bond issue costs.		

If a balance sheet were prepared immediately after the above bond issue, it would present the bonds as a long-term liability of the unrestricted fund in the following manner:

9% Bonds Payable	$400,000	
Add Unamortized Bond Premium	35,400	$435,400

Note that unamortized bond premium is added to the face amount of bonds outstanding, whereas unamortized bond discount was deducted in the previous illustration. The balance sheet also will include the unamortized bond issue costs of $23,600 in a noncurrent "deferred charges" or "other assets" classification and will report the $12,000 of accrued interest payable among the current liabilities.

The amount of bond interest expense to be recorded each month is influenced by the premium or discount recorded at the time the bonds are issued. Amortization of bond discount is regarded as an addition to periodic interest expense, whereas the amortization of bond premium is treated as a reduction of interest expense. This system is followed in order to obtain at least a rough approximation of the effective (actual) interest cost of the bonds. In practice, bond discount and premium may be amortized (allocated) evenly throughout the life of the bond issue by application of the straight-line, or average, method. (A theoretically superior procedure, called the *compound-interest* or *effective-yield method,* is also used in actual practice.) Bond issue costs are usually amortized to expense by application of the straight-line method.

Bond Interest and Amortization

Refer to the Issuance at a Discount discussion earlier in this chapter, where the proceeds of the $400,000, 6 percent bond issue amount to only $370,500. The resulting $29,500 of bond discount should be amortized by charges to interest expense over the 236-month life of the bond issue: the 236 months between the issue date and the maturity date. The idea is that, because the hospital received only $370,500 but must repay $400,000 at maturity, the $29,500 represents a cost that is properly allocable to the period that presumably benefits from the resources the bond issue provided. It is a matter of cost allocation and of matching costs and revenues on a periodic basis. A similar procedure applies to the $17,700 of bond issue costs.

Interest and Discount

At the end of each of the 236 months during which the bonds will be outstanding, adjusting entries will be made to amortize $125 ($29,500 ÷ 236) of bond discount and $75 ($17,700 ÷ 236) of bond issue costs. The required entries for August 31, 19X1, will illustrate the procedure:

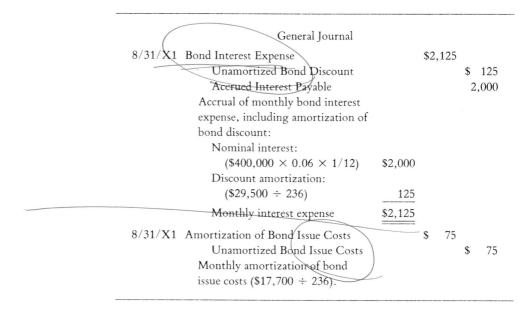

General Journal

8/31/X1 Bond Interest Expense $2,125
            Unamortized Bond Discount $ 125
            Accrued Interest Payable   2,000
         Accrual of monthly bond interest
         expense, including amortization of
         bond discount:
            Nominal interest:
               ($400,000 × 0.06 × 1/12) $2,000
            Discount amortization:
               ($29,500 ÷ 236)   125
            Monthly interest expense $2,125

8/31/X1 Amortization of Bond Issue Costs $ 75
            Unamortized Bond Issue Costs $ 75
         Monthly amortization of bond
         issue costs ($17,700 ÷ 236).

Amortization of Bond
Discount Increases Bond
Interest Expense

Notice that the amortization of bond discount is a part of the debit to bond interest expense, which roughly approximates the effective monthly interest cost. Amortization of bond issue costs, however, is charged to a separate expense account. Such costs, being in the nature of prepaid expenses, should not be confused or combined with bond discount.

The same entries, of course, will be made on September 30, 19X1. Then, on October 1, 19X1, when Supercare Hospital pays six months' interest on the bonds, the interest payment entries are the following:

Voucher Register

10/1/X1 Accrued Interest Payable $12,000
            Accounts Payable $12,000
         Voucher for payment of semiannual
         bond interest.

Cash Disbursements Journal

10/1/X1 Accounts Payable $12,000
            Cash—General Checking
               Account $12,000
         Checks issued to pay semiannual
         bond interest.

Recall that the accrued interest payable account was credited for $8,000 in the bond issue entry on August 1, 19X1, and was credited for $2,000 on August 31 and again on September 30, 19X1, in the month-end adjusting entries. The resulting credit balance of $12,000 is eliminated by the debit in the preceding voucher register entry of October 1, 19X1.

You also should recognize that the entire $29,500 of bond discount and the $17,700 of bond issue costs will have been charged to expense by the maturity date of the bonds. So, when the maturity date arrives and the bonds are retired, the entries are as follows:

	Voucher Register		
4/1/XX	Bonds Payable	$400,000	
	Accounts Payable		$400,000
	Voucher issued for		
	retirement of bonds.		
	Cash Disbursements Journal		
4/1/XX	Accounts Payable	$400,000	
	Cash—General		
	Checking Account		$400,000
	Checks issued to retire		
	bonds.		

In certain circumstances, all or part of a bond issue may be retired prior to its normal maturity date. This matter will be pursued later in this chapter.

Let us return for a moment to 19X1 and summarize all the entries that are made during the year for the $400,000 bond issue. These 19X1 entries are summarized in the general ledger accounts presented in Figure 20–1. Take note of the year-end account balances. The 19X1 income statement of Supercare Hospital will report $10,625 of bond interest expense and $375 of bond issue cost amortization (an expense). The December 31, 19X1, balance sheet will present the bonds as a long-term liability as follows:

Summary of Entries During Year of Bond Issuance

6% Bonds Payable	$400,000	
Less Unamortized Bond Discount	28,875	$371,125

Figure 20–1 Accounting for
Bonds Issued at a Discount

Cash—General Checking Account				Unamortized Bond Issue Costs				Accounts Payable			
(1)	378,500	(3)	17,700	(2)	17,700	(5)	75	(3)	17,700	(2)	17,700
		(9)	12,000			(7)	75	(9)	12,000	(8)	12,000
						(11)	75				
						(13)	75				
						(15)	75				
				Bal.	17,325						

Accrued Interest Payable				Bonds Payable				Unamortized Bond Discount			
(8)	12,000	(1)	8,000			(1) 400,000		(1)	29,500	(4)	125
		(4)	2,000							(6)	125
		(6)	2,000							(10)	125
		(10)	2,000							(12)	125
		(12)	2,000							(14)	125
		(14)	2,000					Bal.	28,875		
		Bal.	6,000								

Bond Interest Expense				Amortization of Bond Issue Costs			
(4)	2,125			(5)	75		
(6)	2,125			(7)	75		
(10)	2,125			(11)	75		
(12)	2,125			(13)	75		
(14)	2,125			(15)	75		
Bal.	10,625			Bal.	375		

Posting references:
(1) 8/1/X1 bond issue—cash receipts journal.
(2) 8/1/X1 payment of bond issue costs—voucher register.
(3) 8/1/X1 payment of bond issue costs—cash disbursements journal.
(4) 8/31/X1 interest accrual and discount amortization—general journal.
(5) 8/31/X1 amortization of issue costs—general journal.
(6) 9/30/X1 interest accrual and discount amortization—general journal.
(7) 9/30/X1 amortization of issue costs—general journal.
(8) 10/1/X1 payment of semiannual interest—voucher register.
(9) 10/1/X1 payment of semiannual interest—cash disbursements journal.
(10) 10/31/X1 interest accrual and discount amortization—general journal.
(11) 10/31/X1 amortization of issue costs—general journal.
(12) 11/30/X1 interest accrual and discount amortization—general journal.
(13) 11/30/X1 amortization of issue costs—general journal.
(14) 12/31/X1 interest accrual and discount amortization—general journal.
(15) 12/31/X1 amortization of issue costs—general journal.

This balance sheet also will report $17,325 of unamortized bond issue costs as an asset and $6,000 of accrued interest payable as a current liability.

Refer to Issuance at a Premium earlier in this chapter, where the proceeds of the $400,000, 9 percent bond issue amount to $435,400. At the end of each of the 236 months during which the bonds will be outstanding, adjusting entries such as the following will be made to amortize $150 ($35,400 ÷ 236) of bond premium and $100 ($23,600 ÷ 236) of bond issue costs:

Interest and Premium

General Journal

8/31/X1	Bond Interest Expense		$2,850	
	Unamortized Bond Premium		150	
	Accrued Interest Payable			$3,000
	Accrual of monthly bond interest expense and premium amortization:			
	Nominal interest:			
	($400,000 × 0.09 × 1/12)	$3,000		
	Premium amortization:			
	($35,400 ÷ 236)	150		
	Monthly interest expense	$2,850		
8/31/X1	Amortization of Bond Issue Costs		$ 100	
	Unamortized Bond Issue Costs			$ 100
	Monthly amortization of bond issue costs ($23,600 ÷ 236).			

Notice that the amortization of bond premium reduces the amount to be debited to bond interest expense to obtain an approximation of the true monthly interest cost.

The same entries, of course, will be made on September 30, 19X1. Then, on October 1, 19X1, when Supercare Hospital pays six months' interest on the bonds, the interest payment entries are as follows:

Interest Payment Entries

Voucher Register

10/1/X1	Accrued Interest Payable	$18,000	
	Accounts Payable		$18,000
	Voucher issued for payment of semiannual bond interest: ($400,000 × 0.09 × 6/12).		

Cash Disbursements Journal

10/1/X1	Accounts Payable	$18,000	
	Cash—General Checking Account		$18,000
	Checks issued to pay semiannual bond interest.		

Following this, the previously described monthly adjusting entries will be made on October 31, November 30, and December 31, 19X1. All the 19X1 entries for the $400,000 of 9 percent bonds issued at a premium are summarized in Figure 20–2.

Notice the year-end balances in Figure 20–2. The December 31, 19X1, balance sheet will present the bonds as a long-term liability as follows:

Bonds Issued at Premium Reported as Long-Term Liability

9% Bonds Payable	$400,000	
Add Unamortized Bond Premium	34,650	$434,650

This balance sheet also will report $23,100 of unamortized bond issue costs as an asset and $9,000 of accrued interest payable as a current liability. The 19X1 income statement of Supercare Hospital will report $14,250 of bond interest expense and $500 of bond issue cost amortization (an expense).

Early Extinguishment of Debt

The normal retirement of term bonds at the scheduled maturity date was illustrated earlier. Let us examine here the procedure to follow when term bonds are reacquired and retired prior to the scheduled retirement date. Accounting for the refunding of bond

Figure 20-2 Accounting for Bonds Issued at a Premium

Cash—General Checking Account		
(1) 447,400	(3)	23,600
	(9)	18,000

Unamortized Bond Issue Costs	
(2) 23,600	
Bal. 23,100	

Accounts Payable			
(3)	23,600	(2)	23,600
(9)	18,000	(8)	18,000

Unamortized Bond Issue Costs detail:
(5)	100
(7)	100
(11)	100
(13)	100
(15)	100

Accrued Interest Payable		
(8) 18,000	(1)	12,000
	(4)	3,000
	(6)	3,000
	(10)	3,000
	(12)	3,000
	(14)	3,000
	Bal.	9,000

Bonds Payable	
	(1) 400,000

Unamortized Bond Premium			
(4)	150	(1)	35,400
(6)	150		
(10)	150		
(12)	150		
(14)	150		
		Bal.	34,650

Bond Interest Expense	
(4)	2,850
(6)	2,850
(10)	2,850
(12)	2,850
(14)	2,850
Bal.	14,250

Amortization of Bond Issue Costs	
(5)	100
(7)	100
(11)	100
(13)	100
(15)	100
Bal.	500

Posting references:
(1) 8/1/X1 bond issue—cash receipts journal.
(2) 8/1/X1 payment of bond issue costs—voucher register.
(3) 8/1/X1 payment of bond issue costs—cash disbursements journal.
(4) 8/31/X1 interest accrual and premium amortization—general journal.
(5) 8/31/X1 amortization of issue costs—general journal.
(6) 9/30/X1 interest accrual and premium amortization—general journal.
(7) 9/30/X1 amortization of issue costs—general journal.
(8) 10/1/X1 payment of semiannual interest—voucher register.
(9) 10/1/X1 payment of semiannual interest—cash disbursements journal.
(10) 10/31/X1 interest accrual and premium amortization—general journal.
(11) 10/31/X1 amortization of issue costs—general journal.
(12) 11/30/X1 interest accrual and premium amortization—general journal.
(13) 11/30/X1 amortization of issue costs—general journal.
(14) 12/31/X1 interest accrual and premium amortization—general journal.
(15) 12/31/X1 amortization of issue costs—general journal.

issues, that is, the replacement of an outstanding bond issue with a new bond issue, and for the operation of bond sinking funds, however, will not be covered in this book.

A hospital may sometimes reacquire its own bonds in the market prior to maturity when bond prices and other factors make such action desirable. To illustrate, refer to the facts of the earlier example in which a $400,000 bond issue is sold at a premium on August 1, 19X1. Assume also that Supercare Hospital reacquires $80,000 (face value) of these bonds at 98 and accrued interest on June 1, 19X7, with brokerage and other reacquisition costs of $115 being paid. At the reacquisition date, the relevant accounts on the hospital's books have the following balances:

Accrued Interest Payable ($3,000 × two months)	$ 6,000 Cr.
Bonds Payable	400,000 Cr.
Unamortized Bond Premium ($35,400) − ($150 × 70 months)	24,900 Cr.
Unamortized Bond Issue Costs ($23,600) − ($100 × 70 months)	16,600 Dr.

The 70 months used in these computations of account balances are the number of months between the bond issue date (August 1, 19X1) and the bond reacquisition date (June 1, 19X7).

Recording a Reacquisition of Bonds

The entry to record the reacquisition requires the recognition of a gain (or loss) measured by the difference between the amount paid for the reacquired bonds (exclusive of accrued interest) and their book value at the date of reacquisition. The book value of the bonds reacquired and retired is computed as follows:

Book value of all bonds outstanding:		
Face value	$400,000	
Unamortized premium	24,900	
Unamortized issue costs	(16,600)	
Total		$408,300
Percentage of bonds reacquired: ($80,000 ÷ $400,000)		0.20
Book value of bonds reacquired		$ 81,660

The amount paid (exclusive of interest) to reacquire these bonds is $78,515 (98 percent of $80,000, plus $115 of brokerage fees and other costs of reacquisition). So, the gain on the reacquisition is $3,145 ($81,660 − $78,515). The necessary entries to record the reacquisition and retirement of the bonds are the following:

Journal Entries for Bond Retirement

Voucher Register

6/1/X7	Bonds Payable	$80,000	
	Accrued Interest Payable	1,200	
	Unamortized Bond Premium	4,980	
	Unamortized Bond Issue Costs		$ 3,320
	Gain on Reacquisition of Bonds		3,145
	Accounts Payable		79,715

Voucher issued for reacquisition and retirement of 20% of bond issue:

Face value (20% × $400,000)	$80,000
Unamortized premium: (20% × $24,900)	4,980
Unamortized issue costs: (20% × $16,600)	(3,320)
Book value of bonds reacquired	$81,660
Reacquisition cost: ($80,000 @ 98)	$78,400
Brokerage fees	115
Total	78,515
Accrued interest: (20% × $6,000)	1,200
Cash disbursement	$79,715

Cash Disbursements Journal

6/1/X7	Accounts Payable	$79,715	
	Cash—General Checking Account		$79,715

Check issued for reacquisition and retirement of 20% of bond issue.

After this reacquisition, accounting continues as before until maturity with respect to the remaining $320,000 of bonds. The monthly amount of amortization and interest, however, will be reduced by 20 percent. The monthly interest expense will be $2,280, monthly premium amortization will be $120, and monthly amortization of bond issue costs will be $80 (rather than $2,850, $150, and $100, respectively). Similarly, the monthly addition to accrued interest payable will be $2,400 ($320,000 × 0.09 × 1/12).

Reporting Gains and Losses on Early Retirement of Bonds

It should be noted that gains and losses on the early extinguishment of debt are reported in the income statement as extraordinary items. A simplified illustration of the presentation follows:

Revenues (assumed)	$800,000
Less expenses (assumed)	750,000
Income before extraordinary items	50,000
Add extraordinary gain (disclosed details)	3,145
Net income for the year	$ 53,145

Serial Bonds

The illustrations prior to this point have assumed that the bonds in question have been term bonds; that is, that all bonds in the issue have the same maturity date. Some hospital bond issues, however, are serial bonds that mature in periodic installments. To illustrate, assume a simplified case in which Supercare Hospital issues $400,000 of 5 percent serial bonds on January 1, 19X1, at 94. These bonds pay interest annually on January 1, and mature at the rate of $80,000 annually, starting January 1, 19X2. Issue costs were $14,400.

The Bonds Outstanding Method of Amortization

Figure 20–3 summarizes annual discount amortization and bond interest expense as computed by the "bonds outstanding" method. This method, rather than the straight-line method described earlier in this chapter, is used because the face amount of bonds outstanding each year varies. It provides for an amortization pattern that corresponds to the amount of bonds outstanding. Bond issue costs are amortized in the same pattern.

To illustrate the entries to be made for serial bonds, let us assume that Supercare Hospital makes entries for amortization and interest accruals only once each year on December 31. All of the necessary entries for 19X1 are summarized in Figure 20–4.

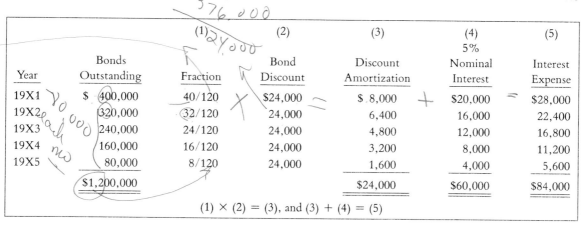

Year	Bonds Outstanding	(1) Fraction	(2) Bond Discount	(3) Discount Amortization	(4) 5% Nominal Interest	(5) Interest Expense
19X1	$ 400,000	40/120	$24,000	$ 8,000	$20,000	$28,000
19X2	320,000	32/120	24,000	6,400	16,000	22,400
19X3	240,000	24/120	24,000	4,800	12,000	16,800
19X4	160,000	16/120	24,000	3,200	8,000	11,200
19X5	80,000	8/120	24,000	1,600	4,000	5,600
	$1,200,000			$24,000	$60,000	$84,000

(1) × (2) = (3), and (3) + (4) = (5)

Figure 20–3 Summary of Discount Amortization and Interest Expense, Bonds Outstanding Method

	Cash Receipts Journal		
1/1/X1	Cash—General Checking Account	$376,000	
	Unamortized Bond Discount	24,000	
	Bonds Payable		$400,000
	Issuance of 5% serial bonds.		
	Voucher Register		
1/1/X1	Unamortized Bond Issue Costs	$ 14,400	
	Accounts Payable		$ 14,400
	Voucher issued for payment of bond issue costs.		
	Cash Disbursements Journal		
1/1/X1	Accounts Payable	$ 14,400	
	Cash—General Checking Account		$ 14,400
	Check issued for payment of bond issue costs.		
	General Journal		
12/31/X1	Bond Interest Expense	$ 28,000	
	Unamortized Bond Discount		$ 8,000
	Accrued Interest Payable		20,000
	Accrual of bond interest expense and amortization of bond discount:		
	Nominal interest: ($400,000 × 5%)	$20,000	
	Discount amortization: [$24,000 × (40 ÷ 120)]	8,000	
	19X1 interest expense	$28,000	

Figure 20–4 Entries for Serial Bonds

12/31/X1	Amortization of Bond Issue Costs	$ 4,800	
	Unamortized Bond Issue Costs		$ 4,800
	Amortization of bond issue costs for 19X1		
	[$14,400 × (40 ÷ 120)].		

Voucher Register

1/1/X2	Accrued Interest Payable	$ 20,000	
	Bonds Payable	80,000	
	Accounts Payable		$100,000
	Vouchers issued for payment of 19X1 accrued interest and for		
	retirement of bonds due January 1, 19X2.		

Cash Disbursements Journal

1/1/X2	Accounts Payable	$100,000	
	Cash—General Checking Account		$100,000
	Checks issued for payment of 19X1 accrued interest and for		
	retirement bonds due January 1, 19X2.		

General Journal

12/31/X2	Bond Interest Expense	$ 22,400	
	Unamortized Bond Discount		$ 6,400
	Accrued Interest Payable		16,000
	Accrual of bond interest and amortization of bond discount:		
	Nominal Interest:		
	($320,000 × 5%)	$16,000	
	Discount amortization:		
	[$24,000 × (32 ÷ 120)]	6,400	
	19X2 interest expense	$22,400	
12/31/X2	Amortization of Bond Issue Costs	$ 3,840	
	Unamortized Bond Issue Costs		$ 3,840
	Amortization of bond issue costs for 19X2		
	[$14,400 × (32 ÷ 120)].		

Figure 20–4 Entries for Serial Bonds *(continued)*

Current less than 1year - L/T is over a year

Questions

Q20–1. How are current and long-term liabilities different?

Q20–2. Briefly identify each of the following:

Contract between boy & bondholder
a. Bond indenture.

register to identify the owner
b. Registered bond.

The owner is not identified
c. Coupon bond.

amount periodic over the life of the
d. Serial bond. issue

e. Term bond.

falls due on a single date

f. Callable bond. _bond can be called in by the Hosp_

g. Secured bond. _Pledged by assets_

h. Revenue bond. _Pledged by revenues_

i. Debentures. _unsecured_

Q20–3. How should (a) unamortized bond discount, (b) unamortized bond premium, and (c) unamortized bond issue costs be presented in the hospital's balance sheet? _(A) Deduction from face of bond (B) addition to the face of bond (C) deferred charge classification_

Q20–4. On January 1, 19X1, a hospital issued serial bonds with a total face value of $1 million. These bonds mature annually in $200,000 amounts, beginning January 1, 19X2. Indicate how these bonds should be presented in the hospital balance sheet as of December 31, 19X1. _$200,000 Current $800,000 L.T._

Q20–5. A hospital bond issue, dated April 1, 19X1, is actually issued for cash on June 1, 19X1. The purchasers of these bonds will pay the hospital for two months of accrued interest. Why? _The purchasers pay for 2 mos because the hosp will pay for 6 mos_

Q20–6. Distinguish between the nominal (or coupon) rate of interest and the effective rate of interest for a hospital bond issue. _nominal rate of interest promised effective is actual rate paid_

Q20–7. For what reasons might a hospital bond issue sell at a price that is higher or lower than face value? _if the rate is higher or lower than the nominal currently_

Q20–8. If a hospital bond issue is sold at a discount, will the monthly charge to bond interest expense be greater or less than the nominal amount of interest per month? Explain. _greater – discount must be amortized._

Q20–9. A hospital bond issue is sold at a premium on January 1, 19X1. Interest on the bonds is payable annually on December 31. Will the annual interest expense recorded on the hospital's books be greater or less than the amount of annual interest actually paid to the bondholders? Explain. _Less_

Q20–10. If the market rate of interest is higher than the nominal (or coupon) rate of interest specified in a hospital bond issue, will the hospital's bonds sell at a price that is higher or lower than face value? Explain.

if interest is higher than nominal the Hosp sells lower so that purchaser can obtain an effective rate

Exercises

E20–1. On 1/1/X1, Sandy Hospital issued 500 of its 9 percent, $1,000 bonds at a rate of 95. Interest is payable semiannually on 7/1 and 1/1, and the bonds mature in 10 years. The hospital paid bond issue costs of $20,000.

_500 × 1,000 = 500,000_
_500,000 × 95 = 475,000_
25,000 (disc)

_LT 500,000 – 22,500 = 477,500. –_

_25,000 × (9/10 yr) = 22,500_

Required: What amount of long-term debt should be reported for the bonds in the hospital's 12/31/X1 balance sheet?

E20–2. On 1/1/X1, Skippy Hospital issued 2,000 of its 10 percent, $1,000 bonds for $2,080,000. These bonds mature in 10 years, but were callable at 101 any time after 12/31/X5. The interest is payable semiannually on 7/1 and 1/1. On 7/1/X6, the hospital called all of the bonds and retired them.

Required: What was the gain (loss) on this early extinguishment of debt?

E20–3. On 1/1/X1, Sally Hospital issued $500 of 8 percent, five-year serial bonds at 94. The bonds mature at the rate of $100 annually, beginning 1/1/X2. Interest is payable annually on 1/1.

Required: What is the amount of 19X2 bond interest expense?

E20–4. On 10/1/X1, Scott Hospital issued $1,000 (face value) of 7.2 percent, five-year term bonds at 100 and accrued interest. Issue costs were $55. Interest is payable semiannually, 5/1 and 11/1, and the bonds mature 5/1/X6. On 1/1/X2, $250 (face value) of these bonds were reacquired at 104 and accrued interest.

Required: What was the gain (loss) on the reacquisition of the bonds?

E20–5. On 9/1/X1, Stepout Hospital issued $4,000 (face value) of five-year, 9.6 percent bonds at 111 and accrued interest. Interest is payable semiannually, 4/1 and 10/1, and the bonds mature 4/1/X6. On 2/1/X2, $1,000 of these bonds are reacquired at 108 and accrued interest.

Required: What was the gain (loss) on the reacquisition of the bonds?

E20–6. On 9/1/X1, Stepup Hospital issued $4,000 (face value) of five-year, 4.8 percent bonds at 94.5 and accrued interest. Interest is payable semiannually on 4/1 and 10/1, and the bonds mature on 4/1/X6.

Required: What is the 19X1 bond interest expense?

Problems

P20–1. Saltville Hospital issued $1 million of five-year, 6 percent bonds at 100 and accrued interest on August 1, 19X1. Issue costs were $56,000. Interest is payable semiannually, April 1 and October 1. The maturity date of the bonds is April 1, 19X6. On February 1, 19X2, $200,000 of these bonds are reacquired at 98 and accrued interest.

Required: Prepare entries to record all matters relating to the bond issue from August 1, 19X1, through February 1, 19X2.

P20–2. Saltick Hospital issued $500,000 (face value) of 6 percent, 10-year bonds at 97.7 and accrued interest on October 1, 19X1. Bond issue costs amounted to $20,700. The bonds, dated May 1, 19X1, pay interest semiannually on May 1 and November 1. The hospital's fiscal year ends on December 31. On January 1, 19X2, the hospital reacquires 20 percent of these bonds by purchase in the open market at 92 and accrued interest, with brokerage and other reacquisition costs of $280 being paid.

Required: (1) Prepare a chart, such as the one in Figure 20–1, showing entries for all matters relating to this bond issue through December 31, 19X1. (2) Indicate how all matters relating to this bond issue should be presented in the hospital's 19X1 financial statements. (3) Prepare the necessary entry to record the reacquisition of 20 percent of the bonds on January 1, 19X2. (4) Compute the amount of bond interest expense for January 19X2.

P20–3. Salty Hospital issued $500,000 (face value) of 6 percent, 10-year bonds at 102.3 and accrued interest on October 1, 19X1. Bond issue costs amounted to $16,100. The bonds, dated May 1, 19X1, pay interest semiannually on May 1 and November 1. The hospital's fiscal year ends on December 31. On January 1, 19X2, the hospital reacquires 20 percent of these bonds by purchase in the open market at 101 and accrued interest, with brokerage and other reacquisition costs of $260 being paid.

Required: (1) Prepare a chart, such as the one in Figure 20–2, showing entries for all matters relating to this bond issue through December 31, 19X1. (2) Indicate how all matters relating to this bond issue should be presented in the hospital's 19X1 financial statements. (3) Prepare the necessary entry to record the reacquisition of 20 percent of the bonds on January 1, 19X2. (4) Compute the amount of bond interest expense for January 19X2.

P20–4. Saltrock Hospital issued $500,000 (face value) of 6 percent serial bonds on January 1, 19X1, at 94. These bonds pay interest annually on January 1 and mature at the rate of $100,000 annually, starting January 1, 19X2. Issue costs amounted to $15,000. The hospital's fiscal year ends on December 31, at which time annual entries are made for amortization and accruals.

Required: (1) Prepare a table, such as the one illustrated in Figure 20–3, to summarize discount amortization and interest expense for the 19X1–19X5 period. (2) Prepare the necessary entries for 19X1 and 19X2 only. (3) Indicate how all matters relating to these bonds should be presented in the hospital's 19X2 financial statements.

P20–5. Saltmine Hospital issued $600,000 (face value) of 8 percent serial bonds on January 1, 19X1, at 106. These bonds pay interest annually on January 1 and mature at the rate of $120,000 annually, starting January 1, 19X2. Issue costs amounted to $18,000. The hospital's fiscal year ends on December 31, at which time annual entries are made for amortization and accruals.

Required: (1) Prepare a table, such as the one in Figure 20–3, to summarize premium amortization and interest expense for the 19X1–19X5 period. (2) Prepare the necessary journal entries for 19X1 and 19X2 only. (3) Indicate how all matters relating to these bonds should be presented in the hospital's 19X2 financial statements.

P20–6. Saltless Hospital issued $600,000 (face value) of 6 percent, 10-year bonds at 94 and accrued interest on June 1, 19X1. Bond issue costs were $18,000. The bonds, dated June 1, 19X1, pay interest annually on June 1. The hospital's fiscal year ends on December 31. On January 1, 19X3, Saltless Hospital reacquires $150,000 (face value) of these bonds by purchase in the open market at 90 and accrued interest, with brokerage and other reacquisition costs of $300 being paid.

Required: Prepare the necessary journal entries at (1) June 1, 19X1, (2) June 30, 19X1, (3) June 1, 19X2, (4) January 1, 19X3.

Statement of Cash Flows

21

An income statement presents the results of a hospital's operations in terms of revenues earned and expenses incurred during a given time period. The balance sheet presents the hospital's financial position in terms of the assets, liabilities, and fund balances existing at a given point in time. The statement of changes in fund balances provides a summary analysis of the factors causing increases and decreases in the individual fund balances over a given period of time. For many years, these three financial statements were considered sufficient for the purposes of external financial reporting.

In 1971, the American Institute of Certified Public Accountants required that a fourth statement (a *statement of changes in financial position*) be included in the external reporting of the financial affairs and activities of an economic enterprise.[1] This position subsequently was affirmed and specifically made applicable to hospital financial reporting by the Institute's Committee on Health Care Institutions.[2] The statement of changes in financial position generally was designed to present the sources and uses of working capital during a given period of time within the unrestricted (general) fund. In some instances, the statement was presented in a cash (or cash equivalents) format rather than in a working capital format.

Recently, however, the FASB issued Statement No. 95, which supersedes APB Opinion No. 19.[3] Statement 95 requires all business enterprises to include a *statement of cash flows* (SCF), rather than a statement of changes in financial position, as an essential component of a complete set of financial statements. The AICPA Health

---

[1]APB Opinion No. 19, "Reporting Changes in Financial Position" (New York: AICPA, 1971).

[2]*Hospital Audit Guide* (New York: AICPA, 1978), p. 38.

[3]Statement No. 95, "Statement of Cash Flows" (Stamford, Connecticut: FASB, 1987).

Figure 21–1 Hopeful Hospital
Comparative Income Statements,
Years Ended December 31, 19X2
and 19X1

	19X2	19X1
Gross patient service revenues	$9,490	$8,870
Less deductions from revenues	890	780
Net patient service revenues	8,600	8,090
Other operating revenues	633	519
Total operating revenues	9,233	8,609
Less operating expenses:		
Nursing services	3,188	2,995
Other professional services	2,030	1,920
General services	1,610	1,540
Fiscal and administrative services	1,460	1,370
Depreciation	540	465
Other	315	292
Total operating expenses	9,143	8,582
Operating income	90	27
Nonoperating income (net)	195	154
Net income	$ 285	$ 181

Care Committee will undoubtedly make Statement No. 95 applicable to not-for-profit healthcare entities as well. In this chapter, we examine the nature of this required statement and illustrate the procedures for its preparation.

Nature of the Statement of Cash Flows

What the Statements Reveal

Comparative income statements and balance sheets for Hopeful Hospital are presented in Figures 21–1 and 21–2. (The changes in the unrestricted fund balance are assumed to consist only of net income as shown within the fund balance section of the balance sheets. Consequently, a separate statement of changes in fund balance is not presented here.)

Clearly, these statements provide a considerable amount of important information concerning the operating results and financial position of the hospital. Intelligent decision making, whether by the hospital's management or by interested external parties, requires such information. Is the information provided in these statements alone sufficient to the needs of management and external users? Is the information complete? Does it clearly reflect all significant operating, investing, and financing activities of the hospital during 19X1 and 19X2? Do income statements and balance sheets alone adequately disclose the flow of cash resources into and out of the hospital enterprise? In each instance, the answer is *no*.

Figure 21–2 Hopeful Hospital Comparative Balance Sheets — Unrestricted Fund, December 31, 19X2 and 19X1

Assets	19X2	19X1
Cash	$ 124	$ 280
Accrued interest receivable	45	30
Accounts receivable, net of allowance for uncollectible accounts of $210 at 12/31/X2 and $160 at 12/31/X1	1,536	1,340
Inventories	175	140
Prepaid expenses	32	40
Total current assets	1,912	1,830
Long-term investments	1,010	600
Plant assets, net of accumulated depreciation of $1,850 at 12/31/X2 and $1,340 at 12/31/X1	5,250	4,920
Total assets	$8,172	$7,350

Liabilities and Fund Balance	19X2	19X1
Accounts payable	$ 302	$ 370
Accrued expenses payable	208	220
Deferred revenues	77	60
Total current liabilities	587	650
Bonds payable	3,000	2,400
Total liabilities	3,587	3,050
Fund balance, January 1	4,300	4,119
Add net income for the year	285	181
Fund balance, December 31	4,585	4,300
Total liabilities and fund balance	$8,172	$7,350

Certain important aspects of the operating, financing, and investing activities of Hopeful Hospital are not disclosed by or made clearly apparent from an examination of its income statements and balance sheets alone. For example, consider the following information drawn from the balance sheets in Figure 21–2:

	19X2	19X1
Long-term investments	$1,010	$600

One might conclude from this presentation that new long-term investments costing $410 were purchased during 19X2. As you will shortly see, however, Hopeful Hospital purchased new long-term investments costing $450 and sold long-term investments (which had cost $40) for $49! Thus, the apparent $410 increase in long-term investments actually is the net difference between the costs of investments purchased and sold during 19X2.

Similar offsetting transactions typically are found in many of the other balance sheet accounts. These offsetting transactions, however, ordinarily are not determinable from the information provided in the balance sheet and income statement alone. If these financial statements are not to be misleading, such "hidden" information must be fully disclosed in some manner.

Purpose of the Statement of Cash Flows

The necessary disclosure is accomplished through the preparation of a statement of cash flows. It provides a summary of all significant cash flows relating to the operating, financing, and investing activities of the hospital. As noted above, many of these cash flows simply are not readily determinable (if at all) through an examination of balance sheet and income statement information alone.

Cash flow information has important implications for the hospital's creditors, reimbursement and planning agencies, and other external groups, as well as for internal management decisions. It can be used in estimating the cash flows that will be generated in the future and the growth potential of the hospital in terms of its ability to pay its existing obligations, finance expansion, and meet added indebtedness. Cash flow information also may indicate the need for external financing and clarify the difference between net income and cash flow from operating activities. The statement of cash flows is most useful, of course, when presented in comparative form for two or more years.

It should be noted that the term *cash,* in the context of the statement of cash flows, is defined as cash plus cash equivalents, that is, short-term investments that are highly liquid, readily marketable, and convertible into definitely known amounts of cash. Some examples of cash equivalents include demand deposits in bank savings accounts, commercial paper, treasury bills, and money market funds. Generally, only investments in securities having original maturities of three months or less should be classified as cash equivalents. It also should be understood that the statement of cash flows should present the *gross* amounts of both cash receipts and cash disbursements from the hospital's operating, investing, and financing activities.

Categories of Cash Flows

In the statement of cash flows, cash receipts and cash disbursements are classified into three categories: *operating activities, investing activities,* and *financing activities.* The types of cash flow transactions to be reported in each of these three categories are indicated at a later point in this chapter.

Figure 21–3 presents a summary of the financial activity of Hopeful Hospital for the year ended December 31, 19X2. This summary worksheet begins with the December 31, 19X1, postclosing balances you saw earlier in the hospital's December 31, 19X1, balance sheet (Figure 21–2). The following two columns of the worksheet provide a summary of the 19X2 transactions; the next two columns show the adjustments required at the end of 19X2; and the last two columns contain the preclosing account balances at the end of 19X2. These preclosing balances appeared in the hospital's 19X2 financial statements illustrated in Figures 21–1 and 21–2.

To assist you in your study of this worksheet, the 19X2 transactions and adjustments are presented here in general journal form:

Illustration Data

(1)	Accounts Receivable	$ 9,490	
	Patient Service Revenues		$ 9,490
	Gross revenues from services to patients.		
(2)	Cash	8,404	
	Deductions from Revenues	840	
	Accounts Receivable		9,244
	Revenue deductions and cash collections on patients' accounts.		
(3)	Cash	49	
	Gain on Sale of Investments		9
	Long-Term Investments		40
	Sale of long-term investments (cost: $40) for $49.		
(4)	Cash	54	
	Loss on Sale of Plant Assets	16	
	Accumulated Depreciation	30	
	Plant Assets		100
	Sale of plant assets (cost: $100; accumulated depreciation: $30) for $54.		

(5) Cash   3,830
          Other Operating Revenues   650
          Nonoperating Revenues   180
          Bonds Payable   3,000
          Other cash receipts, including proceeds
          from new 6% bond issue.

(6) Nursing Services Expenses   3,000
     Other Professional Services Expenses   1,900
     General Services Expenses   1,100
     Fiscal and Administrative Services
       Expenses   1,400
     Other Operating Expenses   300
          Accounts Payable   7,700
          Vouchers issued for operating expenses
          (including employee salaries and wages
          of $4,500) other than supplies.

(7) Inventories   935
     Long-Term Investments   450
     Plant Assets   940
     Bonds Payable   2,400
          Accounts Payable   4,725
          Other vouchers issued for purchase of
          inventory, purchase of long-term
          investments, purchase of plant assets,
          and retirement of 7% bonds.

(8) Accounts Payable   12,493
          Cash   12,493
          Checks issued in payment of vouchers
          issued for employee salaries and wages,
          and all vouchers recorded in entry 7
          above.

(9) Nursing Services Expenses   200
     Other Professional Services Expenses   130
     General Services Expenses   510
     Fiscal and Administrative Services
       Expenses   60
          Inventories   900
     Cost of supplies used.

(10) Depreciation Expense   540
          Accumulated Depreciation   540
       Depreciation expense for 19X2.

(11)	Accrued Interest Receivable	15	
	Nonoperating Revenues		15
	Adjustment for increase in accrued interest receivable.		
(12)	Deductions from Revenues	50	
	Allowance for Uncollectible		
	Accounts		50
	Adjustment for required increase in allowance for uncollectible accounts.		
(13)	Other Operating Expenses	8	
	Prepaid Expenses		8
	Adjustment for decrease in prepaid expenses.		
(14)	Accrued Expenses Payable	12	
	Nursing Services Expenses		12
	Adjustment for decrease in accrued expenses (assuming that expense items are nonlabor and relate solely to nursing services).		
(15)	Other Operating Revenues	17	
	Deferred Revenues		17
	Adjustment for increase in balance of deferred revenues.		

Recognize that certain liberties have been taken in these entries in an effort to simplify and reduce the size of the illustration. It is assumed, for example, that there were no accrued salaries and wages payable either at the beginning or end of 19X2. As you trace the journal entries through the worksheet (Figure 21–3), however, you should concern yourself only with acquiring a general knowledge of Hopeful Hospital's 19X2 financial activities.

Equation for the Statement of Cash Flows

The basic accounting equation, discussed in Chapter 1, can be stated as follows: $A = L + E$. In other words, assets equal liabilities plus hospital equity. Now, let us expand this equation to read as follows:

$$CE + OA = L + E$$

Here, CE means cash and cash equivalents, and OA represents all other assets (assets other than cash and cash equivalents). Remem-

	12/31/X1 Balances		19X2 Transactions		12/31/X2 Adjustments		12/31/X2 Balances	
	Dr.	Cr.	Dr.	Cr.	Dr.	Cr.	Dr.	Cr.
Cash	280		(2) 8,404	(8)12,493			124	
			(3) 49					
			(4) 54					
			(5) 3,830					
Accrued interest receivable	30				(11) 15		45	
Accounts receivable	1,500		(1) 9,490	(2) 9,244			1,746	
Allowance for uncollectible accounts		160				(12) 50		210
Inventories	140		(7) 935	(9) 900			175	
Prepaid expenses	40					(13) 8	32	
Long-term investments	600		(7) 450	(3) 40			1,010	
Plant assests	6,260		(7) 940	(4) 100			7,100	
Accumulated depreciation		1,340	(4) 30			(10)540		1,850
Accounts payable		370	(8)12,493	(6) 7,700				302
				(7) 4,725				
Accrued expenses payable		220				(14) 12		208
Deferred revenues		60				(15) 17		77
Bonds payable		2,400	(7) 2,400	(5) 3,000				3,000
Fund balance		4,300						4,300
Patient service revenues				(1) 9,490				9,490
Deductions from revenues			(2) 840		(12) 50		890	
Other operating revenues				(5) 650	(15) 17			633
Nursing services expenses			(6) 3,000			(14) 12	3,188	
			(9) 200					
Other professional services expenses			(6) 1,900				2,030	
			(9) 130					
General services expenses			(6) 1,100				1,610	
			(9) 510					
Fiscal and administrative services expenses			(6) 1,400				1,460	
			(9) 60					
Depreciation expense					(10)540		540	
Other operating expenses			(6) 300		(13) 8		308	
Gain on sale of investments				(3) 9				9
Loss on sale of plant assets			(4) 16				16	
Nonoperating revenues				(5) 180		(11) 15		195
Totals	8,850	8,850	48,531	48,531	642	642	20,274	20,274

Figure 21–3 Hopeful Hospital Worksheet, Year Ended December 31, 19X2

ber, as noted earlier, that cash equivalents include some, but not all, short-term investments. So, OA (other assets) includes short-term investments that are not cash equivalents, receivables, inventories, prepaid expenses, long-term investments, plant assets, and so on. Purchases and sales of short-term investments that are not cash equivalents are reported as investing activities in the statement of cash flows.

Now, let us subtract OA (other assets) from each side of the equation:

$$CE = L + E - OA$$

Given this equation, how can the value of the left-hand side of the equation increase? The answer is easy: by increasing the value of the right-hand side of the equation. Given this equation, how can the value of the left-hand side of the equation decrease? By decreasing the value of the right-hand side of the equation.

Cash inflows normally result from an increase in the value of the right-hand side of the equation—that is, an increase in liabilities (L), an increase in equity (E), or a *decrease* in other assets (OA). So, *increases* in liabilities (L), *increases* in equity (E), and *decreases* in other assets (OA) generally produce cash inflows (or, at least, defer cash outflows into the future, thereby preserving current cash balances).

Cash Inflows

Why is an increase in liabilities (L) considered to be a source or inflow of cash? Obviously, if the hospital issues bonds or borrows money from a bank (either for the short or long term), cash inflows result. But what about an increase in, say, accounts payable to suppliers? How can this be viewed as a cash inflow? Well, the hospital has acquired assets (inventory) without an immediate expenditure of cash. This temporary "saving" (retention) of cash is treated as an equivalent of cash inflow. As indicated later, however, certain increases in liabilities may not result in cash inflows.

The Temporary Retention of Cash from Increasing Liabilities

An increase in hospital equity (E) generally arises from an excess of revenues over expenses (net income), and net income eventually results in a net cash inflow. In a very few instances, as noted later, certain increases in hospital equity (E) may not result in cash inflows.

Decreases in noncash assets ordinarily generate cash inflows. If long-term investments or plant assets are sold, for example, the sales proceeds increase the hospital's cash balances.

Cash outflows normally result from a decrease in the value of the right-hand side of the equation—that is, a decrease in liabilities (L), a decrease in equity (E), or an *increase* in other assets (OA).

Cash Outflows

Why is a decrease in liabilities (L) considered to be a use or outflow of cash? Obviously, if the hospital makes payments on accounts payable, repays the principal amount of bank loans, or retires long-term debt, cash outflows result. As indicated later, however, there may be certain transactions that decrease liabilities but do not require disbursements of cash.

A decrease in hospital equity (E) generally arises from an excess of expenses over revenues (net loss), and the net loss eventually results in a net cash outflow. In a very few instances, as noted

Equity Decreased by Net Losses

later, certain decreases in hospital equity (E) may not result in cash outflows.

Increases in noncash assets ordinarily require cash outflows. If new long-term investments or plant assets are purchased, for example, such purchases generally result in cash disbursements.

Classification of Cash Flows

As noted earlier, cash receipts and cash disbursements are classified within the statement of cash flows into three types of economic activity: operating activities, investing activities, and financing activities.

Operating Activities

Hospital *operating activities* are those directly or indirectly related to the provision of healthcare services to patients. Cash flows from operating activities generally result from revenue and expense transactions that enter into the determination of the hospital's net income (or net loss).

Cash Flows from Operating Activities

Cash inflows from operating activities include collections of accounts receivable arising from healthcare services provided to inpatients and outpatients, cash receipts related to other operating revenues, and certain cash receipts (interest and dividend income, for example) that are related to nonoperating revenues. Cash outflows from operating activities include cash disbursements for employee salaries and wages, inventory items and purchased services, interest on borrowings, taxes to governmental agencies, and other types of operating and nonoperating expenses. These cash inflows and outflows may arise from revenues and expenses that were recognized in a prior period, ones recognized in the current period, or some that will be recognized in one or more future periods.

Investing Activities

The investing activities of a hospital generally consist of transactions in which the hospital purchases and sells investments in securities (that are not cash equivalents) and plant assets. Investing activities may also include lending money and collecting the principal amount. (Receipts of interest income on such loans are classified as cash inflows from operating activities.)

Financing Activities

Financing activities generally are transactions that involve the acquisition and repayment of resources obtained through short-term and long-term borrowings in the form of bonds payable, mortgages payable, and notes payable (interest payments on these debts are treated as cash outflows relating to operating activities). Investor-owned hospitals include the proceeds from issuance of equity securities and the payment of dividends to stockholders as financing activities.

Figure 21–4 presents a statement of cash flows for Hopeful Hospital. Observe that the cash flows during the year ended December 31, 19X2, are classified into the three types of economic activity: operating, investing, and financing. The net cash outflow for the year is $156, which accounts for the decrease in cash indicated in Figure 21–2. Also note that this schedule provides a reconciliation of net income and the net cash inflows from operating activities.

During 19X2, Hopeful Hospital had a net cash inflow from operating activities of $531:

1. Cash received from patients and third-party payers (see transaction 2 under Illustration Data), $8,404.
2. Cash received from other operating revenue sources (see transaction 5), $650.
3. Cash received from nonoperating revenue sources (see transaction 5), $180.
4. Cash payments to employees (see transactions 6 and 8), $4,500.
5. Cash payments to suppliers of goods and services (see the computation that follows), $4,203.

In this illustration, the dollar amounts for the first four items are given. (Recall that we have assumed that there were no accrued salaries and wages payable at either the beginning or the end of 19X2.) The dollar amount of Item 5, however, requires a computation:

Cash payments on accounts payable (see transaction 8 under Illustration Data)	$12,493
Less:	
Payments of vouchers issued for purchase of long-term investments, purchase of plant assets, and retirement of bonds payable (see transaction 7).	(3,790)
Payments of vouchers issued for employee salaries and wages (see transactions 6 and 8).	(4,500)
Cash payments to suppliers of goods and services	$ 4,203

Form and Content of the Statement of Cash Flows

Net Cash Flow from Operating Activities

Figure 21-4 Hopeful Hospital
Statement of Cash Flows—
Unrestricted Fund (Direct
Method), Year Ended December
31, 19X2

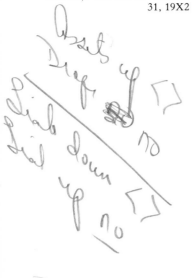

Cash Flows from Operating Activities:		
Cash received from patients and third-party payers	$ 8,404	
Cash received from other operating revenue sources	650	
Cash received from nonoperating revenue sources	180	
Cash payments to employees	(4,500)	
Cash payments to suppliers of goods and services	(4,203)	
Net cash inflow from operating activities		
(see Schedule A)		$ 531
Cash Flows from Investing Activities:		
Cash payments for purchase of plant assets	(940)	
Cash payments for purchase of long-term		
investments	(450)	
Proceeds from sale of plant assets	54	
Proceeds from sale of long-term investments	49	
Net cash outflow from investing activities		(1,287)
Cash Flows from Financing Activities:		
Proceeds from issuance of 6% bonds payable	3,000	
Cash payment for retirement of 7% bonds payable	(2,400)	
Net cash inflow from financing activities		600
Net decrease in cash		$ (156)
Schedule A:		
Net income		$ 285
Depreciation expense		540
Increase in accrued interest receivable		(15)
Increase in accounts receivable		(196)
Increase in inventories		(35)
Decrease in prepaid expenses		8
Decrease in accounts payable		(68)
Decrease in accrued expenses payable		(12)
Increase in deferred revenues		17
Gain on sale of long-term investments		(9)
Loss on sale of plant assets		16
Net cash inflow from operating activities		$ 531

Computing Cash Flows
from Operating Activities

There may be situations where other dollar amounts of cash flows from operating activities must be computed. Consider, for example, the following facts:

Accounts receivable, net, 12/31/X1	$1,340
Accounts receivable, net, 12/31/X2	1,536
Net patient service revenues for 19X2	8,600

The computation of cash received from patients and third-party payers is as follows:

Accounts receivable, net, 12/31/X1	$1,340
Net patient service revenues for 19X2	8,600
Total	9,940
Accounts receivable, net, 12/31/X2	1,536
Cash received from patients and third-party payers during 19X2	$8,404

Figure 21–4 illustrates the use of the *direct method* of reporting cash flow from operating activities. Under this method, cash receipts and disbursements are presented by major classes of revenues and expenses. In Schedule A, the resulting net cash flow from operating activities is proven by a reconciliation of net income to the net cash flow. This reconciliation is required by FASB Statement No. 95 when the direct method of presentation is employed.

An alternative to the direct method is the *indirect method* of reporting cash flow from operating activities. Under the indirect method, the reconciliation is moved up into the body of the statement, and is substituted for the presentation of cash inflows and outflows from operating activities. Additional discussion concerning this matter appears later in this chapter.

Placement of Reconciliation Using the Indirect Method

In its 19X2 statement of cash flows, Hopeful Hospital reports a net cash outflow ($1,287) from investing activities composed of:

Cash Flow from Investing Activities

1. Cash payments for purchase of plant assets (see transaction 7 under Illustration Data), $940.
2. Cash payments for purchase of new long-term investments (see transaction 7), $450.
3. Cash proceeds from sale of plant assets (see transaction 4), $54.
4. Cash proceeds from sale of long-term investments (see transaction 3), $49.

All of the dollar amounts for cash flows from investing activities are given in this illustration. In some instances, however, one or more of the dollar amounts must be computed.

Assume, for example, the following facts:

Long-term investments, 12/31/X1	$ 600
Long-term investments, 12/31/X2	1,010
Purchase of long-term investments during 19X2	450
Gain on sale of long-term investments during 19X2	9
Proceeds from sale of long-term investments during 19X2	?

The necessary computation is as follows:

Long-term investments, 12/31/X1	$ 600
Purchase of long-term investments during 19X2	450
Total	1,050
Less long-term investments, 12/31/X2	1,010
Cost of long-term investments sold during 19X2	40
Gain on sale of long-term investments	9
Proceeds from sale of long-term investments	$ 49

Cash Flow from Financing Activities

Hopeful Hospital had a net cash inflow from its financing activities during 19X2:

1. Proceeds from issue of 6 percent bonds (see transaction 5 under Illustration Data), $3,000.
2. Cash payment to retire 7 percent bonds (see transaction 7), $2,400.

Borrowing of Donor-Restricted Funds as Part of Cash Flows

Although not included in this illustration, cash flows from the financing activities of a hospital also may include borrowings by the unrestricted (general) fund from donor-restricted funds and repayments of such borrowings.

Reconciliation Schedule

Schedule A, presented at the bottom of Figure 21–4, consists of a reconciliation of net income and the net cash flow from Hopeful Hospital's operating activities. Increases in current assets other than cash or cash equivalents are treated as deductions from net income; decreases in these accounts are added to net income. Increases in current liabilities (other than short-term borrowings) are treated as additions to net income; decreases are deducted from net income.

The logic for this procedure was discussed earlier in this chapter. Why, however, were depreciation expense and the loss on sale of plant assets added to net income? Why was the gain on sale of long-term investments deducted from net income?

Depreciation expense ($540) and the loss on sale of plant assets ($16) were deducted in determining net income. Neither, however, required the use of cash (or cash equivalents). Net income, therefore, is an understatement of the amount of cash inflow generated from operations. Thus, these two items must be added back to net income. The gain on the sale of long-term investments ($9) was included in net income. The gain, however, did not provide (increase) cash; the proceeds of sale did. Net income, therefore, is an overstatement (by $9) of the amount of cash inflow from operations. Thus, the gain must be deducted from net income.

Figure 21–5 presents a statement of cash flows under the indirect method for Hopeful Hospital's Unrestricted Fund. In effect, Schedule A is substituted for the operating cash flows reported in Figure 21–4.

Exchange (Noncash) Transactions

Hospitals sometimes enter into significant financing and investing transactions that do not directly or immediately affect cash. A plant asset, for example, may be acquired in exchange for a long-term note payable. Here, we have a transaction that results in an increase in a noncash asset (but no decrease in cash) and an increase in a liability (but no increase in cash).

Another example is the receipt of a plant asset donated in kind. The entry for this transaction is a debit to plant assets and a direct credit to the Unrestricted (General) Fund Balance account. As a result, we have an increase in a noncash asset (but no decrease in cash) and an increase in hospital equity (but no increase in cash). Transactions of these types, if significant, are disclosed in a schedule or note accompanying the statement of cash flows.

Questions

Q21–1. If a hospital's annual financial report includes a balance sheet, an income statement, and statement of changes in fund balances, why should a statement of cash flows also be included?

Q21–2. State the equation for the statement of cash flows. Cash = Liab + Fund Bal − Noncash assets

Q21–3. In the context of the statement of cash flows, list the three major possible sources of cash inflows. Give an example of each.

Figure 21-5 Hopeful Hospital Statement of Cash Flows — Unrestricted Fund (Indirect Method)

Cash Flows from Operating Activities:		
Net income	$ 285	
Depreciation expense	540	
Increase in accrued interest receivable	(15)	
Increase in accounts receivable	(196)	
Increase in inventories	(35)	
Decrease in prepaid expenses	8	
Decrease in accounts payable	(68)	
Decrease in accrued expenses payable	(12)	
Increase in deferred revenues	17	
Gain on sale of long-term investments	(9)	
Loss on sale of plant assets	16	
Net cash inflow from operating activities		$ 531
Cash Flows from Investing Activities:		
Cash payments for purchase of plant assets	(940)	
Cash payments for purchase of long-term investments	(450)	
Proceeds from sale of plant assets	54	
Proceeds from sale of long-term investments	49	
Net cash outflow from investing activities		(1,287)
Cash Flows from Financing Activities:		
Proceeds from issuance of 6% bonds payable	3,000	
Cash payment for retirement of 7% bonds payable	(2,400)	
Net cash inflow from financing activities		600
Net decrease in cash		$ 156

Q21-4. In the context of the statement of cash flows, list the three major possible sources of cash outflows. Give an example of each.

Q21-5. Under the indirect method, depreciation expense is added back to net income to obtain the net cash flow from operating activities. Is depreciation expense a source of cash inflows? Explain.

Q21-6. What is the purpose of a statement of cash flows?

Q21-7. Explain what is meant by
a. Operating activities.
b. Investing activities.
c. Financing activities.

Q21-8. Distinguish between the direct and indirect methods of reporting cash flows from operating activities. Which do you prefer? Explain.

Q21–9. A hospital acquired an item of equipment in exchange for a long-term note payable. How should this transaction be reported in the statement of cash flows?

Q21–10. Do all expenses in the income statement represent cash outflows in the current period? Do all revenues in the income statement represent cash inflows in the current period? Explain.

Exercises

E21–1. Gras Hospital reported a net income of $87,400 for 19X1. The income statement included the following items, among others:

Loss on sale of long-term investments	$ 13,900
Depreciation expense	141,600
Gain on sale of plant assets	8,300

In the hospital's 19X1 statement of cash flows, what amount should be reported as "net cash inflow from operating activities"?

E21–2. Refer to Exercise 1, but assume that Gras Hospital reported a net loss of $87,400 for 19X1. In the hospital's 19X1 statement of cash flows, what amount should be reported as "net cash inflow from operating activities"?

E21–3. Carole Hospital's balance sheets provide the following information:

	12/31/X2	12/31/X1
Long-term investments	$288,300	$262,700

During 19X2, the hospital sold certain long-term investments at a gain of $14,600 and purchased new long-term investments at a cost of $87,500. In the hospital's 19X1 statement of cash flows, what amount should be reported as a cash inflow from its investing activities?

E21–4. The following information was drawn from the general ledger of Frumer Hospital:

	12/31/X2	12/31/X1
Accounts receivable	$400,000	$340,000
Inventory	30,000	45,000
Prepaid expenses	5,000	4,000
Accounts payable to suppliers	50,000	46,000
Accrued wages payable	10,000	12,000
Revenues	850,000	

Employee compensation	$560,000
Cost of supplies used	25,000
Depreciation expense	15,000
Other expenses	200,000

Required: Prepare the cash flow from the operating activities section of the 19X2 statement of cash flows, assuming the direct method of reporting operating cash flows.

E21–5. Refer to the data of E21–4.

Required: Prepare the cash flow from the operating activities section of the 19X2 statement of cash flows, assuming the indirect method of reporting operating cash flows.

Problems   P21–1. Barbara Hospital provides you with the following comparative balance sheets at December 31, 19X2, and 19X1:

	12/31/X2	12/31/X1
Cash	$ 180	$ 100
Other current assets	420	400
Long-term investments	440	450
Plant and equipment	7,900	7,600
Accumulated depreciation	(1,740)	(1,550)
Total	$ 7,200	$ 7,000
Current liabilities	$ 534	250
7% bonds payable	2,800	3,000
Fund balance	3,866	3,750
Total	$ 7,200	$ 7,000

The following additional information is available:
1. The 19X2 income statement reports a net income of $116.
2. Long-term investments that had cost $60 were sold for $75 in 19X2.
3. In 19X2, plant and equipment was purchased for $500.
4. Depreciation expense for 19X2 was $280.
5. During 19X2, plant and equipment items were sold for $100.

Required: Prepare, in good form, a statement of cash flows for Barbara Hospital for the year ended December 31, 19X2.

P21–2. Linda Hospital provides you with the following comparative balance sheets at December 31, 19X2 and 19X1:

	12/31/X2	12/31/X1
Cash	$ 160	$ 30
Other current assets	160	70
Long-term investments	400	350
Plant and equipment	2,000	1,860
Accumulated depreciation	(900)	(780)
Total	$1,820	$1,530
Current liabilities	$ 90	$ 40
8% long-term notes payable	—	500
7% long-term notes payable	600	—
Fund balance	1,130	990
Total	$1,820	$1,530

The 19X2 income statement shows a net income of $80. Long-term investments were purchased at a cost of $90; other investments were sold for $54. Plant and equipment that had cost $100 (and was 60 percent depreciated) was sold for $32. In 19X2, $60 was transferred from the hospital's plant replacement and expansion fund to the unrestricted fund for the purchase of plant assets.

Required: Prepare, in good form, a statement of cash flows for Linda Hospital for the year ended December 31, 19X2.

P21–3. Tracy Hospital's preclosing trial balance at December 31, 19X1, is as follows:

	Dr.	Cr.
Cash	$ 310	
Accrued interest receivable	40	
Accounts receivable	1,460	
Allowance for uncollectible accounts		$ 170
Inventories	180	
Prepaid expenses	35	
Long-term investments	990	
Plant assets	6,100	
Accumulated depreciation		1,300
Accounts payable		390
Accrued expense payable		210
Deferred revenue		50
Bonds payable		2,500
Fund balance		4,825

Patient service revenues		$ 8,900
Deductions from revenues	$ 800	
Other operating revenues		670
Nursing services expense	3,200	
Other professional services expense	2,100	
General services expense	1,600	
Fiscal and administrative services		
expense	1,500	
Depreciation expense	570	
Other expenses	320	
Nonoperating revenues		190
	$19,205	$19,205

The following information relates to 19X2 activities:
1. Patient service revenues totaled $9,600.
2. Collections were as follows on accounts receivable:

Cash	$8,600
Deductions from revenues	750
Credited to accounts receivable	$9,350

3. The hospital sold long-term investments (cost $50) for $58.
4. The hospital sold plant assets (cost $250; accumulated depreciation $170) for $65.
5. Other cash receipts were as follows:

Other operating revenues	$ 680
Nonoperating revenues	170
Proceeds of new bond issue	3,500

6. Operating expenses vouchered were as follows:

Nursing services	$3,100
Other professional services	2,000
General services	900
Fiscal and administrative services	1,500
Other operating expenses	260

7. Depreciation expense for the year was $550.
8. Vouchers issued for other items were as follows:

Purchase of inventory	$ 900
Purchase of long-term investments	500
Purchase of plant assets	1,500
Retirement of long-term debt (bonds payable)	2,500

9. Checks issued in payment of vouchers totaled $12,300.

10. Cost of supplies used during the year was as follows:

Nursing services $210
Other professional services 140
General services 490
Fiscal and administrative services 70

11. Accrued interest receivable at December 31, 19X2, is $55.
12. The allowance for uncollectible accounts at December 31, 19X2, should be adjusted to a balance of $195.
13. Prepaid expenses at December 31, 19X2, total $49.
14. Accrued expenses payable at December 31, 19X2, total $234 (make the necessary adjustment through nursing services expense).
15. Deferred revenues at December 31, 19X2, total $75 (make the necessary adjustment through other operating revenues).

Required: (1) Prepare a summary worksheet, such as the one in Figure 21–3, for the year ended December 31, 19X2. (2) Prepare a statement of cash flows, such as the one in Figure 21–4, for the year ended December 31, 19X2.

P21–4. Bennett Hospital provides you with the following comparative balance sheets:

	12/31/X2	12/31/X1
Cash	$ 140	$ 290
Accrued interest receivable	50	40
Accounts receivable	1,800	1,600
Allowance for uncollectible accounts	(200)	(180)
Inventories	170	130
Prepaid expenses	60	70
Long-term investments	1,000	750
Plant assets	7,000	6,800
Accumulated depreciation	(1,900)	(1,300)
Total	$ 8,120	$ 8,200
Accounts payable	$ 300	$ 290
Accrued expenses payable	210	240
Deferred revenues	80	90
Bonds payable	3,000	3,000
Fund balance	4,530	4,580
Total	$ 8,120	$ 8,200

The following additional information is available:

1. During 19X2, certain long-term investments were sold at a loss of $40, and new long-term investments were purchased for $400.
2. During 19X2, certain plant assets (cost $250; accumulated depreciation $240) were sold for $22.
3. During 19X2, an old $3,000, 7 percent bond issue was retired at face value, and a new $3,000, 6 percent bond issue was sold at face value.
4. The 19X2 income reported a net loss of $50.

Required: Prepare a statement of cash flows for 19X2.

Principles of Budgeting

22

The preparation and use of a budget is essential to the successful management of today's hospital. The budget is an absolute requirement in the administration of all hospitals, regardless of size, type, or other characteristics. Securing adequate financing and keeping expense levels below revenue levels are universal and increasingly complex problems that cannot be solved merely by reacting on a day-to-day basis to changing conditions and events. Objectives must be established, long-range plans must be developed, and controls must be instituted, to ensure that objectives and plans are fulfilled. A well-conceived program of budgetary planning and control, closely integrated with the accounting system, is one of the most important tools available to hospital management.

Budgeting is a major topic; entire books have been written on the subject. It deserves more space than can be given to it in this volume. In this one chapter, however, we can introduce you to some of the general principles and basic procedures of budgeting as practiced by hospitals. The purpose of this chapter is therefore limited to the presentation of a broad view of hospital budgeting, with selected illustrations of budgetary procedures.

Comprehensive Budgeting

A budget, simply stated, is a formal plan for future operations expressed in quantitative terms and serving as a basis of measurement for subsequent control of such operations. It is a written document in which the objectives and plans of the hospital are translated into dollars and various nonmonetary statistical terms. The dietary department budget for a given future period of time, for example, may be expressed as $900,000 and as 225,000 served meals. Budgeting is the process by which these forecasts are developed and used not only as a device for planning but also as a measurement tool for managerial review and control.

Components of the Master Budget

The term *comprehensive budget* refers to the total management plan for the hospital as a whole and for each of its departmental subdivisions. It is an overall master budget composed of individual budgets for revenues, expenses, assets, and liabilities. This includes all sources of revenues, all types of expenses, cash flow, levels of receivables and inventories, requirements for purchasing and personnel, plant asset additions, and debt retirement schedules. The comprehensive budget brings together all these individual budgets, consolidating them into a coordinated and complete plan for the conduct of operations so as to achieve desired objectives. Comprehensive budgeting permits the development of projected financial statements as goals to be attained at various points in the future.

Prerequisites for Effective Budgeting

A number of conditions are essential to the development and operation of an effective budgetary program. Some of the fundamental prerequisites are briefly discussed below.

Effective budgeting requires a sound organizational structure in which authority and lines of responsibility are clearly identified and understood at all levels of management. Every employee must know for what and to whom he or she is responsible. Each must be granted sufficient authority to perform assigned tasks. A departmentalization of activities must exist in which department managers and supervisors know the scope of their responsibility and authority within the overall organizational framework of the hospital. Such relationships are best presented by formal organization charts such as those illustrated earlier in this book.

Budgets are developed in a manner that conforms to the existing pattern of authority and responsibility as reflected by the organization chart. Individual plans are established for the achievement of specified objectives for each area of responsibility. Each department manager or supervisor is responsible for the development of the departmental plan and for controlling departmental operations so as to conform to that plan. These individual plans are combined and coordinated into the comprehensive budget for the hospital as a whole.

Appropriate Chart of Accounts

Effective budgeting requires an appropriate chart of accounts, that is, one designed to conform to the plan of organization. It should provide for the accumulation of revenues and expenses according to the organizational units responsible for producing the revenues and incurring the expenses. The revenues associated with each unit are subclassified by activity source; the expenses of each unit are subclassified by object of expenditure.

This facilitates the budgeting process, because historical revenue and expense data are accumulated in the same classifications in which future revenues and expenses are budgeted. The classification of historical data and budgeted data thus conforms to the same chart of accounts which, in turn, conforms to the plan of organization.

Adequate Statistical Data

The availability of reliable nonmonetary statistical data relating to the volume and scope of services in prior periods is as essential for effective hospital budgeting as historical financial information. In budgeting, analyses are made of previously accumulated general statistics such as number of admissions, patient days of service, percentage of occupancy, and average length of stay as a basis for projecting the future level of activity in overall terms.

Studies of Service Statistics

Once a forecast is made of the expected general level of activity, studies are made of historical departmental occasions (units) of service statistics, such as meals served, laboratory examinations, nursing hours, and pounds of laundry. This permits a projection of the probable volume of service, in statistical terms, in each department or organizational unit of the hospital. To be useful in projecting future service levels, of course, the statistics must be accurately compiled and classified in a manner parallel to and consistent with the chart of accounts and organizational structure.

Support of Management

To be successful, a budgetary program must have the full support of management at all levels, starting with the hospital's chief executive officer. Token support by top management personnel is not sufficient to obtain the cooperation and interest that is necessary at lower levels. Although impetus must come from the very top of the hospital organization, budgets should not be developed at that level alone. All department managers and supervisors should participate actively in formulating the budgets by which their future performances will be evaluated.

Formal Budgeting Procedures

Effective results will not be achieved if budgeting is approached in a haphazard, disorganized manner. Although the budget is a cooperative endeavor, a specific individual must be assigned responsibility for the development of the various departmental inputs and for their integration into a coordinated and comprehensive master plan. This individual, sometimes called the *budget officer,* generally is the chairman of the hospital's budget committee. Among other things, this committee prepares a budget manual for the guidance of department managers and supervisors, establishes a budget calendar as a time schedule for completion of each step in the budgeting procedure, and reviews, amends, and presents departmental budgets for approval. And, as a result, the committee produces a comprehensive budget for presentation to the hospital's governing board.

Budgeting Operating Results

To know whether the operating results are satisfactory, hospital revenues and expenses must be budgeted. Management control of operating results can be effective only if the hospital's managers are aware of what revenues and expenses *ought* to be, as well as what they actually are. Let us turn our attention, then, to the procedure by which the operating budget is developed.

Revenue Budgeting

Revenue is the very lifeblood of any organization, and it is particularly vital to the hospital enterprise, which generally has a rather narrow operating income margin. Because relatively small miscalculations of anticipated revenues may result in operating losses, careful attention must be given to the preparation of an accurate revenue budget. The revenue budget is the foundation of the entire budgetary program; all other budgets are formulated on the basis of the revenue budget.

Patient Service Revenues. The budgeting of revenues from services to patients begins by gathering historical revenue dollars and nonmonetary statistics of volume of service. These data should be scheduled by months and should embrace a sufficient number of years to disclose significant trends. The data should be classified by individual revenue centers, with subclassification into inpatient and outpatient totals where appropriate.

After a thorough study and analysis of this information, an evaluation should be made of the factors likely to have a material influence on the volume and types of revenue-producing services to be provided during the coming budget period. This procedure permits a realistic projection of statistical data that, when multiplied by the charges to be made for the various services, results in a budget of gross revenues from services to patients.

The revenue to be derived from room, board, and routine nursing services obviously is dependent on the daily rates for such services and the occupancy of the hospital's inpatient accommodations. Given the rates to be charged, the budgeting problem is one of forecasting occupancy in terms of patient days of service for the

	Total	January	December
Historical Data			
Patient Days:			
19X1	14,262	1,284	1,192
19X2	15,140	1,363	1,238
19X3	14,980	1,348	1,216
19X4	15,474	1,393	1,257
19X5 (current year)[a]	15,250	1,310	1,240
Revenue Dollars:			
19X1	$577,896	$52,567	$48,729
19X2	638,302	58,241	52,850
19X3	642,642	57,977	52,252
19X4	684,724	61,835	55,640
19X5 (current year)[a]	686,250	59,553	56,234
Average Revenue per Patient Day:			
19X1	$ 40.52	$ 40.94	$ 40.88
19X2	42.16	42.73	42.69
19X3	42.90	43.01	42.97
19X4	44.25	44.39	44.26
19X5 (current year)[a]	45.00	45.46	45.35
19X6 Revenue Budget			
Patient Days	15,400	1,320	1,250
× 19X5 Average Revenue per Patient Day	$ 45.00	$ 45.46	$ 45.35
Unadjusted Revenue Dollars[b]	$693,000	$60,000	$56,700
Adjustments:			
(none)			
19X6 Revenue Budget	$693,000	$60,000	$56,700

[a]Actual to date plus estimate for remainder of year.
[b]Rounded to nearest $100.

Figure 22–1 Wellrun Hospital Comparative Historical Data and 19X6 Revenue Budget, Daily Inpatient Service—Medical and Surgical Acute Nursing Unit #1

budget period. This forecast is developed for each nursing unit for each month of the period to facilitate subsequent budget versus actual comparisons on a monthly basis and to permit the preparation of monthly cash budgets.

Basis of the Forecast of Patient Days

The forecast of patient days is based on an analysis of historical data, adjusted for trends and the probable impact of variations in the factors that affect occupancy. Factors include changes in several areas: certain characteristics of the population served, hospital capacity, types of services offered, medical practices, characteristics of the medical staff, capabilities of other hospitals in the area, and insurance coverages.

An illustration of the budgeting of daily inpatient service revenues for a medical and surgical nursing unit appears in Figure 22–1. The format provides for a tabulation of historical data (patient days, revenue dollars, and average revenue per patient day) for a five-year period, 19X1 through 19X5. Because the 19X6 budget is developed before the end of the 19X5 year, the 19X5 data include estimates for the remaining month or so of that year. An analysis of these data leads to the budgeting of 15,400 patient days of service for 19X6. Because we assume that statistics for patient days are not accumulated according to accommodation type, budgeted patient days are multiplied by the 19X5 average revenue per patient day to obtain an unadjusted budget of revenue dollars, or $693,000. This assumes no change in room rates and no change in accommodation mix (the relative proportions of private and semi-private occupancies, for example). If changes in these factors were anticipated, the impact of such changes would be shown as adjustments (either plus or minus) to the $693,000 budget.

Departmental Revenue Forecasts from Professional Services

The budgeting of revenues from other professional services is a similar procedure. Many of these services, however, are provided to both inpatients and outpatients. In such cases, historical dollar and statistical occasions of service data must be available in inpatient and outpatient categories or classifications so that a separate revenue budget may be developed for each patient group.

After a careful study of the historical data and an evaluation of the effects of anticipated changes in underlying factors, forecasts of activity are made for each of the patient service departments or revenue centers. These departmental activity forecasts are made in terms of statistical occasions or units of service such as hours in operating rooms, procedures or films in radiology, and examinations in the laboratory. In most cases, however, these general statistics can be refined into more specific or weighted units of measurement. Where this can be done, the resulting revenue budgets tend to be more accurate and more useful to department heads in planning personnel requirements, determining equipment needs, and evaluating productivity.

It should be noted that the numbers employed in the illustrations in this chapter are not necessarily realistic. Relatively small numbers are used for clarity and ease of exposition.

Figures 22–2 and 22–3 illustrate the development of inpatient and outpatient revenue budgets for the laboratory department of Wellrun Hospital for 19X6. The inpatient revenue budget anticipates 106,000 occasions of service. This, when multiplied by the 19X5 average revenue per occasion of service, produces an unadjusted revenue dollar budget of $689,000. A rate increase, however, is scheduled to go into effect on January 1, 19X6, and it is estimated that this will provide $55,100 of additional revenues. Also, a new

	Total	January	December
Historical Data			
Occasions of Service:			
19X1	105,642	10,035	8,980
19X2	102,075	9,697	8,676
19X3	106,908	10,156	9,087
19X4	105,259	9,905	8,947
19X5 (current year)[a]	106,400	10,100	9,050
Revenue Dollars:			
19X1	$642,303	$61,414	$53,611
19X2	603,263	57,988	51,015
19X3	659,622	63,069	55,340
19X4	686,024	65,571	57,887
19X5 (current year)[a]	691,600	66,155	57,920
Average Revenue per Occasion of Service:			
19X1	$ 6.08	$ 6.12	$ 5.97
19X2	5.91	5.98	5.88
19X3	6.17	6.21	6.09
19X4	6.52	6.62	6.47
19X5 (current year)[a]	6.50	6.55	6.40
19X6 Revenue Budget			
Occasions of Service	106,000	10,000	9,000
× 19X5 Average Revenue per Occasion of			
Service	$ 6.50	$ 6.55	$ 6.40
Unadjusted Revenue Dollars[b]	$689,000	$65,500	$57,600
Adjustments:			
Rate Increase	55,100	5,200	4,600
New Laboratory Procedure	3,900	400	200
19X6 Revenue Budget	$748,000	$71,100	$62,400

[a]Actual to date plus estimate for remainder of year.
[b]Rounded to nearest $100.

Figure 22–2 Wellrun Hospital Comparative Historical Data and 19X6 Revenue Budget, Other Professional Services—Laboratory Department Inpatients

procedure (examination) is to be added to the services of the laboratory, and this adjustment increases the revenue budget to $748,000. Similar adjustments may be noted in Figure 22–3 for the outpatient revenue budget.

Deductions from Patient Service Revenues. After budgeting gross revenues from services to patients, budgets are developed for the amounts of such revenues that will not be collected due to bad debts, contractual adjustments, and the provision of charity care. These budgets of revenue deductions are based on an analysis of historical data with suitable modifications being made for trends and changes in factors such as hospital operating policies, reimbursement contract provisions, availability of specific-purpose

Deductions for
Uncompensated Care

Figure 22-3 Wellrun Hospital
Comparative Historical Data and
19X6 Revenue Budget, Other
Professional Services—Laboratory
Department Outpatients

	Total	January	December
Historical Data			
Occasions of Service:			
19X1	14,677	1,321	1,027
19X2	13,908	1,252	974
19X3	14,482	1,303	1,014
19X4	14,156	1,274	991
19X5 (current year)[a]	14,620	1,316	1,020
Revenue Dollars:			
19X1	$101,858	$ 9,300	$7,076
19X2	95,409	8,689	6,623
19X3	102,967	9,356	7,149
19X4	106,028	9,631	7,393
19X5 (current year)[a]	108,919	9,870	7,550
Average Revenue per Occasion of Service:			
19X1	$ 6.94	$ 7.04	$ 6.89
19X2	6.86	6.94	6.80
19X3	7.11	7.18	7.05
19X4	7.49	7.56	7.46
19X5 (current year)[a]	7.45	7.50	7.40
19X6 Revenue Budget			
Occasions of Service	14,800	1,330	1,030
× 19X5 Average Revenue per Occasion of Service	$ 7.45	$ 7.50	$ 7.40
Unadjusted Revenue Dollars[b]	$110,300	$10,000	$7,600
Adjustments:			
Rate Increase	11,900	1,100	600
New Laboratory Procedure	1,200	100	100
19X6 Revenue Budget	$123,400	$11,200	$8,300

[a]Actual to date plus estimate for remainder of year.
[b]Rounded to nearest $100.

grants for charity work, and economic conditions in the community. Each category of deductions should be separately budgeted and classified into inpatient and outpatient totals.

Figure 22-4 illustrates the budgeting of 19X6 contractual adjustments related to inpatient services for Wellrun Hospital. Note that the contractual adjustments are budgeted as a percentage of budgeted gross inpatient service revenues. (Other types of revenue deductions also may be budgeted on a percentage basis.) Because no significant changes are expected either in the provisions of third-party contracts or in patient mix, the percentages experienced in 19X5 are used in developing the 19X6 budget. If material changes

	Total	January	December
Historical Data			
Gross Inpatient Service Revenues:			
19X1	$7,462,893	$671,660	$622,403
19X2	7,855,107	714,815	698,246
19X3	8,172,783	727,378	701,494
19X4	7,906,449	711,580	696,338
19X5 (current year)[a]	8,256,000	751,300	738,100
Contractual Adjustments—Inpatients:			
19X1	$ 276,127	$ 25,523	$ 21,784
19X2	274,929	25,019	23,740
19X3	277,875	24,003	22,448
19X4	245,099	22,771	20,890
19X5 (current year)[a]	247,700	23,300	21,400
Percentage Adjustments to Gross Revenues:			
19X1	3.7%	3.8%	3.5%
19X2	3.5	3.5	3.4
19X3	3.4	3.3	3.2
19X4	3.1	3.2	3.0
19X5 (current year)[a]	3.0	3.1	2.9
19X6 Budget			
Budgeted Gross Inpatient Service Revenues for 19X6 ——	$8,589,200	$773,000	$687,100
× 19X5 Contractual Adjustments Percentage	3.0%	3.1%	2.9%
Unadjusted Contractual Adjustments Budget[b]	$ 257,700	$ 24,000	$ 19,900
Adjustments: (none)			
19X6 Contractual Adjustments Budget—Inpatients	$ 257,700	$ 24,000	$ 19,900

[a]Actual to date plus estimate for remainder of year.
[b]Rounded to nearest $100.

Figure 22–4 Wellrun Hospital Comparative Historical Data and 19X6 Revenue Deductions
Budget, Contractual Adjustments—Inpatients

were anticipated, the impact of such changes would be shown as adjustments (plus or minus) in the computations.

Other Revenues.   The budgeting of other operating revenues and nonoperating revenues should not be taken lightly. These revenues often are substantial in amount and should be estimated as accurately as possible. Because historical data may not be available or may not be indicative of the amounts to be received in the future, the budgeting of certain of these revenues may be difficult. Where reasonable certainty cannot be obtained, it is prudent to make conservative estimates.

Each of these revenue items is budgeted on the best basis available. The revenue from educational programs, for example, is budgeted on the basis of expected enrollments and tuition fees to be charged. Budgets of revenues to become available from unrestricted gifts and specific-purpose funds may be determined from an analysis of past experience, existing contracts, fund-raising programs, and requests made to granting organizations. Rentals of hospital space to doctors and employees may be estimated from a study of lease agreements. The budgets of cafeteria sales and gift shop sales often are related to projected patient days and outpatient visits.

A similar relationship also may be found with respect to telephone and television service, nonpatient sales of supplies, and medical record transcript fees. Budgeting investment income requires an analysis of the hospital's current investments and an estimate of the changes likely to occur in the amounts of such investments during the budget period.

Expense Budgeting

A basic management objective is to hold expenses at a level consistent with anticipated revenues in order to maintain the very necessary financial integrity of operating results. This requires expense budgeting, and, because employee compensation accounts for more than 50 percent of hospital operating expenses, special attention must be given to the development of accurate budgets for salaries and wages. Supplies, purchased services, and other nonlabor costs are significant, however, and they also should be budgeted with appropriate care.

Salaries and Wages

Salary and wage budgets should be developed in the classifications provided in the hospital's chart of accounts, assuming that the chart conforms to the organization plan that is required for responsibility accounting. Each departmental cost center supervisor should be responsible for the preparation of the salary and wage budget relating to personnel over whose employment and performance he or she has primary control. These department heads or supervisors should be supplied with adequate information concerning forecasted levels of activity, authorized numbers of employees in each job classification, and the approved rates of pay for each position. Staffing levels should be carefully monitored and controlled in relation to service volume.

Estimating Personnel Requirements to Control Labor Costs

Given a firm projection of the amount of work to be done, these supervisors are asked to determine the number of personnel in each classification that are needed to meet expected workloads in an efficient manner. In this way, major emphasis is placed on the control of labor costs at the lowest levels of organization where decision authority and responsibility for the performance of personnel exists. Although much of the salaries and wages paid by hospitals is relatively fixed within wide ranges of activity, the number of employees and the manner in which their services are utilized can vary considerably in certain areas that experience large variations in volume of activity.

In addition to a cost center classification, the labor budget also must be broken down by months of the year. This permits a determination of the amounts and times of cash disbursements for salaries and wages needed for cash budgeting purposes. It also permits the necessary month-by-month comparison of budgeted and actual costs during the budget period. The labor hours budgeted for each cost center also should be classified by months for comparison with actual hours in subsequent budget versus actual reports. Comparisons on a dollar basis alone are not nearly so indicative of employee utilization and efficiency as comparisons made on the basis of hours.

Figure 22–5 illustrates a worksheet for development of the salaries and wages budget for the radiology department of Wellrun Hospital. A similar worksheet is prepared for each department or cost center of the hospital. The worksheet lists each authorized position by job classification code and employee name. Note that Wellrun Hospital has an 03 position vacant but expects to fill this position before the budget period begins. The current compensation rate for each position is indicated along with the budgeted increase and the date the increase becomes effective.

Worksheet for Salaries and Wages Estimates

The scheduled work hours at straight-time pay are entered for each position. Assuming a 40-hour work week, the number of scheduled hours normally is 2,080 (40 hours × 52 weeks). Employee Buzby, however, is scheduled for an additional 200 hours (4 overtime hours per week for 50 weeks). This employee will be paid time and a half for these excess hours, so the premium pay of $360 (200 hours × 1/2 × $3.60) is listed as one of the adjustments on the worksheet. Note that vacation hours are included in the scheduled work hours column.

In addition to the adjustment for the dollar amount of premium pay, adjustments also are listed for estimated work hours and dollar amounts relating to vacation relief, holiday relief, and on-call requirements. In each case, the costs are determined by multiplying the budgeted hourly rate by the number of hours required for each month. These hours and computed dollar amounts are distributed to the months during which vacations are scheduled, holidays occur, and on-call duty may be necessary.

Types of Adjustments Required

Code	Authorized Positions Name	Current Rate*	Budgeted Amount*	Increase Eff. Date	Scheduled Work Hours	Vacation Hours	Total	January	February	March	April	November	December
01	Hartmann, J.	$1,800 PM	$150 PM	11/1	2,080	120	$21,900	$1,800	$1,800	$1,800	$1,800	$1,950	$1,950
02	Noble, B.	1,500 PM	90 PM	4/1	2,080	80	18,810	1,500	1,500	1,500	1,590	1,590	1,590
02	Biagioni, L.	1,500 PM	90 PM	2/1	2,080	80	18,990	1,500	1,590	1,590	1,590	1,590	1,590
03	Thomas, P.	1,000 PM	60 PM	12/1	2,080	80	12,060	1,000	1,000	1,000	1,000	1,000	1,060
03	Heitger, E.	1,000 PM	60 PM	3/1	2,080	80	12,600	1,000	1,000	1,060	1,060	1,060	1,060
03	Hansen, J.	800 PM	40 PM	2/1	2,080	80	10,040	800	840	840	840	840	840
03	(position vacant)	800 PM	—	—	2,080	80	9,600	800	800	800	800	800	800
04	Baker, R.	700 PM	30 PM	4/1	2,080	80	8,670	700	700	700	730	730	730
04	Buzby, T.	3.60 PH	—	—	2,280	80	8,208	684	684	684	684	684	684
	Totals				18,920	760	120,878	9,784	9,914	9,974	10,094	10,244	10,304
	Adjustments												
	Premium Pay						360	30	30	30	30	30	30
	Vacation Relief				600		3,000	1,400					
	Holiday Relief				90		540	45			90		270
	On Call				2,400		4,800	400	400	400	400	400	400
	Total Adjustments				3,090	—	8,700	1,875	430	430	520	430	700
	19X6 Salaries and Wages Budget—Dollars						$129,578	$11,659	$10,344	$10,404	$10,614	$10,674	$11,004
	19X6 Salaries and Wages Budget—Hours				22,010	760		2,100	1,650	1,810	1,780	1,760	1,850

*PM = Per Month
PH = Per Hour

Figure 22-5 Wellrun Hospital Salaries and Wages Budget Worksheet, Radiology Department—19X6

Budgets also must be prepared for payroll-related costs such as FICA taxes, unemployment taxes, and workmen's compensation insurance. The budgeting of these expense items involves application of the insurance or tax rates to the budgeted amounts of salaries and wages subject to those rates. Other employee benefits such as the hospital's share of employee insurance and pension programs are budgeted on the basis of the payroll budget and the provisions of such programs.

In budgeting the nonlabor expenses, each cost center supervisor should be supplied by the accounting department with an analysis of the major categories of supplies and other expenses that have been charged to the center in the last few years. This analysis should show dollars and, where feasible, units such as dozens, pounds, and gallons. In addition, the historical dollars should be compared to historical statistical data such as patient days of service or departmental occasions of service, as appropriate.

Supplies and Other Nonlabor Expense

Nonlabor expenses generally are more responsive than salaries and wages to changes in service volume, particularly in departments that render services directly to patients. As volume increases, nonlabor expenses tend to increase proportionately; as volume declines, these expenses tend to decrease at about the same rate. Assuming that a close relationship of this kind exists for Wellrun Hospital's laboratory department, the budgeting of that department's supplies and other nonlabor expenses for 19X6 may proceed as illustrated in Figure 22–6. Note, however, that the tentative dollar budget must be adjusted for the effects of expected cost price changes and for the effects of changes in the types of patient services provided and supply usage patterns.

A close correlation between nonlabor expenses and activity level, such as that assumed in Figure 22–6, will not be found in all departments of the hospital. This is likely to be the case in many of the hospital's indirect service departments. The amount of supplies used by the housekeeping department in servicing a given area, for example, probably would not vary greatly with changes in the number of patient days. Given no change in cleaning methods and assuming no changes in supply prices, the cost of housekeeping supplies should vary mainly with the square footage serviced.

When nonlabor expenses are not closely related to volume, these expenses must be budgeted on an item-by-item basis in each department or cost center. A careful study is made of historical dollars by major category of expense. And, taking into account expected price changes, changes in the types of services provided,

Estimating Nonlabor Expenses by Historical Expenditures

Figure 22–6 Wellrun Hospital
Supplies and Expense Budget,
Laboratory Department—19X6

	Total	January	December
Inpatients			
19X5 Supplies and Expense	$128,744	$11,587	$ 9,656
÷ 19X5 Occasions of Service	106,400	10,100	9,050
19X5 Expense Per Occasion of Service	$1.21	$1.15	$1.07
x 19X6 Budgeted Occasions of Service	106,000	10,000	9,000
Unadjusted 19X6 Dollar Budget*	128,300	11,500	9,600
Adjustments:			
Estimated 8% Price Increase	10,300	900	800
New Laboratory Procedure	2,400	200	200
19X6 Supplies and Expense Budget—			
Inpatients	141,000	12,600	10,600
Outpatients			
19X5 Supplies and Expense	13,597	1,198	908
÷ 19X5 Occasions of Service	4,620	1,316	1,020
19X5 Expense Per Occasion of Service	$ 0.93	$ 0.91	$0.89
x 19X6 Budgeted Occasions of Service	14,800	1,330	1,030
Unadjusted 19X6 Dollar Budget*	13,800	1,200	900
Adjustments			
Estimated 8% Price Increase	1,100	100	100
New Laboratory Procedure	600	100	100
19X6 Supplies and Expense Budget—			
Outpatients	15,500	1,400	1,100
Total 19X6 Supplies and Expense Budget	$156,500	$14,000	$11,700

*Rounded to nearest $100.

and changes in the methods of providing those services, each department manager determines for each expense item the amount the department should incur to accomplish the department's objective, usually with written justification for each amount budgeted.

Repairs and routine maintenance work to be performed may be estimated by the hospital engineer on the basis of experience, knowledge of current costs, and condition of the facilities. Heat, light, power, and other utilities are budgeted in terms of past and projected usage and expected future prices and service rates. Budgets for rent and insurance expense may be developed from an analysis of lease agreements and insurance policies. Items such as depreciation and interest are budgeted on the basis of plant asset records, plans for asset acquisitions and retirements, current debt service schedules, and plans for new borrowings.

Summarizing the Operating Budget

It should be understood that the expense and revenue budgets prepared by department heads and supervisors are preliminary in nature. The initial drafts of these budgets are consolidated by the hospital's budget officer into a projected income statement for the budget year. This tentative operating plan, after careful evaluation by the budget committee, is likely to undergo several revisions (1) to secure the desired relationship between revenues and expense for the hospital as a whole, (2) to achieve the necessary degree of coordination among the many departmental segments of the plan, and (3) to obtain compatibility between the operating plan and the hospital's financial position objectives, requirements, and limitations.

Department heads who disagree with budget committee amendments should be given an opportunity to present their views for further consideration by the committee. All such differences should be resolved to the fullest extent possible so that the resulting final budget is generally accepted and supported by those responsible for its implementation.

The final 19X6 operating budget for Wellrun Hospital is illustrated in projected income statement form in Figure 22–7. As the figure indicates, detailed information relating to the condensed totals in the statement are provided in supporting schedules (Schedules A through O). All revenue and expense items should be budgeted in as much detail as is practicable and useful. Here, however, we present illustrations only of Schedules B (Figure 22–8) and J (Figure 22–9). Note that the departmental budgets include statistical units as well as dollars.

Budgeting Financial Position

As stated earlier, the operating budget is not developed in final form until its impact on the hospital's financial position is determined. The tentative operating budget, in other words, must be translated into balance sheet terms. This requires the development of a projected balance sheet for the end of each month of the budget year. The revenue budget, which was prepared on an accrual basis, is converted to a cash basis to permit a forecast of monthly cash receipts and accounts receivable figures. The expense budget, which also was prepared on an accrual basis, is similarly converted to a cash basis to permit estimates of monthly cash disbursements, inventory, and accounts payable figures.

When this information is combined with the hospital's plans for plant asset acquisitions and retirements, investments and sales of securities, retirement of debt, and new borrowings, monthly balance sheets can be projected for the budget year. This will indicate whether the budgets for operations, plant and equipment, debt retirement, and other plans are compatible with the hospital's current and projected financial resources. If not, appropriate adjustments must be made in one or more of the preliminary budgets.

	Detail Schedule[a]	19X6 Total	January	December
Gross revenue from services to patients:				
Nursing services	A	$6,082,300	$552,400	$487,600
Other professional services	B	2,506,900	220,600	199,500
Total		8,589,200	773,000	687,100
Less deductions from revenue:				
Bad debts	C	94,200	8,200	9,300
Contractual adjustments	D	257,700	24,000	19,900
Charity service	E	421,300	38,200	32,700
Total deductions from revenues:		773,200	70,400	61,900
Net revenues from services to patients		7,816,000	702,600	625,200
Other operating revenues:				
Cafeteria sales	F	307,400	30,800	24,900
Other	G	606,600	53,300	52,800
Total other operating revenues		914,000	84,100	77,700
Total operating revenues		8,730,000	786,700	702,900
Less operating expenses:				
Nursing services	H	3,038,400	255,200	241,500
Other professional services	I	1,580,500	142,300	139,400
General services	J	1,176,000	115,800	100,700
Fiscal services	K	604,800	54,400	48,000
Administrative services	L	740,000	66,600	59,400
Unassigned expenses	M	1,260,300	100,200	104,300
Total operating expenses		8,400,000	734,500	693,300
Operating income		330,000	52,200	9,600
Add nonoperating revenues:				
General contributions	N	105,000	6,300	5,200
Other	O	42,000	3,100	2,500
Total nonoperating revenues		147,000	9,400	7,700
Net income		$ 477,000	$ 61,600	$ 17,300

[a]Only Schedules B and J are illustrated:
see Figures 22-8 and 22-9.

Figure 22-7 Wellrun Hospital 19X6 Operating Budget

Possible adjustments include increases in hospital service rates, changes in tentative expense budgets, increases in the amounts of planned borrowings, and postponements of planned additions to plant assets.

Assuming that all necessary coordinating adjustments have been made, Figure 22-10 provides a simplified illustration of Wellrun Hospital's projected balance sheets in condensed form for the 19X6 budget year. This chapter, however, is intended only as an introduction to budgeting, with emphasis on the operating budget. Consequently, the budgeting of each balance sheet item will not be described here; our attention is limited largely to the development of the cash budget.

		19X6		January		December	
	Statistical Units	Units	Dollars	Units	Dollars	Units	Dollars
Inpatient revenues:							
Laboratory	Examinations	106,000	$ 748,000	9,600	$ 67,300	8,400	$ 59,800
Radiology	Procedures	54,000	815,300	4,900	73,400	4,300	65,200
Pharmacy	Requisitions	43,000	346,200	3,800	31,200	3,400	27,700
Anesthesia	Hours	9,300	239,100	900	23,100	700	17,900
Total inpatient revenues			2,148,600		195,000		170,600
Outpatient revenues:							
Laboratory	Examinations	14,800	12,400	1,300	7,400	1,100	11,400
Radiology	Procedures	9,100	136,500	800	9,300	700	8,600
Pharmacy	Requisitions	8,600	72,300	800	6,500	800	6,500
Anesthesia	Hours	1,000	26,100	100	2,400	100	2,400
Total outpatient revenues			358,300		25,600		28,900
Total revenues			$2,506,900		$220,600		$199,500

Figure 22–8 Wellrun Hospital, Other Professional Services Revenues, 19X6 Budget—Schedule B

		19X6		January		December	
	Statistical Units	Units	Dollars	Units	Dollars	Units	Dollars
Administrative office:							
Salaries and wages	Hours	6,300	$ 28,500	600	$ 2,600	500	$ 2,400
Supplies and expenses	Hours	6,300	8,100	600	700	500	600
Total			36,600		3,300		3,000
Dietary:							
Salaries and wages	Hours	40,000	97,100	3,600	8,800	3,400	8,200
Supplies and expenses	Number of meals	325,000	511,800	31,400	47,100	29,800	44,300
Total			608,900		55,900		52,500
Plant operation and maintenance:							
Salaries and wages	Hours	14,600	53,700	1,300	4,300	1,200	4,800
Supplies and expenses	Square feet	315,000	288,100	315,000	25,900	315,000	22,300
Total			341,800		30,200		27,100
Housekeeping:							
Salaries and wages	Hours	28,000	71,900	2,500	7,500	2,400	6,800
Supplies and expenses	Square feet	260,000	44,600	260,000	12,300	260,000	4,300
Total			116,500		19,800		11,100
Laundry:							
Salaries and wages	Hours	15,200	49,400	1,400	4,500	1,300	4,700
Supplies and expenses	Pounds	148,000	22,800	13,300	2,100	13,600	2,300
Total			72,200		6,600		7,000
Total salaries and wages			300,600		27,700		26,900
Total supplies and expenses			875,400		88,100		73,800
Total general services expenses			$1,176,000		$115,800		$100,700

Figure 22–9 Wellrun Hospital General Services Expenses, 19X6 Budget—Schedule J

	1/31/X6	2/28/X6	3/31/X6		12/31/X6
Current assets:					
Cash	$ 95,100	$ 37,400	$ 49,800		$ 74,500
Short-term investments	105,000	105,000	180,000		45,000
Receivable from patients (net)	694,600	682,400	699,000		715,000
Inventories	100,600	110,000	112,800		118,000
Total current assets	995,300	934,800	1,041,600		952,500
Plant and equipment (net)	7,442,500	7,416,900	7,383,500		7,366,500
Total assets	$8,437,800	$8,351,700	$8,425,100		$8,319,000
Current liabilities:					
Notes payable	$ 120,000	$ –0–	$ –0–		$ 35,000
Accounts payable	83,000	93,200	94,500		98,600
Payroll taxes withheld and accrued	143,300	136,200	148,900		134,700
Accrued interest payable	16,500	25,000	37,500		60,300
Current portion of long-term debt	500,000	500,000	500,000		500,000
Total current liabilities	862,800	754,400	780,900		828,600
Long-term debt (bonds payable)	2,000,000	2,000,000	2,000,000		1,500,000
Total liabilities	2,862,800	2,754,400	2,780,900		2,328,600
Fund balance, 12/31/X5	5,513,400	5,513,400	5,513,400		5,513,400
Add net income to date	61,600	83,900	130,800		477,000
Fund balance, end of month	5,575,000	5,597,300	5,644,200		5,990,400
Total liabilities and fund balance	$8,437,800	$8,351,700	$8,425,100		$8,319,000

Figure 22–10 Wellrun Hospital Projected Balance Sheets, 19X6 Budget Year

Purpose of the Cash Budget

A cash budget is a detailed estimate of future cash receipts from all sources and cash disbursements for all purposes. By budgeting these cash flows, the cash balance at various future places in time can be predicted in a reasonably accurate manner. In this way, the need for additional funds can be foreseen, and plans can be made for the investment of excess funds, if any. Cash budgeting also tends to provide assurance that money will be available in the amounts and at the times needed but, at the same time, avoids the holding of idle cash balances in excessive amounts.

To illustrate cash budgeting procedure, assume the 19X6 operating budget previously presented in Figure 22–7 and the December 31, 19X5, balance sheet in Figure 22–11. The completed 19X6 cash budget for Wellrun Hospital appears in Figure 22–12.

Budgeting Cash Receipts

It is assumed that the December 31, 19X5, accounts receivable (net of allowances for uncollectible accounts) originated from charges made for services rendered during the previous three months:

19X5	Net Charges to Patients				12/31/X5 Receivables
October	$680,000	×	10%	=	$ 68,000
November	660,000	×	30%	=	198,000
December	690,000	×	60%	=	414,000
					$680,000

A study must be made of the hospital's collection experience in order to determine the pattern in which its receivables generally are collected in cash. Let us assume that Wellrun Hospital's analysis shows that about 40 percent of a given month's net charges (to inpatients and outpatients) is collected in the same month, an additional 30 percent is collected in the first following month, another 20 percent is collected in the second following month, and the remaining 10 percent is collected in the month after that. Thus, at December 31, 19X5, 10 percent of October charges, 30 percent of November charges, and 60 percent of December charges remain

Determining the Receivables Collection Pattern

Current assets:		
Cash	$ 94,700	
Short-term investments	55,000	
Receivables from patients (net)	680,000	
Inventories	105,700	
Total current assets		$ 935,400
Plant and equipment (net)		7,502,500
Total assets		$8,437,900
Current liabilities:		
Notes payable	$120,000	
Accounts payable	88,800	
Payroll taxes withheld and accrued	137,500	
Accrued interest payable	78,200	
Current portion of long-term debt	500,000	
Total current liabilities		$ 924,500
Long-term debt (bonds payable)		2,000,000
Total liabilities		2,924,500
Fund balance		5,513,400
Total liabilities and fund balance		$8,437,900

Figure 22-11 Wellrun Hospital Balance Sheet, December 31, 19X5

	19X6 Total	January	February	March	Second Quarter	Third Quarter	Fourth Quarter
Beginning cash balance	$ 94,700	$ 94,200	$ 95,100	$ 37,400	$ 49,800	$ 106,800	$ 71,400
Budgeted cash receipts:							
Collections on patients accounts receivable	7,781,000	688,000	683,200	695,800	1,999,900	1,771,300	1,942,800
Other operating revenues	914,000	84,100	76,300	81,200	242,100	201,700	228,600
Nonoperating revenue	147,000	9,900	7,900	8,800	44,700	35,100	41,100
Other receipts							
Proceeds from sales of investment accurities	275,000					275,000	
Proceeds from sales of plant assets	32,000	20,000					12,000
Short-term borrowings	95,000				95,000		
Total budgeted cash reciepts	9,244,000	802,000	767,400	785,800	2,381,700	2,283,100	2,224,500
Estimated cash available	9,338,700	896,200	862,500	823,200	2,431,500	2,389,900	2,295,900
Budgeted cash disbursements:							
Salaries and wages (net)	4,258,800	372,300	354,300	387,300	1,132,200	974,900	1,037,800
Payroll taxes withheld and accrued	1,640,300	137,500	143,300	136,200	440,400	367,000	415,900
Supplies	1,008,500	88,800	83,000	93,200	267,700	223,000	252,800
Interest	157,200	75,000	4,800			75,000	2,400
Other expenses	824,400	77,500	69,700	81,700	214,400	178,600	202,500
Other disbursements							
Purchases of new investment securities	265,000	50,000		75,000	100,000		40,000
Purchases of new plant and equipment	430,000		50,000		170,000		210,000
Repayment of short-term borrowings	180,000		120,000				60,000
Retirement of long-term debt	500,000					500,000	
Total budgeted cash disbursements	9,264,200	801,100	825,100	773,400	2,324,700	2,318,500	2,221,400
Ending cash balance	$ $74,500	$ 95,100	$ 37,400	$ 49,800	$ 106,800	$ 71,400	$ 74,500

Figure 22-12 Wellrun Hospital 19X6 Cash Budget

uncollected and in receivables, as shown in the three months of net charges listed earlier.

Assuming that this collection pattern is valid for 19X6, month-end balances of receivables and cash collections on patients' accounts may be budgeted for the first three months of the year, as illustrated in Figure 22–13. These are the budgeted cash collections and receivables balances that appear in Figures 22–10 and 22–12 for January, February, and March of 19X6. Budgeted amounts for other months of the year would be developed in the same way.

Cash receipts relating to other operating and nonoperating revenues also should be accurately budgeted on the best basis available. This often requires an account-by-account analysis of each revenue source of major significance, giving consideration to projected accrued and deferred revenues. In Figure 22–12, however, it is assumed that these revenue items are collected largely in the month that they are earned and recorded as revenues. Note, for example, that the operating budget in Figure 22–7 includes $84,100

Receivable originating in:	Collected During			Uncollected At		
	January	February	March	January 31	February 28	March 31
October, 19X5— $680,000 x 10%	$ 68,000					
November, 19X5— $660,000 x 20%	132,000					
$660,000 x 10%		$ 66,000		$ 66,000		
December, 19X5— $690,000 x 30%	207,000					
$690,000 x 20%		138,000		138,000		
$690,000 x 10%			$ 69,000	69,000	$ 69,000	
January, 19X6— $702,600 x 40%	281,000					
$702,600 x 30%		210,800		210,800		
$702,600 x 20%			140,500	140,500	140,500	
$702,600 x 10%				70,300	70,300	$ 70,300
February, 19X6— $671,000 x 40%		268,400				
$671,000 x 30%			201,300		201,300	
$671,000 x 20%					134,200	134,200
$671,000 x 10%					67,100	67,100
March, 19X6— $712,400 x 40%			285,000			
$712,400 x 30%						213,700
$712,400 x 20%						142,500
$712,400 x 10%						71,200
Budgeted cash collections on patients' accounts	$688,000	$683,200	$695,800			
Budgeted end-of-month accounts receivable				$694,600	$682,400	$699,000

Figure 22–13 Budgeting Cash Collections and Month-End Receivables Balances

of other operating revenues and $9,400 of nonoperating revenues for January of 19X6. These amounts also appear in Figure 22–12 in the cash budget for that month. This procedure likely will be satisfactory when there are no material variations from month to month in the amounts of accrued and deferred revenues.

The other cash receipts in Figure 22–12 are budgeted on the basis of management plans for the sale of investment securities, for the occasional sales of plant assets, and for new short-term borrowings. Certain of these plans, of course, are based on the results of the cash budgeting process. So, the budgeting of cash receipts from these sources generally is postponed until all other segments of the cash budget have been formulated.

Budgeting Cash Disbursements

The estimates for cash disbursements are derived from previously established budgets for departmental salaries and wages, supplies and other expenses, and plant asset acquisitions. With knowledge of payroll periods, the monthly cash requirements for salaries and wages are easily determined. The budgeted amount of a month's payroll plus the estimated accrued payroll at the beginning of the month minus the accrued payroll at the end of the month produces the necessary figures. Taxes and other payroll withholdings are excluded from the budgeted monthly payroll disbursement and are instead included in budgeted cash disbursements of the month in which such taxes and withholdings are to be remitted to governmental and other agencies.

Cash for Supplies and Services

Cash requirements also must be estimated by months with regard to the purchase of supplies and payments for insurance, interest, and purchased services such as utilities and telephone. (Of course, depreciation expense is omitted from the budget of cash expenditures unless it is being "funded," as described in Chapter 18.) These determinations may be based on budgets for purchasing, insurance expiration and debt retirement schedules, and other relevant data provided by the operating budget. Cash requirements for planned investments in securities and new plant assets must also be estimated.

A number of simplifying assumptions were made in developing Wellrun Hospital's budget for 19X6 cash disbursements. The general procedure followed appears in Figure 22–14 for the first three months of 19X6. The same types of computations would be made for other months.

Operating Expenses

Figure 22–14 begins with total monthly operating expenses that are drawn from the operating budget (Figure 22–12). Monthly gross salaries and wages are assumed, for the purposes of this illustration, to be 65 percent of total operating expenses. In actual practice, of course, the operating budget would provide the monthly salaries and wages figures. The same is true of supplies expense, but here we simply assume that this expense item is a flat 12 percent of total operating expenses budgeted for each month. The depreciation expense amounts appearing in Figure 22–14 are assumed, although in an actual case the information would be available in the detailed operating budget. The hospital's share of payroll taxes is assumed to be 8 percent of gross salaries and wages. Finally, monthly interest expense figures are deducted. In this illustration, the amounts of interest expense include $12,500 interest on the bonds ($2,500,000 × 6 percent × 1/12) and $800 interest on the short-term notes payable (that were retired at the end of February).

After deducting the expense items just mentioned, an amount labeled "other expenses" remains in each column of Figure 22–14. It is assumed for purposes of this example that these amounts are paid in the same month that they are budgeted as expenses. It would be useful to trace these figures back to the cash disbursements section of Figure 22–12.

		19X6	
	January	February	March
Total operating expenses	$734,500	$698,300	$763,900
Less salaries and wages (assumed 65% of operating expenses)	477,400	454,200	496,500
Balance	257,100	244,100	267,400
Less supplies expense (assumed 12% of operating expenses)	88,100	83,800	91,700
Balance	169,000	160,300	175,700
Less depreciation expense	40,000	41,000	41,800
Balance	129,000	119,300	133,900
Less payroll taxes (assumed 8% of salaries and wages)	38,200	36,300	39,700
Balance	90,800	83,000	94,200
Less interest expense	13,300	13,300	12,500
Other expenses (assumed paid in same month)	$ 77,500	$ 69,700	$ 81,700
Payroll taxes withheld (assumed 22% of salaries and wages)	$105,100	$ 99,900	$109,200
Accrued payroll taxes (above)	38,200	36,300	39,700
Total payroll taxes withheld and accrued (assumed paid in following month)	$143,300	$136,200	$148,900
Salaries and wages (above)	$477,400	$454,200	$496,500
Less payroll taxes withheld (above)	105,100	99,900	109,200
Net salaries and wages (assumed paid in same month)	$372,300	$354,300	$387,300
Supplies expense (above)	$ 88,100	$ 83,800	$ 91,700
Desired ending inventory (assumed 120% of following month's budgeted supplies expense)	100,600	110,000	112,800
Total	$188,700	$193,800	$204,500
Less opening inventory	105,700	100,600	110,000
Purchases of supplies (assumed paid in following month)	$ 83,000	$ 93,200	$ 94,500

Figure 22–14 Budgeting Cash Disbursements (Dollar Amounts Rounded to Nearest $100)

The next section of Figure 22–14 shows the computation of total payroll taxes withheld and those accrued during each month. It is assumed that withholdings are 22 percent of gross salaries and wages and that the hospital's share of payroll taxes is 8 percent of gross salaries and wages. It also is assumed that these amounts are paid (that is, remitted to governmental agencies) in the following month, as may be seen in the cash budget shown in Figure 22–12.

Payroll Taxes

Figure 22–14 also includes a computation of the net salaries and wages of each month. It is assumed that the full amount of the net payroll is paid each month, and that there is no accrued payroll at the beginning or end of any month. You will want to locate these net payroll figures in the cash disbursements section of Figure 22–12.

Finally, Figure 22–14 shows the computation of required monthly purchases of supplies, assuming that Wellrun Hospital's policy is to maintain month-end inventories in a dollar amount equal to 120 percent of the next month's budgeted supplies expense. In this budget it is assumed that all purchases of supplies during any given month are paid for in the following month. This computation provides cash disbursement amounts for the cash bud-

Payments for Supplies

get illustrated in Figure 22–12 and accounts payable figures for the budgeted balance sheets shown in Figure 22–10.

The budgeted interest payments in Figure 22–12 were developed on the assumption that the bonds pay interest semiannually on January 1 and July 1. It also is assumed that $500,000 (face amount) of the bonds are retired annually on July 1. The remaining interest payments in the cash budget are assumed interest payments on the hospital's short-term notes payable. The other disbursements listed in the budget reflect management plans for the purchase of investment securities, the purchase of new plant assets, and the repayment of short-term borrowings.

Adjusting Quarterly Budgets

Finally, notice that Wellrun Hospital's cash budget is detailed by months for the first quarter of the year and by quarters only for the remainder of the year. This is often the practice because it may be impractical to try to prepare a detailed monthly cash budget that projects beyond three months into the future. As the year progresses, however, these quarterly budgets are adjusted to more current expectations and are revised into detailed monthly budgets. On the other hand, some hospitals have found it possible and useful to budget cash on a daily basis for a month into the future; that is, as a new month approaches, the cash budget for that month is converted to a detailed daily budget.

This chapter has been concerned almost entirely with the planning aspect of budgeting. The uses of the budget as a means of controlling a hospital's operating results and financial position are described in Chapter 24.

Questions

Q22–1. What are the five major prerequisites for effective budgeting?

Q22–2. Define the term *budget*. Why is budgeting essential to the successful management of a hospital?

Q22–3. What is meant by *comprehensive budgeting*?

Q22–4. Describe, in general terms, how you would go about developing a budget for daily patient service revenues for a nursing unit.

Q22–5. On what factors is the budget for deductions from patient service revenues based?

Q22–6. Indicate briefly the bases on which the following "other revenues" might be budgeted:
  a. Tuition from educational programs.
  b. Rental income.
  c. Cafeteria sales.
  d. Income from unrestricted fund investments.
  e. Unrestricted contributions.

Q22–7. Describe, in general terms, how you would go about developing a budget for the salaries and wages of a laboratory department of a hospital.

Q22–8. Describe, in general terms, how you would go about developing a budget for supplies and other nonlabor expenses for the dietary department of a hospital.

Q22–9. Why are the tentative departmental budgets consolidated into a projected income statement and converted into a projected balance sheet?

Q22–10. Describe, in general terms, how you would go about developing a budget of cash receipts and disbursements for a hospital's unrestricted fund.

Exercises

E22–1. A healthcare entity has cash of $5,500 and accounts receivable of $71,000 on February 28. The entity sells a single product to its customers. The entity's sales are billed on the last day of each month, and customers are allowed a 3 percent discount if payment is made within 10 days after the billing date. Sixty percent of billings are normally collected within the discount period, 25 percent are collected by the end of the month following sale (but not within the discount period), 9 percent are collected during the second month following the month of sale, and 6 percent eventually prove to be uncollectible. The following shows budgeted sales:

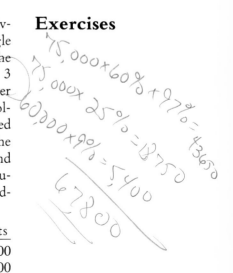

	Dollars	Units
March	$60,000	12,000
April	75,000	15,000
May	65,000	13,000
June	70,000	14,000

Each month's ending inventory is budgeted in units to equal 130 percent of the next month's budgeted sales units.

Required: Budgeted cash receipts during the month of May are the following:
a. $49,050
b. $62,400
c. $67,800
d. $69,150

E22–2. Refer to the data of Exercise 22–1. The entity purchases its product on account at $3 per unit, paying for the purchases of each month (net of a 1 percent discount) on the tenth day of the following month. Purchase discount opportunities are never missed.

Required: Budgeted payments (net of discounts) on accounts payable during May are the following:
a. $36,828
b. $44,550
c. $50,193
d. $63,558

E22–3. Helms Hospital's ledger shows a $5,000 balance in accounts receivable at August 31. Inpatient service revenues are budgeted as follows:

September	$ 6,000
October	8,000
November	10,000
December	20,000

Past experience indicates that 50 percent of revenues are collected in the month following the month of service, 30 percent are collected in the second month following the month of service, 15 percent are collected in the third month following the month of service, and the remainder proves to be uncollectible.

Required: What amount of cash receipts should be budgeted for the month of December?

Problems   P22–1. The July 1 accounts receivable of Vigor Hospital originate from charges made to patients during the previous three months as follows:

Handwritten notes:
April Sales — 15,000
May 13,000 × 130% = 16,900
31,900
April
15,000 × 130% = −19,500
12,400
× 3.00
37,200 × 1%
−372
36,828

900
2400
5000
8300

September 15%
October 30%
November 50%

Month	Charges	Accounts Receivable
June	$300,000	$300,000
May	320,000	96,000
April	270,000	27,000

The hospital's past experience shows that about 70 percent of charges in any month are collected in the following month. An additional 20 percent are collected in the next following month, 8 percent are collected in the third month, and the remaining 2 percent prove to be uncollectible.

Required: Calculate the probable collections on accounts receivable during July for purposes of cash budgeting.

P22–2. Verywell Hospital provides you with the following information:

	March	April	May	June	July
Revenues	$100,000	$120,000	$90,000	$80,000	$110,000
Purchases of supplies	10,000	15,000	12,000	8,000	20,000
Other expenses	80,000	93,000	69,000	64,000	79,000

Eighty percent of revenues are collected in the month following the month in which services are rendered. The remaining 20 percent are collected in the second following month. Fifty percent of purchases are made for cash. The remainder is paid, net of a 1 percent discount, in the month following the month of purchase. Other expenses are paid in cash in the month incurred. Depreciation of $5,000 per month is included in the "other expenses" given above. Depreciation, however, is not funded by the hospital. A short-term bank loan of $40,000 falls due on July 1, and the hospital plans to purchase new equipment for $75,000 cash on June 1. The cash balance at April 30 is $25,000.

Required: Prepare a cash budget for May, June, and July, showing the projected cash balance at the end of each month.

P22–3. Various information relating to the laboratory department of Vigilant Hospital is presented:

1. The hospital establishes charges for services at an amount that will approximate costs as nearly as possible. Total budgeted income for a department should be within a range of $2,000 of total budgeted expenses. A relative unit system is used in the laboratory depart-

ment. For the fiscal year ending June 30, 19X4, the average charge per unit is budgeted at $1.48.

2. Deductions from revenues should be assumed to be 10 percent of gross revenues.

3. In budget preparation, it is assumed that the laboratory department will continue to grow at the same rate, as far as the number of relative units of service is concerned, as it has in the past two years.

4. The two pathologists are guaranteed a base salary of $50,000 each, plus a pool of 10 percent of net revenue (gross revenue less revenue deductions) that is divided equally.

5. The budget committee of the hospital has instructed you to allow for a 5 percent salary increase to all eligible personnel except the pathologists. These increases are to become effective for each employee on the first of the month following the anniversary of each employee's employment date.

6. Because of the increased workload, the budget committee has approved the addition of one new technologist to begin at the approved starting rate.

7. Overtime, vacation and holiday relief, and on-call pay should be computed at 15 percent of the technologists' and aides' salaries. The indirect cost ratio for the laboratory department is 25 percent of direct expenses.

8. The nonsalary direct expenses for the laboratory department in the year ended June 30, 19X3, amounted to $50,000. It is expected that the 19X3–X4 nonsalary direct expenses will increase approximately 27 cents per unit of service.

	Year Ended June 30		
	19X1	19X2	19X3
Units of service	165,300	181,820	200,000
Gross charges	$175,218	$189,093	$204,000
Deductions	17,500	18,900	20,300
Net charges	157,718	170,193	183,700

Selected wage range for year ending June 30, 19X4:

Job Code		Range in Dollars per Month
23	Secretary	$325–$450
44	Laboratory technologists	375– 525
67	Aides	300– 400

Analysis of personnel, July 1, 19X3, yields the following:

Job Code	Authorized Positions Name	Current Annual Rate	Monthly Rate	Employment Date
01	Apple, Pathologist	$50,000		7/1/X1
01	Orange, Pathologist	50,000		9/1/X1
23	P. Pine	4,800	$400	1/15/X1
44	G. Gerber	6,120	510	8/5/X1
44	D. Dudley	6,000	500	7/9/X1
44	R. Ratterman	5,520	460	9/14/X2
44	S. Smith	4,680	390	12/13/X2
67	O. Otteson	4,560	380	6/12/X2
67	T. Thompson	4,080	340	7/13/X2

Required: Prepare an annual revenue and expense budget for the laboratory department of Vigilant Hospital for the year ending June 30, 19X4.

P22–4. The following is information relating to the radiology department of Vanity Hospital concerning the preparation of a budget of revenues and expenses for the year ending December 31, 19X3:

1. A relative unit value system has been adopted to account for the activities of the radiology department. Below is a schedule of these relative unit values:

	19X1 Actual	19X2 Actual	19X3 Budget
January	10,500	11,000	11,500
February	10,000	10,500	11,000
March	12,500	12,500	13,500
April	11,500	12,000	13,000
May	13,500	14,500	15,000
June	14,500	14,500	15,500
July	10,500	11,000	12,000
August	13,000	13,500	14,000
September	15,500	16,000	16,500
October	14,500	15,500	16,500
November	12,500	14,000	14,500
December	10,000	11,000	11,500
	148,500	156,000	164,500

2. A review of management's overall plans does not indicate any changes that will affect the radiology department in the coming year.

3. The average revenue per relative unit value for the budget year is estimated to be 85 cents.

4. Deductions from revenues should be assumed to be 2 percent of gross revenues.

5. Salary increases in accordance with approved personnel policies are indicated here:

Position	Name	Present Salary	Date of Increase	Monthly Increase
Supervisor	Alton	$7,680	2/1/X3	$40
Sr. technician	Baker	7,020	7/1/X3	30
Sr. technician	Carson	5,820	7/1/X3	30
Jr. technician	Dowd	4,320	3/1/X3	20
Jr. technician	Early	4,440	10/1/X3	20
Jr. technician	French	4,080	1/1/X3	10
Student technician	Gordon	3,840	7/1/X3	10
Student technician	Hadley	3,780	1/1/X3	10

6. An allowance of 5 percent of each monthly budgeted salary should be provided for on-call and overtime pay.

7. Supplies and expenses for the budget year have been determined to be 15 cents per relative unit value.

8. Radiologists' fees are determined at 40 percent of net income, and indirect expenses have been determined to be 8 percent of direct expenses excluding radiologists' fees.

Required: Prepare a revenue and expense budget for the radiology department in dollar detail for the first three months of 19X3. Show all computations, rounding out all figures to the nearest dollar.

Cost Finding

23

In a typical accounting system, controllable expenses are classified and accumulated according to the organizational units or departments with which they are directly associated and by which they are incurred. The expenses recorded in the accounts of a given medical and surgical nursing unit, for example, consist largely of the salaries and wages paid to the employees of the unit and the costs of supplies consumed in the unit's activities. These expenses clearly are related to the operation of the nursing unit, and the unit supervisor can exercise a high degree of control over the amounts in which such expenses are incurred. This is accomplished mainly by controlling the labor hours and quantities of supplies used.

The operation of the nursing unit, however, requires services from other departments of the hospital. Meals for patients, for example, must be prepared and served by the dietary department. Cleaning and linen services are obtained from the housekeeping and laundry departments. Utilities and repair services are provided to the nursing unit by the plant operation and maintenance department. The expenses related to the provision of these and other departmental services, however, are not recorded in the nursing unit expense accounts but in the expense accounts of the departments providing the services.

In addition, certain other hospital expenses such as depreciation, insurance, and employee benefits often are recorded as unassigned expenses, because they are not routinely recorded as direct expenses of any particular organizational unit. Yet, the incurrence of these expenses is necessary to the operation of all organizational units of the hospital.

The emphasis of the general accounting process, then, is on expense control through the classification and accumulation of expenses according to the organizational units primarily responsible for incurring the expenses. No attempt is made within the formal accounting records to measure the full cost of operating any particular organizational unit or department. The departmental expense accounts in the general ledger include only those direct, controllable expenses incurred by each department. Departmental expense accounts do not include the costs of services, if any, provided by other departments of the hospital. The departmental expense accounts also exclude an appropriate share of the costs that are recorded in the unassigned expense classification.

Need for Cost Finding

Full cost information, however, is needed by hospital management for many important purposes. To develop the necessary full cost information, a procedure known as *cost finding* is performed at least annually, preferably monthly. This chapter provides an introductory discussion of the nature of cost finding and a somewhat simplified illustration of the techniques involved in a cost-finding procedure for a hospital of modest size. Should your interest in this subject extend beyond the materials of this chapter, a reading of the AHA's *Cost Finding and Rate Setting for Hospitals*[1] manual is recommended.

Nature of Cost Finding

General cost finding may be defined as a procedure in which unassigned expenses and the expenses of nonrevenue-producing departments are allocated to the revenue-producing departments of the hospital for the purpose of determining the full costs of providing various healthcare services to patients. It is a procedure that is performed apart from, and supplemental to, the formal accounting system. Cost-finding results are not recorded in the accounts of the hospital, nor do they appear in its income statement. The results of the cost-finding procedure are presented, however, in a cost report, as illustrated later in this chapter.

The prerequisites for a satisfactory cost-finding procedure include a sound organizational structure, an appropriate classification of accounts, and statistical data that adequately measure the amounts of service provided by each nonrevenue-producing department to all other departments of the hospital. These statistics, however, need not always be complete, actual counts; estimates derived from a sampling process frequently are used. And in certain cases, the use of weighted statistics may be necessary to produce more accurate and equitable allocations to the various departments.

[1]*Cost Finding and Rate Setting by Hospitals* (Chicago: American Hospital Association, 1968).

A major objective of general cost finding is to provide full cost information for use in setting service rates. Also, cost finding may be employed to determine the amount of reimbursable costs and to aid in the negotiation of reimbursement contracts with third-party payers. This should not be regarded, however, as the sole purpose of the cost-finding procedure. Cost finding, like responsibility accounting and budgeting, is a basic tool of management and is valuable for managerial decision-making in other areas to which full cost information is relevant.

Objectives and Uses of Cost Finding

Methods of Cost Finding

Several different methods of cost finding have been developed over the years. Those most widely used at the present time are (1) the step-down method and (2) the double-distribution method. To illustrate these two methods in a greatly simplified manner, let us assume Handy Hospital has the following: one item of unassigned expense; three nonrevenue-producing departments to be called Departments 1, 2, and 3; and three revenue-producing departments to be referred to as Departments A, B, and C. A trial balance of the hospital's expenses is presented in Figure 23–1.

Let us also assume that the nonrevenue-producing departments (Departments 1, 2, and 3) rendered services during 19X2 to each other and to the revenue-producing departments (Departments A, B, and C) as shown in Figure 23–2. Department 1, for example, rendered 25 percent of its services to Department 2, 15 percent to Department 3, 30 percent to Department A, 20 percent to Department B, and 10 percent to Department C. The indicated percentages are derived from an analysis of statistical data such as number of employees, labor hours, pounds of laundry, and square footage.

Unassigned expense	$ 80,000
Department 1	100,000
Department 2	60,000
Department 3	40,000
Department A	200,000
Department B	250,000
Department C	150,000
Total	$880,000

Figure 23–1 Handy Hospital Trial Balance of Expenses, Year Ended December 31, 19X2

Figure 23–2 Handy Hospital, Services Rendered by Nonrevenue-Producing Departments, Year Ended December 31, 19X2

| | Departments Rendering Services | | |
Departments Receiving Services:	Dept. 1	Dept. 2	Dept. 3
Department 1	—	10%	—
Department 2	25%	—	20%
Department 3	15	20	—
Department A	30	40	35
Department B	20	—	45
Department C	10	30	—
Totals	100%	100%	100%

Step-Down Method

A cost-finding worksheet that illustrates the step-down method appears in Figure 23–3. Column 1 consists of the trial balance of expenses shown in Figure 23–1. The objective of the cost-finding is to allocate unassigned expense to all departments and to allocate the expenses of the nonrevenue-producing departments to each other and to the revenue-producing departments so that, at the end of the allocation process, all expenses will be located in Departments A, B, and C. As a result, the total cost of the patient services provided by Handy Hospital's revenue-producing departments is determined.

Column 2 of the worksheet shows the allocation of un-assigned expense to the nonrevenue-producing and revenue-producing departments. It is assumed here that the appropriate allocation basis is departmental direct expenses as shown here:

Department	Direct Expenses	Percentage of Total Direct Expenses	×	Unassigned Expenses	=	Allocated Expense
1	$100,000	12.50%		$80,000		$10,000
2	60,000	7.50		80,000		6,000
3	40,000	5.00		80,000		4,000
A	200,000	25.00		80,000		20,000
B	250,000	31.25		80,000		25,000
C	150,000	18.75		80,000		15,000
	$800,000	100.00%				$80,000

Other Possible Allocation Bases

Depending on the nature of the unassigned expense item, it may be more appropriate to use other allocation bases, such as number of employees, gross salaries and wages, or square footage in the various departments. It also is assumed that the unassigned expense in this illustration is properly allocable to all departments.

Sequence of Allocations

The next step is to allocate the expenses of the nonrevenue-producing departments to each other and to the revenue-producing

	(1) Trial Balance	(2) Unassigned Expense	(3) Subtotal	(4) Dept. 1	(5) Subtotal	(6) Dept. 2	(7) Subtotal	(8) Dept. 3	(9) Full Cost Totals*
Unassigned expense	$ 80,000	$ 80,000							
Nonrevenue-producing departments:									
Department 1	100,000	$ 10,000	$110,000	$110,000					
Department 2	60,000	6,000	66,000	$ 27,000	$ 93,500	$ 93,500			
Department 3	40,000	4,000	44,000	16,500	60,500	20,778	$ 81,278	$ 81,278	
Revenue-producing departments:									
Department A	200,000	20,000	220,000	33,000	253,000	41,556	294,556	$ 35,559	$330,115
Department B	250,000	25,000	275,000	22,000	297,000		297,000	45,719	342,719
Department C	150,000	15,000	165,000	11,000	176,000	31,166	207,166		207,166
Totals	$880,000	$ 80,000	$880,000	$110,000	$880,000	$ 93,500	$880,000	$ 81,278	$880,000

*For revenue-producing departments only.

Figure 23–3 Handy Hospital Cost-Finding Worksheet: Step-Down Method, Year Ended December 31, 19X2

departments. In what sequence, however, should Departments 1, 2, and 3 be allocated? Generally, the department that renders the greatest amount of service to the greatest number of other departments and receives the least in services from other departments is the first department whose expenses are allocated. The department that provides the next greatest amount of service to the next greatest number of other departments and receives the next least in services from other departments is the second department whose expenses are allocated, and so on. The nonrevenue-producing department whose expenses are allocated last is the one that renders the least service to the smallest number of other departments and receives the greatest amount of service from other departments.

When the sequence of allocation cannot be determined on this basis, the sequence may be established on the basis of accumulated expenses. In such cases, the department having the largest amount of expense is allocated first, the department having the next largest amount of expense is allocated second, and so on.

This means that the allocation sequence will not be identical in all hospitals, nor will it necessarily be consistent from year to year in the same hospital. Similarly, the allocation bases employed will differ among hospitals and may not necessarily be consistent from year to year in a given hospital. When an allocation sequence that is more logical and defensible can be determined or when improved allocation bases become available, appropriate changes should be considered in the cost-finding procedure.

In Figure 23–3, it is assumed that the nonrevenue-producing departments are properly allocable in this sequence:

1. Department 1
2. Department 2
3. Department 3

Notice, in column 4, the allocation of the expenses of Department 1. The allocation, based on the percentages provided in Figure 23–3, is 25 percent to Department 2, 15 percent to Department 3, 30 percent to Department A, 20 percent to Department B, and 10 percent to Department C. The allocation to Department 2, for example, is 25 percent of $110,000, or $27,500. Note also that the expenses of Department 1 are allocated to all departments to which Department 1 renders services. This includes other nonrevenue-producing departments as well as the revenue-producing departments.

Once the expenses of a nonrevenue-producing department have been allocated under the step-down method of cost finding, that department is considered to be closed. That department therefore will not receive any allocation of the expenses of the other nonrevenue-producing departments whose expenses are yet to be allocated. Thus, Department 1 is now closed; it will receive no allocation of the expenses of Departments 2 and 3. This is the procedure even though Departments 2 and 3 may have rendered services to Department 1 during 19X2.

The allocation of the accumulated expenses ($60,000 + $6,000 + $27,500 = $93,500) of Department 2 is shown in column 6 of Figure 23–3. As noted earlier, although Department 2 rendered 10 percent of its services to Department 1, no allocation of Department 2 expenses is made to Department 1. So, the allocation of Department 2 expenses is made as follows:

Department	Percent of Dept. 2 Services Received[2]	Fraction ×	Accum. Expenses of Dept. 2	= Expense Allocation
3	20%	2/9	$93,500	$20,778
A	40	4/9	93,500	41,556
C	30	3/9	93,500	31,166
	90%	9/9		$93,500

[2]See Figure 23–2.

	(1) Unassigned Expenses	(2) Nonrevenue Dept. 1	(3) Producing Dept. 2	(4) Departments Dept. 3	(5) Dept. A	(6) Revenue Producing Dept. B	(7) Departments Dept. C	(8) Total
Trial balance, December 31, 19X2	$ 80,000	$100,000	$ 60,000	$ 40,000	$200,000	$250,000	$150,000	$880,000
Allocation of unassigned expenses	–80,000	+10,000	+6,000	+4,000	+20,000	+25,000	+15,000	-0-
Subtotals	$ -0-	110,000	66,000	44,000	220,000	275,000	165,000	880,000
Initial allocation of Department 1		–110,000	+27,500	–16,500	+33,000	+22,000	+11,000	-0-
Subtotals		-0-	93,500	60,500	253,000	297,000	176,000	880,000
Initial allocation of Department 2		+9,350	–93,500	+18,700	+37,400	-0-	+28,050	-0-
Subtotals		9,350	-0-	79,200	290,400	297,000	204,050	880,000
Initial allocation of Department 3		-0-	+15,840	–79,200	+27,720	+35,640	-0-	-0-
Subtotals		9,350	15,840	-0-	318,120	332,640	204,050	880,000
Final allocation of Department 1		–9,350	+2,337	+1,403	+2,805	+1,870	+935	-0-
Subtotals		$ -0-	18,177	1,403	320,925	334,510	204,985	880,000
Final allocation of Department 2			–18,177	+4,039	+8,079	-0-	+6,059	-0-
Subtotals			$ -0-	5,442	329,004	334,510	211,044	880,000
Final allocation of Department 3				–5,442	+2,381	+3,061	-0-	-0-
				$ -0-				
Full cost totals					$331,385	$337,571	$211,044	$880,000

Figure 23–4 Handy Hospital Cost-Finding Worksheet: Double-Distribution Method, Year Ended December 31, 19X2

Similarly, in column 8, the $81,278 of accumulated expenses in Department 3 are allocated only to the revenue-producing departments because both of the other nonrevenue-producing departments (Departments 1 and 2) have previously been closed. The allocation of Department 3 expenses is 35/80 to Department A and 45/80 to Department B. As indicated in Figure 23–2, Department 3 rendered no services to Department C during 19X2.

The results of the cost finding are shown in column 9. Here, you see that Handy Hospital's total expenses of $880,000 are located in the revenue-producing departments only. The full costs of operating these departments are found to be $330,115 for Department A, $342,719 for Department B, and $207,166 for Department C. The step-down method of cost finding, however, does not produce full cost information about the nonrevenue-producing departments.

Double-Distribution Method

A cost-finding worksheet using the double-distribution method is presented for Handy Hospital in Figure 23–4. Under this method, greater recognition is given to the fact that nonrevenue-producing departments render services to each other as well as to revenue-producing departments. Nonrevenue-producing departments are not closed after their expenses have been allocated. Instead, they remain open to receive expense allocations from other nonrevenue-producing departments. As a result, after an initial allocation of the accumulated expenses of the nonrevenue-producing departments, a second round of expense allocations must be made.

The second-round allocations usually are made in accordance with the step-down method. That is, when a department is closed in the second round, it remains closed. There are other variations of the double-distribution method of cost finding, but these variations are not described here.

The worksheet illustrated in Figure 23–4 is arranged in a vertical format (the Figure 23–3 worksheet is arranged in a horizontal format). In Figure 23–4, the unassigned expenses are allocated in exactly the same way as they were in the step-down method. The initial allocation of Department 1 expenses also is the same as in the step-down method. Under the step-down method, however, Department 1 would now be considered permanently closed and would receive no subsequent allocations from Departments 2 and 3.

Reopening Departments for Additional Expense Allocations

But, as you can see in Figure 23–4, after an initial allocation of the accumulated expenses of Department 2, Department 1 is reopened to receive 10 percent of Department 2 expenses. (Figure 23–2 indicates that Department 2 provides 10 percent of its services to Department 1.) Similarly, Department 2 is closed after the initial allocation of its accumulated expenses but is reopened when the expenses of Department 3 are initially allocated.

So, after the initial round of expense allocations for Departments 1, 2, and 3, expenses remain in each of these departments. This necessitates a second and final round of expense allocations. These final allocations are made in conformity with the step-down procedure. In other words, once a department's expenses are allocated in the final round, the department is permanently closed.

The results of a double-distribution cost finding will differ somewhat from the results of the step-down method. A comparison is presented in Figure 23–5. It also should be recognized that the double-distribution method, unlike the step-down method, tends to provide a reasonable approximation of the full costs of operating the nonrevenue-producing departments.

Cost-Finding: An Extended Illustration

Now that you have had an opportunity to examine the cost-finding procedure in highly simplified form, let us turn to a more realistic example. The step-down method is used in this illustration for ease of exposition and also because it is a widely employed method in actual practice.

The statistical and accounting data relate to Happy Hamlet Hospital, a hypothetical short-term, general hospital of modest size.

Full Costs of Services Provided by:	Double-Distribution Method	Step-Down Method
Department A	$331,385	$330,115
Department B	337,571	342,719
Department C	211,044	207,166
Totals	$880,000	$880,000

Figure 23–5 Handy Hospital Comparison of Cost-Finding Results

Because of space and other limitations, certain liberties have been taken with respect to dollar amounts, statistics, and the number of departments involved in the illustration. It also should be understood that differences among hospitals affect the cost-finding procedure and the results it produces. Although the illustrated procedure is relevant and generally applicable to all hospitals, the illustration does not include certain of the more troublesome problems that may arise in an actual cost-finding procedure.

Worksheet A

Happy Hamlet Hospital's cost finding begins with the placement of a trial balance of expenses and certain revenues on a worksheet (generally referred to as Worksheet A), as shown in column 3 of Figure 23–6. Note that the trial balance relates to the six months ended June 30, 19X3, and includes the following:

1. Departmental cost center expenses:
   a. Salaries
   b. other expenses
2. Unassigned expenses, classified by major type
3. Certain "other operating" revenues that represent recoveries of specific operating-expense items

Examples of other types of expense recoveries include tuition fees from educational programs, telephone revenues, nonpatient room rentals, and sales of scrap. To keep the illustration relatively simple, Worksheet A includes only three items under expense recoveries (lines 23 through 25).

Making Adjustments

Columns 4 through 7 of Worksheet A are used to make various reclassifications and adjustments for cost-finding purposes. The number and types of reclassifications and adjustments depend on the manner in which direct expenses are accumulated in the accounts and on the hospital's need for detailed full cost data.

In this illustration, we assume that the direct expenses ($245,000) of all nursing units have been recorded by Happy Hamlet Hospital in a single cost center (see account 6021 on line 3). Let us assume, however, that management wishes to obtain from the

Acct. No.		Ledger Balances Salaries	Ledger Balances Other	Ledger Balances Total	Adj. Salaries Add	Adj. Salaries Deduct	Adj. Other Add	Adj. Other Deduct	Adjusted Salaries	Adjusted Other	Adjusted Total	Worksheet B Line Number
	Nursing services:											
6010	Administrative office	$ 8,000	$ 1,000	$ 9,000					$ 8,000	$ 1,000	$ 9,000	8
6021	Nursing units	220,000	25,000	245,000		(1)220,000		(1)25,000				13
6210	Operating rooms	12,000	6,000	18,000					12,000	6,000	18,000	20
6230	Emergency rooms	8,000	5,000	13,000					8,000	5,000	13,000	9
6250	Central supply	10,000	9,000	19,000					10,000	9,000	19,000	
	Other professional services:											
7011	Laboratory	20,000	10,000	30,000					20,000	10,000	30,000	14
7040	Radiology	28,000	12,000	40,000					28,000	12,000	40,000	15
7070	Pharmacy	14,000	11,000	25,000					14,000	11,000	25,000	10
7120	Outpatient clinic	9,000	6,000	15,000					9,000	6,000	15,000	19
7180	Medical records	8,000	4,000	12,000				(2) 2,000	8,000	2,000	10,000	11
	General services:											
8050	Dietary	46,000	40,000	86,000					46,000	40,000	86,000	7
8060	Plant operation and maintenance	25,000	38,000	63,000					25,000	38,000	63,000	4
8090	Housekeeping	23,000	8,000	31,000					23,000	8,000	31,000	5
8110	Laundry	17,000	7,000	24,000					17,000	7,000	24,000	6
8200	Fiscal and administrative services	88,000	12,000	100,000				(3) 3,000	88,000	9,000	97,000	3
	Unassigned expenses:											
8510	Depreciation		50,000	50,000						50,000	50,000	1
8710	Employee benefits		48,240	48,240						48,240	48,240	2
	Expense recoveries:											
5061	Cafeteria sales		(17,000)	(17,000)						(17,000)	(17,000)	21
5085	Medical record transcript fees		(2,000)	(2,000)				(2)(2,000)				
5171	Purchase discounts		(3,000)	(3,000)				(3)(3,000)				
	Totals	$536,000	$270,240	$806,240								
	Nursing units—adult and pediatric				(1)196,000		(1)22,000		196,000	22,000	218,000	17
	Newborn nursery				(1) 24,000		(1) 3,000		24,000	3,000	27,000	18
	Totals				$220,000	$220,000	$ 25,000	$ 25,000	$536,000	$270,240	$806,240	

Figure 23–6 Happy Hamlet Hospital Cost Finding—Worksheet A, Six Months Ended June 30, 19X3

cost finding the full costs of (a) adult and pediatric nursing units and (b) the newborn nursery. In other words, the single cost center must be reclassified into two cost centers. An entry (number 1) therefore is made on the worksheet to reclassify the $245,000 of expense as follows:

Nursing Units—Adult and Pediatric:		
Salaries	$196,000	
Other Expense	22,000	
Newborn Nursery:		
Salaries	24,000	
Other Expense	3,000	
Nursing Units:		
Salaries		$220,000
Other Expense		25,000

This entry eliminates account 6021 from line 3 of the worksheet and establishes two new cost centers on lines 29 and 30. Were full cost data required in more detail from the cost finding, additional nursing-unit cost centers could easily be established on Worksheet A (for example, separate cost centers could be set up for medical and surgical units, pediatric units, psychiatric units, obstetric units, and intensive care units).

As another example, assume that a hospital routinely records the direct expenses of operating an electrocardiology unit in expense accounts of the laboratory department. This practice may be satisfactory for the purpose of month-to-month expense control but not for the purposes of cost finding. Management may wish to determine the full cost of providing EKG services.

If so, a Worksheet A reclassification entry is required to remove the direct EKG expenses from the laboratory expenses and establish them in an EKG cost center. The direct expenses associated with the newly created cost centers generally can be estimated from an analysis of payroll and other records.

On the other hand, reclassification entries may be needed to combine two or more responsibility accounting cost centers into a single cost center for cost finding. Assume, for example, that a hospital operates a school of nursing whose direct expenses are recorded in several cost centers. An entry might be made on the worksheet to combine the direct expenses of these centers into a

Reclassifying Entries to Combine Accounting Cost Centers

		(1) Adjusted Balances	(2) Depreci- ation	(3) Employee Benefits	(4) Subtotals	(5) F & A Services	(6) Plant O & M
1	Depreciation	50,000	$50,000				
2	Employee benefits	48,240		$48,240			
3	Fiscal and administrative services	97,000	$ 900	$ 7,920	$105,820	$105,820	
4	Plant operation and maintenance	63,000	2,500	2,250	67,750	$ 9,993	$77,743
5	Housekeeping	31,000	200	2,070	33,270	4,907	$ 334
6	Laundry	24,000	1,400	1,530	26,930	3,972	2,335
7	Dietary	86,000	4,200	4,140	94,340	13,915	7,006
8	Nursing service—adm. office	9,000	200	720	9,920	1,463	334
9	Central supply	19,000	1,600	900	21,500	3,171	2,669
10	Pharmacy	25,000	500	1,260	26,760	3,947	834
11	Medical records	10,000	400	720	11,120	1,640	667
12	Cost of meals sold						
13	Operating rooms	18,000	3,000	1,080	22,080	3,257	5,004
14	Laboratory	30,000	800	1,800	32,600	4,808	1,334
15	Radiology	40,000	1,400	2,520	43,920	6,478	2,335
16	Cost of drugs sold						
17	Nursing units—adult & pediatric	218,000	29,000	17,640	264,640	39,037	48,386
18	Newborn nursery	27,000	1,400	2,160	30,560	4,508	2,336
19	Outpatient clinic	15,000	1,500	810	17,310	2,553	2,502
20	Emergency rooms	13,000	1,000	720	14,720	2,171	1,668
21	Cafeteria sales	(17,000)			(17,000)		
	Totals	$806,240	$50,000	$48,240	$806,240	$105,820	$77,748

Figure 23–7 Happy Hamlet Hospital Cost-Finding Worksheet B,
Six Months Ended June 30, 19X3

single cost center for nursing education. This facilitates the cost-finding procedure.

Entry 2 on Worksheet A reduces the direct expenses of the medical records department for the $2,000 of revenues obtained from medical record transcript fees. Entry 3 similarly credits fiscal and administrative services for the $3,000 of purchase discounts earned. In some cases, it may be appropriate to offset cafeteria sales to employees and guests against the direct expenses of the dietary department. Happy Hamlet Hospital, however, follows an alternative procedure to be described subsequently in the chapter.

The adjusted balances, taking into account the reclassifications and adjustments, are extended into columns 8 through 10 of Worksheet A. Column 11 indicates the line numbers of Worksheet B (Figure 23–7) to which the adjusted totals shown in column 10 are transferred.

Worksheets B and B-1   Worksheet B, illustrated in Figure 23–7, begins with the entry of adjusted balances in column 1 (from Worksheet A, Figure 23–6). Note that the sequence in which the cost centers are listed is not the

(7) Hskpg.	(8) Laundry	(9) Dietary	(10) Nursing Adm. Off.	(11) Central Supply	(12) Pharmacy	(13) Medical Records	(14) Subtotals	(15) Net Cost of Meals Sold	(16) Total Costs
$38,511									
$ 1,162	$34,399								
3,486	$ 200	$118,947							
166	40		$11,923						
1,328	6,000		$ 720	$35,388					
415	30				$31,986				
332	20					$13,779			
		$ 27,000					$ 27,000	$27,000	
2,490	6,500		896	$ 4,320	$ 2,668		47,215	$ 609	$ 47,824
664	70				552		40,028	536	40,544
1,162	400				644		54,939	709	55,648
					18,400		18,400		18,400
24,069	16,739	91,947	9,211	29,493	7,422	$10,610	541,554	6,952	548,506
1,162	2,200		440	405	440	1,102	43,172	557	43,729
1,245	800		304	180	736	1,378	27,008	348	27,356
830	1,400		352	990	1,104	689	23,924	309	24,233
							(17,000)	17,000	
$38,511	$34,399	$118,947	$11,923	$35,388	$31,986	$13,779	$806,240	$27,000	$806,240

Figure 23-7 Happy Hamlet Hospital Cost-Finding Worksheet B,
Six Months Ended June 30, 19X3 *(continued)*

same as the sequence in which they were listed in Worksheet A. The cost centers were listed in Worksheet A in account-number sequence, the same order in which they appear in the hospital's ledger. In Worksheet B, the cost centers are listed in the order in which they will be allocated and closed.

Depreciation. The allocation of depreciation expense ($50,000) is shown in column 2 of Worksheet B. Fiscal and administrative services, for example, received an allocation of $900; plant operation and maintenance was charged with $2,500; and so on. These allocations were determined on the basis of the number of square feet occupied by each department or cost center as indicated in Worksheet B-1 (Figure 23-8). In column 1 of Worksheet B-1, note the listing of square footage (a total of 50,000 square feet) by department or cost center. Because total depreciation expense is $50,000 and there is a total of 50,000 square feet, the unit cost multiplier is $1 ($50,000 ÷ 50,000 square feet). In other words, each department will be allocated $1 of depreciation expense for each square foot it occupies. The fiscal and administrative services

Allocation bases	(1) Depreci-ation Square Feet	(2) Employee Benefits Payroll Dollars	(3) F & A Services Accum. Expenses	(4) Plant O & M Square Feet	(5) Hskpg. Square Feet	(6) Laundry Pounds	(7) Dietary Meals Served	(8) Nursing Adm. Off. Hours	(9) Central Supply Priced Reg.	(10) Pharmacy Priced Reg.	(11) Medical Records Estimated Time	(12) Net Cost of Meals Sold Accum. Expenses
Fiscal and administrative services	900	$ 88,000										
Plant operation and maintenance	2,500	25,000	$ 67,750									
Housekeeping	200	23,000	33,270	200								
Laundry	1,400	17,000	26,930	1,400	1,400							
Dietary	4,200	46,000	94,340	4,200	4,200	2,000						
Nursing services—administrative office	200	8,000	9,920	200	200	400		9,000				
Central supply	1,600	10,000	21,500	1,600	1,600	60,000						
Pharmacy	500	14,000	26,760	500	500	300						
Medical records	400	8,000	11,120	400	400	200						
Cost of meals sold							18,000					
Operating rooms	3,000	12,000	22,080	3,000	3,000	65,000		11,200	$ 9,600	$ 2,900		$ 47,215
Laboratory	800	20,000	32,600	800	800	700				600		40,028
Radiology	1,400	28,000	43,920	1,400	1,400	4,000				700		54,939
Cost of drugs sold										20,000		
Nursing units—adult and pediatric	29,000	196,000	264,640	29,000	29,000	167,400	61,300	115,137	65,540	8,067	77%	541,554
Newborn nursery	1,400	24,000	30,560	1,400	1,400	22,000		5,500	900	500	8	43,172
Outpatient clinic	1,500	9,000	17,310	1,500	1,500	8,000		3,800	400	800	10	27,008
Emergency room	1,000	8,000	14,720	1,000	1,000	14,000		4,400	2,200	1,200	5	23,924
Totals	50,000	$536,000	$717,420	46,600	46,400	344,000	79,300	149,037	$78,640	$34,767	100%	$777,840
Accumulated expenses per Worksheet B	$50,000	$ 48,240	$105,820	$77,743	$38,511	$ 34,399	$118,947	$ 11,923	$35,388	$31,986	$13,779	$ 10,000
Unit cost multiplier (line 25/line 23)	1.00	.09	.1475	1.668	.83	.10	1.50	.08	.45	.92		.0129
Worksheet B column number	2	3	5	6	7	8	9	10	11	12	13	15

Figure 23–8 Happy Hamlet Hospital Cost-Finding Worksheet B-1, Six Months Ended June 30, 19X3

department, for example, uses 900 square feet of space and therefore is charged with $900 of depreciation.

A similar computation is made for each department, and the allocations so determined are entered in column 2 of Worksheet B. This column then is totaled to be sure that the individual allocations add up to $50,000.

This illustration, of course, makes no distinction between depreciation on the hospital building and depreciation of equipment. When a detailed equipment ledger is maintained, equipment depreciation may be more properly allocated, perhaps on the basis of the investment in equipment by each department. Depreciating the hospital building would be a separate allocation based on square footage. Depreciation on an outlying building that houses boilers and generators, for instance, might be allocated entirely to the plant operation department.

Employee Benefits. As seen in Worksheet B-1, employee benefits are allocated on the basis of departmental payroll dollars, as indicated in column 8 of Worksheet A. Dividing $48,240 of benefits by $536,000 of payroll dollars results in a unit cost multiplier of nine cents per dollar of payroll. Or, to put it another way, the amount of employee benefits to be allocated to a department is 9 percent of departmental gross payroll. The fiscal and administrative services payroll is $88,000, for example; the allocation for employee benefits therefore is $7,920 ($88,000 × 9 percent). The computed allocations then are entered in column 3 of Worksheet B. Note that the column adds to the correct total of $48,420.

Fiscal and Administrative Services. The allocation of fiscal and administrative expenses appears in column 5 of Worksheet B. This allocation is based on the accumulated departmental expenses as shown by the subtotals in column 4 of Worksheet B. To determine the unit cost multiplier, the subtotals are entered in column 3 of Worksheet B-1. The accumulated fiscal and administrative expenses of $105,820 ($97,000 + $900 of depreciation + $7,920 of employee benefits) divided by the $717,420 of accumulated expenses in all other departments produces a unit cost multiplier of 14.75 percent. Plant operation and maintenance therefore is charged with $9,993 ($67,750 × 14.75 percent) of fiscal and administrative expenses. A similar computation is made for each department, and the results are entered in column 5 of Worksheet B.

Fiscal and administrative services, in this illustration, are treated as a single cost center. The results of the cost finding might be considerably more accurate and useful, however, if fiscal and administrative services were broken down into several cost centers, each

Depreciating the Hospital Building and Outlying Buildings

Breakdown into Several Cost Centers

being allocated on a different basis. On Worksheet A, for instance, reclassification entries may be made to create separate cost centers for admitting (to be allocated on the basis of admissions), patient accounting (to be allocated on the basis of patient days), personnel (to be allocated on the basis of number of employees), purchasing (to be allocated on the basis of nonlabor expenses), and so on.

Plant Operation and Maintenance.   The plant operation and maintenance cost center, at this stage of the cost finding, has accumulated expenses of $77,743, which are allocated on the basis of square footage, as shown in column 6 of Worksheet B. As computed in column 4 of Worksheet B-1, these allocations were determined by the use of a 1.668 multiplier. The allocation to housekeeping, for example, is $334 (200 square feet × 166.8 percent). Again, where plant operation and maintenance expenses are accumulated in two or more cost centers, different allocation bases might be employed. Plant operation, for instance, might be allocated on the basis of a measure of utility usage, whereas plant maintenance expenses might be allocated on the basis of maintenance hours. Because plant operation and maintenance expenses are substantial, this procedure could improve a cost-finding markedly.

Housekeeping.   As indicated in column 5 of Worksheet B-1, housekeeping expenses are allocated on the basis of square footage, using a unit cost multiplier of 83 cents per square foot. Hours of housekeeping services also may be an equitable allocation basis. As before, the computed allocations are entered in the appropriate column of Worksheet B.

Laundry.   Laundry expenses, as seen in column 6 of Worksheet B-1, are allocated on the basis of 10 cents per pound. Laundry might be allocated on the basis of pieces of laundry rather than of pounds. Where either pieces or pounds are employed as the allocation basis, the number of pieces or pounds may be weighted to take into account that it costs more to process certain laundry items than others.

Dietary.   Total dietary expenses (see column 7 of Worksheet B-1) are prorated at the rate of $1.50 per meal served. Because 18,000 meals were served by the hospital's cafeteria, $27,000 of dietary expense is allocated to a special cost center (line 12, column 9, of Worksheet B) that later will be offset against cafeteria sales (Worksheet B, column 15). The $91,947 balance of dietary expense is charged to the adult and pediatric nursing units. If the cafeteria is established as a separate cost center by an entry on Worksheet A, this likely will improve the cost-finding procedure. In such cases, raw food costs may be allocated apart from other dietary expenses.

Nursing—Administrative Office. As may be noted in Worksheet B-1, these expenses are allocated on the basis of eight cents per hour of nursing service worked in cost centers supervised by the nursing service director. The basis for allocation of nursing education expenses generally is hours of assigned student time. It is assumed, however, that Happy Hamlet Hospital has no school of nursing.

Central Supply. The expenses of central services and supply are allocated on the basis of 45 cents per dollar of priced requisitions. Other bases of allocation, such as percentage estimates of the time spent in servicing other departments, sometimes may be employed.

Pharmacy. Pharmacy expenses also are allocated on the basis of the dollar value of priced requisitions. As indicated in Worksheet B-1, the apportionment is 92 cents per dollar of priced requisitions.

Medical Records. The cost center for medical records is allocated on the basis of percentage estimates of the time spent in maintaining medical records for the various classifications of patients. These percentages are given in Worksheet B-1.

Net Cost of Meals Sold. Because cafeteria sales were $17,000 and the cost of meals sold was $27,000, the net cost of meals sold is $10,000. As shown in column 12 of Worksheet B-1, this $10,000 is allocated on the basis of the accumulated expenses indicated by the subtotals in column 14 of Worksheet B. The apportionment uses a unit cost multiplier of 0.0129. After the computed allocations are entered in column 15 of Worksheet B, the worksheet is completed with the computation and entry of total costs in column 16.

Cost Reports

The results of the cost finding are summarized and reported to the management of Happy Hamlet Hospital in the cost report shown in Figure 23-9. The report assumes the gross revenue data in column 1. Column 2 figures are drawn from column 1, lines 18-20, of Worksheet B (Figure 23-7); column 4 figures are drawn from column 16 of Worksheet B. The indirect costs in column 3 of the cost report may be computed simply by subtracting column 2 figures from column 4 figures; alternatively, the indirect costs of each center may be determined by adding the expense allocations presented in Worksheet B.

The units of service rendered by each center are shown in columns 5 through 7 of the cost report. Column 8 indicates the

Adequacy of Service Rates by Cost Center

Revenue-Cost Centers	(1) Gross Revenues	(2) Direct	(3) Costs Indirect	(4) Total	(5) Units of Service Rendered Units	(6) Statistic	(7)	(8) Average Unit Cost	(9) Net
Operating rooms	$ 42,909	$ 18,000	$ 29,824	$ 47,824	523	Operations		91.44	$ (4,915)
Laboratory	72,346	30,000	10,544	40,544	11,065	Tests		3.66	31,802
Radiology	95,261	40,000	15,648	55,648	2,347	Films		23.71	39,613
Cost of drugs sold	29,408		18,400	18,400	7,208	Prescriptions filled		2.55	11,008
Nursing units—adult and pediatric	581,221	218,000	330,506	548,506	8,244	Patient days		66.53	32,715
Newborn nursery	36,382	27,000	16,729	43,729	1,077	Newborn days		40.60	(7,347)
Outpatient clinic	15,290	15,000	12,356	27,356	2,180	Visits		12.55	(12,066)
Emergency rooms	21,028	13,000	11,233	24,233	1,109	Admissions		21.85	(3,205)
Totals	$893,845	$361,000	$445,240	$806,240					$837,605
Less deductions from revenues									62,569
Excess of revenues over costs and revenue deductions									$ 25,036

Figure 23-9 Happy Hamlet Hospital Cost Report, Six Months Ended June 30, 19X3

average cost per unit of service, determined by dividing the total of column 4 by that of column 6. The excess of gross revenues over total costs (or the excess of total costs over gross revenues) is reported in column 9. This tends to indicate the adequacy of the service rates established in each center.

An additional cost report is illustrated in Figure 23–10. This report presents, on lines 16 through 22, a summary of total costs and gross revenues classified by type of patient: inpatients, newborns, outpatients, and emergency patients. The costs are allocated to these patient groups on the basis of a charge converter or the ratio of costs to charges.

This procedure requires an accounting classification of gross revenues by type of patient. Consider, for example, the laboratory department whose total costs are $40,544 and whose gross revenues are $72,346. The revenue for each type of patient is then multiplied by the cost converter to determine the costs to be allocated as follows:

	Gross Revenues	Cost Converter	Cost Allocation
Inpatients	$64,822	.560418	$36,328
Newborn	1,266	.560418	709
Outpatients	6,258	.560418	3,507
Emergency			
Totals	$72,346		$40,544

Department:	Total Costs	Gross Revenues	Cost Converter	Inpatients Revenues	Inpatients Allocated Costs	Newborn Revenues	Newborn Allocated Costs	Outpatients Revenues	Outpatients Allocated Costs	Emergency Revenues	Emergency Allocated Costs
Operating rooms	$ 47,824	$ 42,909	1.114545	$ 42,265	$ 47,106	$ 1,266	$ 709	$ 644	$ 718		
Laboratory	40,544	72,346	.560418	64,822	36,328	1,143	668	6,258	3,507		
Radiology	55,648	95,261	.584164	70,779	41,346	147	92	23,339	13,634	$ 956	$ 598
Cost of drugs sold	18,400	29,408	.625680	24,526	15,346			3,779	2,364		
Nursing units—adult and pediatric	548,506	581,221	.943713	581,221	548,506						
Newborn nursery	48,729	36,382	1.201941			36,382	43,729				
Outpatient clinic	27,356	15,290	1.789143					15,290	27,356		
Emergency rooms	24,233	21,028	1.152416							21,028	24,233
Totals	$806,240	$893,845		$783,613	$688,632	$38,938	$45,198	$49,310	$47,579	$21,984	$24,831

Type of Patient:	Gross Revenues	Allocated Costs	Net
Inpatients	$783,613	$688,632	$94,981
Newborn	38,938	45,198	(6,260)
Outpatients	49,310	47,579	1,731
Emergency	21,984	24,831	(2,847)
Totals	$893,845	$806,240	$87,605

Figure 23–10 Happy Hamlet Hospital Cost Allocation: Ratio of Costs to Charges Applied to Costs, Six Months Ended June 30, 19X3

In other words, because laboratory costs are 56.0418 percent of laboratory revenues, and $64,822 of revenues were derived from services rendered to inpatients, 56.0418 percent of those revenues (or $36,328) represents the costs allocated to inpatients. The allocations to newborns and outpatients are determined in the same way. (The example assumes that the laboratory provided no services to emergency patients.)

Cost Accounting

This chapter has focused on cost-finding, an exercise performed apart from and supplemental to the formal accounting system. A relatively recent development in accounting for hospitals and certain other healthcare entities, however, is *cost accounting*. In cost accounting, the full costs of providing specific healthcare services are determined *within* the accounting system. The chart of accounts, journals, and ledgers are designed to permit costs to be classified and recorded within the formal accounting records so that supplementary cost-finding exercises (such as those described in this chapter) are not necessary. Implementation of a cost accounting system is a highly complex matter that is far beyond the scope of this book.

Questions

Q23–1. Write a brief definition of general cost finding.

Q23–2. What are the basic prerequisites for a satisfactory cost-finding procedure?

Q23–3. What are the primary purposes of general cost finding?

Q23–4. Distinguish briefly between the step-down and double-distribution methods of cost finding.

Q23–5. In what sequence should the expenses of nonrevenue-producing departments be allocated to each other and to the revenue-producing departments in a general cost-finding procedure?

Q23–6. Suggest a basis for the allocation of each of the following expenses in a cost finding procedure:
a. Depreciation expense—building
b. Depreciation expense—equipment
c. Employee benefits
d. Insurance

Q23–7. Suggest a basis for the allocation of each of the following expenses in a cost finding procedure:
a. Fiscal and administrative services

b. Plant operation and maintenance
c. Housekeeping
d. Laundry
e. Dietary

E23–1. Calico Hospital has a single item of unassigned expense, three nonrevenue-producing departments (departments 1, 2, and 3), and three revenue-producing departments (departments A, B, and C). A trial balance of expenses for the year ended December 31, 19X1, is provided here:

Unassigned expense	$ 60,000
Department 1	120,000
Department 2	80,000
Department 3	40,000
Department A	170,000
Department B	240,000
Department C	160,000
	$870,000

The nonrevenue-producing departments rendered services during 19X1 to each other and to the revenue-producing departments as indicated below:

Departments Receiving Services	Dept. 1	Dept. 2	Dept. 3
Dept. 1	—	15%	—
Dept. 2	30%	—	30%
Dept. 3	10	15	—
Dept. A	25	35	25
Dept. B	20	—	45
Dept. C	15	35	—
	100%	100%	100%

Unassigned expenses should be allocated to the nonrevenue-producing and revenue-producing departments on the basis of departmental direct expenses.

Required: Prepare a cost-finding worksheet, using (1) the step-down method and (2) the double-distribution method.

E23–2. Bingo Hospital has two items of unassigned expense, four nonrevenue-producing departments (departments 1, 2, 3, and 4), and four revenue-producing departments (departments A, B, C, and D). A trial balance of expenses for the quarter ended December 31, 19X1, is shown here:

Unassigned expense (item X)	$ 40,000
Unassigned expense (item Y)	30,000
Department:	
1	100,000
2	80,000
3	50,000
4	30,000
A	150,000
B	220,000
C	110,000
D	90,000
	$900,000

Seventy-five percent of unassigned expense item X is allocable to the nonrevenue-producing departments and 25 percent to the revenue-producing departments, on the basis of departmental direct expenses. Unassigned expense item Y then should be allocated on the basis of accumulated expenses to the nonrevenue-producing and revenue-producing departments. The nonrevenue-producing departments rendered services during 19X1 to each other and to the revenue-producing departments as follows:

Department Receiving Services:	Departments Rendering Services			
	Dept. 1	Dept. 2	Dept. 3	Dept. 4
Dept. 1	—	10%	15%	—
Dept. 2	20%	—	15	10%
Dept. 3	10	10	—	—
Dept. 4	15	20	10	—
Dept. A	30	—	40	25
Dept. B	10	20	—	—
Dept. C	5	20	—	65
Dept. D	10	20	20	—
	100%	100%	100%	100%

Required: (1) Prepare a cost-finding worksheet under the step-down method, and (2) prepare a cost-finding worksheet under the double-distribution method.

P23–1. Cart Hospital's trial balance of expenses and expense recoveries for the six months ended June 30, 19X2, is shown here:

	Ledger Balances		
	Salaries	Other	Total
Nursing services			
Administrative office	$ 10,000	$ 3,000	$ 13,000
Nursing units	200,000	20,000	220,000
Operating rooms	14,000	7,000	21,000
Emergency rooms	6,000	4,000	10,000
Central supply	12,000	10,000	22,000
Other professional services			
Laboratory	23,000	9,000	32,000
Radiology	26,000	11,000	37,000
Pharmacy	15,000	12,000	27,000
Outpatient clinic	8,000	5,000	13,000
Medical records	7,000	3,000	10,000
General services			
Dietary	51,000	44,000	95,000
Plant operation and maintenance	24,000	36,000	60,000
Housekeeping	25,000	9,000	34,000
Laundry	19,000	8,000	27,000
Fiscal and administrative services	79,000	15,000	94,000
Unassigned expenses			
Depreciation		60,000	60,000
Employee benefits		46,000	46,000
Expense recoveries			
Cafeteria sales		(24,000)	(24,000)
Medical record transcript fees		(3,000)	(3,000)
Purchase discounts		(2,000)	(2,000)
Totals	$519,000	$273,000	$792,000

Worksheet A adjustments:
1. The $220,000 of expenses in nursing units is to be reclassified:

	Salaries	Other	Total
Nursing units— adult and pediatric	$171,000	$ 17,000	$188,000
Newborn nursery	29,000	3,000	32,000
Total	$200,000	$ 20,000	$220,000

2. Medical record transcript fees are to be treated as a reduction of the direct expenses of the medical records department.
3. Purchase discounts are to be treated as a reduction of the direct expenses of fiscal and administrative services.

The necessary statistics for a cost-finding procedure are summarized in Figure 23–11.

Required: Complete a cost finding for Cart Hospital for the six months ended June 30, 19X2. This includes Worksheets A, B, and B-1, as illustrated in Figures 23–6, 23–7, and 23–8, respectively.

	Square Feet	Pounds of Laundry	Meals Served	Nursing Adm. Hours	Central Supply Priced Reg.	Pharmacy Priced Reg.	Medical Records
Fiscal and administrative services	900	—					
Plant operation and maintenance	3,500	400					
Housekeeping	300	400					
Laundry	1,600	—					
Dietary	4,400	2,200					
Nursing service—administrative office	200	500					
Central supply	1,800	62,00		9,500			
Pharmacy	600	400					
Medical records	400	300					
Cost of meals sold	—	—	20,000				
Operating rooms	3,000	67,000			$10,000	$ 3,000	
Laboratory	1,000	800		11,400		800	
Radiology	1,400	4,200				1,000	
Cost of drugs sold	—	—				22,000	
Nursing units—adult and pediatric	36,000	168,000	70,000	116,000	68,000	9,000	75%
Newborn nursery	2,400	24,000		6,000	1,000	600	10
Outpatient clinic	1,500	8,800		3,500	500	900	10
Emergency	1,000	15,000		5,000	2,500	2,700	5
Totals	60,000	354,000	90,000	151,400	$82,000	$40,000	100%

Figure 23–11 Cart Hospital Cost-Finding Statistics

P23–2. Oscar Hospital's trial balance of expenses and expense recoveries for the quarter ended March 31, 19X2, is shown here:

| | Ledger Balances | | |
	Salaries	Other	Total
Nursing services			
Administrative office	$ 12,000	$ 4,000	$ 16,000
Nursing units	250,000	48,000	298,000
Operating rooms	15,000	8,000	23,000
Emergency rooms	7,000	4,000	11,000
Central supply	14,000	8,000	22,000
Other professional services			
Laboratory	21,000	9,000	30,000
Radiology	25,000	10,000	35,000
Pharmacy	16,000	11,000	27,000
Outpatient clinic	9,000	5,000	14,000
Medical records	8,000	2,000	10,000
General services			
Dietary	49,000	38,000	87,000
Plant operation and			
maintenance	23,000	41,000	64,000
Housekeeping	22,000	8,000	30,000
Laundry	20,000	7,000	27,000
Fiscal and administrative			
services	55,000	16,000	71,000
Unassigned expenses			
Depreciation		51,000	51,000
Insurance on hospital			
building		12,000	12,000
Employee benefits		48,000	48,000
Expense recoveries			
Cafeteria sales		(26,000)	(26,000)
Telephone service		(3,000)	(3,000)
Purchase discounts		(4,000)	(4,000)
Totals	$546,000	$297,000	$843,000

The $298,000 of expenses accumulated in nursing units is to be reclassified on worksheet A as follows:

	Salaries	Other	Total
Nursing units—adult and pediatric	$218,000	$42,000	$260,000
Newborn nursery	32,000	6,000	38,000
Total	$250,000	$48,000	$298,000

The necessary statistics for a cost-finding procedure appear in Figure 23–12.

Required: Complete a cost finding for Oscar Hospital for the quarter ended March 31, 19X2. This includes worksheets A, B, and B-1, as illustrated in Figures 23–6, 23–7, and 23–8.

	Square Feet	Pounds of Laundry	Meals Served	Nursing Adm. Hours	Central Supply Priced Reg.	Pharmacy Priced Reg.	Medical Records
Fiscal and administrative services	1,000	100					
Plant operation and maintenance	3,600	500					
Housekeeping	400	500					
Laundry	1,500						
Dietary	4,500	3,000					
Nursing service—administrative office	300	500					
Central supply	1,800	60,000		8,600			
Pharmacy	600	500					
Medical records	400	400					
Cost of meals sold			25,000				
Operating rooms	3,000	62,000		12,000	$12,000	$ 4,000	
Laboratory	1,400	800				800	
Radiology	1,200	4,200				1,000	
Cost of drugs sold						23,000	
Nursing units—adult and pediatric	38,000	168,000	75,000	120,000	66,000	9,000	72%
Newborn nursery	2,800	24,000		6,000	1,000	600	12
Outpatient clinic	1,500	8,800		4,000	500	900	12
Emergency	1,000	12,700		9,400	5,500	5,700	4
Totals	63,000	346,000	100,000	160,000	$85,000	$45,000	100%

Figure 23–12 Oscar Hospital Cost-Finding Statistics

P23–3. Refer to the facts of Problem 23–2 and assume the following additional information:

	Gross Revenue	Units of Service	
Operating rooms	$ 48,000	520	Operations
Laboratory	72,000	11,400	Tests
Radiology	96,000	2,400	Films
Cost of drugs sold	30,000	7,200	Prescriptions
Nursing units—adult and pediatric	590,000	8,100	Patient days
Newborn nursery	36,000	1,000	Newborn days
Outpatient clinic	17,000	2,200	Visits
Emergency rooms	20,000	1,300	Admissions
Total	$909,000		

Deductions from revenues for the quarter ended March 31, 19X2, totaled $62,000.

Required: Prepare a cost report similar to that illustrated in Figure 23–12 for Oscar Hospital for the quarter ended March 31, 19X2.

Analysis and Interpretation of Financial Statements

The foregoing chapters of this book were concerned primarily with the fundamental mechanics of the accounting process and with the basic accounting concepts underlying the financial statements of the hospital enterprise. The discussion was directed mainly toward performing accounting operations and developing internal financial reports from the information generated by those operations. In this final chapter, the discussion is directed toward the analysis and interpretation of financial statements for the purpose of evaluating the hospital's financial position and operating results.

To introduce the subject of financial analysis and interpretation, let us briefly examine the Handy Hospital financial statements presented in Figures 24–1 and 24–2. Take a moment to study these statements, noticing the amounts (in thousands of dollars) reported

Gross patient service revenues	$14,517
Less deductions from revenues	1,742
Net patient service revenues	12,775
Other operating revenues	1,225
Total operating revenues	14,000
Less operating expenses:	
Nursing services	4,460
Other professional services	3,361
General services	2,263
Fiscal and administrative services	3,150
Total operating expenses	13,234
Operating income	766
Add nonoperating revenues	128
Net income for the year	$ 894

Figure 24–1 Handy Hospital Income Statement, Year Ended December 31, 19X5

Figure 24–2 Handy Hospital
Balance Sheet, December
31, 19X5

Current assets:	
Cash	$ 296
Temporary investments	110
Receivables (net)	2,450
Inventories	220
Prepaid expenses	24
Total current assets	3,100
Long-term investments	430
Plant and equipment (net)	6,370
Total assets	$9,900
Current liabilities:	
Notes payable	$ 50
Accounts payable	366
Accrued expense payable	651
Other	139
Total current liabilities	1,206
Long-term debt	1,800
Total liabilities	3,006
Unrestricted fund balance	6,894
Total liabilities and fund balance	$9,900

as revenues, expenses, assets, liabilities, and equity. On the basis of the information provided in these statements, what (if anything) can you conclude about Handy Hospital's 19X5 operating results and its financial position at December 31, 19X5? Are the operating results satisfactory? Is the hospital's financial position strong?

If you were a member of Handy Hospital's top management team, what would be your reaction to the reported 19X5 operating results? Are revenues too low? Are expenses too high? Note that the net income for 19X5 is $894,000. Is this "good" or "bad"? Is it exciting or disappointing? How can a hospital executive make judgments about the financial impact of operating results for 19X5?

Similarly, how would you evaluate the hospital's financial position? The balance sheet, for example, reports $2.45 million of receivables. Is this amount too large or about "right"? What does it tell you, if anything, about the quality of the hospital's credit and collection efforts? Also reported in the balance sheet are inventories totaling $220,000. What, if anything, does the balance sheet indicate about the quality of inventory management at Handy Hospital? Is the hospital overinvested in this asset, or are the inventories at a dangerously low level? As a final observation, note that the hospital has $3.006 million of liabilities. Do you regard this as an excessive amount of debt?

As these questions reveal, the accounting function does not end with the accumulation of economic data and the communication of that information in financial statements. Once the financial statements are developed, the information they contain should be analyzed and interpreted to answer the kinds of questions posed in the above paragraphs. The answers can be extremely useful to hospital management and external groups in evaluating a hospital's operations and financial status for decision-making purposes. Hospital accountants, either directly or indirectly, are closely involved in the decision-making process by providing relevant information and by assisting in its proper interpretation.

The Next Step: Analysis and Interpretation of Statements

In the analysis and interpretation of an item of financial information, one must have a basis of comparison. Consider, for example, the following item from Handy Hospital's December 31, 19X5, balance sheet:

Basic Analytical Techniques

Receivables (net)	$2,450

What does this mean? Is the amount too high, too low, or about what it "ought" to be? Standing alone, this bit of information is almost meaningless (except that perhaps we would all agree that $2.45 million is a large amount). There is no way to evaluate a single figure in isolation. It must be compared with, or measured against, something, usually another figure that provides a relevant and useful standard.

It would be helpful, for example, to compare the amount of December 31, 19X5, receivables with that of December 31, 19X4. Or we could compare the actual amount of receivables at December 31, 19X5, with the amount budgeted for that date. Another possibility would be to compare the amount of December 31, 19X5, receivables with the amount of total assets at December 31, 19X5. In addition, the December 31, 19X5, receivables might be compared with net patient service revenues for 19X5. Each of these comparisons would be relevant and useful in evaluating the level of receivables at the end of 19X5.

Such comparisons involve the use of three basic analytical techniques:

Common Accounting Comparison Yardsticks

- Horizontal analysis
- Vertical analysis
- Ratio analysis

This section illustrates each of these techniques.

Horizontal Analysis   *Horizontal analysis* consists of the comparison of two or more figures across a single line of a financial statement. The following is an example:

	19X5	19X4	Increase (Decrease) Amount	Percent
Net patient service revenues	$12,775	$12,045	$730	6.1%

In this analysis, we see that net patient service revenues in 19X5 were higher than in 19X4. The columns on the right indicate the dollar amount of the increase as well as the percentage increase. The

	19X5	19X4	Increase (Decrease) Amount	Percent
Gross patient service revenues	$14,517	$13,534	$ 983	7.3%
Less deductions from revenues	1,742	1,489	253	17.0
Net patient service revenues	12,775	12,045	730	6.1
Other operating revenues	1,225	955	270	28.3
Total operating revenues	14,000	13,000	1,000	7.7
Less operating expenses:				
Nursing services	4,460	4,269	191	4.5
Other professional services	3,361	3,167	194	6.1
General services	2,263	1,953	310	15.9
Fiscal and administrative services	3,150	3,129	21	.7
Total operating expenses	13,234	12,518	716	5.7
Operating income	766	482	284	58.9
Add nonoperating revenues	128	120	8	6.7
Net income for the year	$ 894	$ 602	$ 292	48.5

Figure 24–3 Handy Hospital Comparative Income Statements Horizontal Analysis, Years Ended December 31, 19X5 and 19X4

percentage increase (or decrease) is determined by dividing the dollar amount of change by the base-year figure (the earliest year in the comparison—19X4 in this example), that is, $730 ÷ $12,045 = 6.1 percent. Where the base-year figure is zero or a negative value, the dollar change cannot be expressed as a percentage.

Figures 24–3 and 24–4 illustrate the horizontal analysis technique applied to Handy Hospital's income statement and balance sheet. In each case, both dollar changes and percentage changes are provided to show the absolute as well as the relative changes. Although not illustrated here, a similar analysis could be made of the hospital's statements of changes in fund balances and statements of cash flows. Whatever the statement may be, the purpose of horizontal analysis is to direct the statement reader's attention to those items exhibiting the greatest absolute and relative changes compared to the prior year. Significant changes should be fully investigated and explained.

What Horizontal Analysis Reveals

| | December 31 | | Increase (Decrease) | |
	19X5	19X4	Amount	Percent
Current assets:				
Cash	$ 296	$ 230	$ 66	28.7%
Temporary investments	110	80	30	37.5
Receivables (net)	2,450	2,145	305	14.2
Inventories	220	234	(14)	(6.0)
Prepaid expenses	24	11	13	118.2
Total current assets	3,100	2,700	400	14.8
Long-term investments	430	390	40	10.3
Plant and equipment (net)	6,370	6,010	360	6.0
Total assets	$9,900	$9,100	$ 800	8.8
Current liabilities:				
Notes payable	$ 50	$ 200	$(150)	(75.0)
Accounts payable	366	431	(65)	(15.1)
Accrued expenses payable	651	545	106	19.5
Other	139	124	15	12.1
Total current liabilities	1,206	1,300	(94)	(7.2)
Long-term debt	1,800	1,800	-0-	—
Total liabilities	3,006	3,100	(94)	(3.0)
Unrestricted fund balance	6,894	6,000	894	14.9
Total liabilities and fund balance	$9,900	$9,100	$ 800	8.8

Figure 24–4 Handy Hospital Comparative Balance Sheets Horizontal Analysis, December 31, 19X5 and 19X4

	19X5	19X4	19X3	19X2	19X1
Amounts					
Gross patient service revenues	$14,517	$13,534	$11,630	$10,250	$8,440
Less deductions from revenues	1,742	1,489	1,245	996	738
Net patient service revenues	12,775	12,045	10,385	9,254	7,702
Other operating revenues	1,225	955	846	782	646
Total operating revenues	14,000	13,000	11,231	10,036	8,348
Less operating expenses:					
Nursing services	4,460	4,269	3,916	3,528	3,084
Other professional services	3,361	3,167	3,074	2,997	2,905
General services	2,263	1,953	1,788	1,433	937
Fiscal and administrative services	3,150	3,129	2,144	1,993	1,265
Total operating expenses	13,234	12,518	10,922	9,951	8,191
Operating income	766	482	309	85	157
Add nonoperating revenues	128	120	211	70	43
Net income for the year	$ 894	$ 602	$ 520	$ 155	$ 200
Trend Percentages					
Gross patient service revenues	172.0	160.4	137.8	121.4	100.0
Less deductions from revenues	236.0	201.8	168.7	135.0	100.0
Net patient service revenues	165.9	156.4	134.8	120.2	100.0
Other operating revenues	189.6	147.8	131.0	121.1	100.0
Total operating revenues	167.7	155.7	134.5	120.2	100.0
Less operating expenses:					
Nursing services	144.6	138.4	127.0	114.4	100.0
Other professional services	115.7	109.0	105.8	103.2	100.0
General services	241.5	208.4	190.8	152.9	100.0
Fiscal and administrative services	249.0	247.4	169.5	157.5	100.0
Total operating expenses	161.6	152.8	133.3	121.5	100.0
Operating income	487.9	307.0	196.8	54.1	100.0
Add nonoperating revenues	297.7	279.1	490.7	162.8	100.0
Net income for the year	447.0	301.0	260.0	77.5	100.0

Figure 24–5 Handy Hospital Trend Analysis of Income Statements 19X1–19X5

Uncovering Trends in the Data

When more than two years are included in horizontal analysis, trend percentages can be developed. Examine, for example, the illustration in Figure 24–5 of a trend analysis of Handy Hospital's condensed income statements for a five-year period. In this method of analysis, the figures in the base-year statement are considered to represent 100 percent. The base year in this example is 19X1. The corresponding figures of each succeeding year are expressed as percentages of the base-year figures.

	19X5		19X4	
	Amount	Percent	Amount	Percent
Gross patient service revenues				
Gross patient service revenues	$14,517	100.0%	$13,534	100.0%
Less deductions from revenues	1,742	12.0	1,489	11.0
Net patient service revenues	$12,775	88.0%	$12,045	89.0%
Net patient service revenues (above)	$12,775	91.3%	$12,045	92.7%
Other operating revenues	1,225	8.7	955	7.3
Total operating revenues	14,000	100.0	13,000	100.0
Less operating expenses:*				
Nursing services	4,460	31.8	4,269	32.8
Other professional services	3,361	24.0	3,167	24.4
General services	2,263	16.2	1,953	15.0
Fiscal and administrative services	3,150	22.5	3,129	24.1
Total operating expenses	13,234	94.5	12,518	96.3
Operating income	766	5.5	482	3.7
Add nonoperating revenues	128	0.9	120	0.9
Net income for the year	$ 894	6.4%	$ 602	4.6%
*Natural classification of expenses:				
Salaries and wages	$ 8,364	63.2%	$ 8,024	64.1%
Supplies	1,606	12.1	1,423	11.4
Purchased services	1,945	14.7	1,702	13.6
Depreciation	583	4.4	563	4.5
Interest	138	1.0	120	1.0
Other	598	4.6	686	5.4
Total operating expenses	$13,234	100.0%	$12,518	100.0%

Figure 24–6 Handy Hospital Comparative Income Statements Vertical Analysis, Years Ended December 31, 19X5 and 19X4

The net patient service revenues of 19X5 are 165.9 percent of 19X1 net patient service revenues ($12,775 ÷ $7,702 = 165.9 percent). Such percentages can be extremely useful in bringing out unusual relationships and trends that might go unnoticed in an examination of dollar amounts alone. The technique, of course, can also be applied to balance sheets and other financial statements.

Vertical Analysis

Vertical analysis involves the development of component percentages that express the relationships among related data within a particular statement. This procedure also is referred to as *common-size analysis.* Figures 24–6 and 24–7 illustrate the application of vertical analysis to Handy Hospital's income statement and balance sheet.

	December 31, 19X5		December 31, 19X4	
Cash	Amount	Percent	Amount	Percent
Current assets:				
Cash	$ 296	3.0%	$ 230	2.5%
Temporary investments	110	1.1	80	0.9
Receivables (net)	2,450	24.8	2,145	23.6
Inventories	220	2.2	234	2.6
Prepaid expenses	24	0.2	11	0.1
Total current assets	3,100	31.3	2,700	29.7
Long-term investments	430	4.3	390	4.3
Plant and equipment (net)	6,370	64.4	6,010	66.0
Total assets	$9,900	100.0%	$9,100	100.0%
Current liabilities:				
Notes payable	$ 50	0.5%	$ 200	2.2%
Accounts payable	366	3.7	431	4.7
Accrued expenses payable	651	6.6	545	6.0
Other	139	1.4	124	1.4
Total current liabilities	1,206	12.2	1,300	14.3
Long-term debt	1,800	18.2	1,800	19.8
Total liabilities	3,006	30.4	3,100	34.1
Unrestricted fund balance	6,894	69.6	6,000	65.9
Total liabilities and fund balance	$9,900	100.0%	$9,100	100.0%

Figure 24–7 Handy Hospital Comparative Balance Sheets Vertical Analysis, December 31, 19X5 and 19X4

Total Operating Revenue as Base Figure

In the vertical analysis of an income statement, total operating revenue usually is selected as the base figure for the computation of component percentages. All other figures (with the possible exception noted below) in the statement are expressed as percentages of this base figure. In Figure 24–6, for instance, the 19X5 base figure is $14,000 of total operating revenues, and each other figure in the 19X5 income statement is reported as a percentage of the $14,000 base figure. Similarly, in the 19X4 income statement, the $13,000 of total operating revenue serves as the base figure. All figures in the 19X4 income statement (with the possible exception noted shortly) are expressed as a percentage of this $13,000 base figure.

As can be seen at the top of the income statement in Figure 24–6, deductions from gross patient service revenues may be presented as a percentage of gross patient service revenues (rather than of total operating revenues). Otherwise, the component percentage would be distorted to the extent of other operating revenues to which the deductions are not related. In other words, although

19X5 deductions are 12.4 percent of total operating revenues ($1,742 ÷ $14,000), it is perhaps more meaningful to say that revenue deductions are 12 percent of gross patient service revenues ($1,742 ÷ $14,517), or 12 cents of each dollar of services rendered to patients.

Notice also in Figure 24–6 that operating expenses are reported both in a functional and in a natural (or object of expenditure) classification. In their external reports particularly, hospitals often present operating expenses in a natural classification because that form of classification is better understood by the general public. The percentages indicated for the natural classification in Figure 24–6 are based on total operating expenses simply to illustrate the use of an acceptable alternative base figure.

Natural Classifications for Operating Expenses

Vertical analysis can be quite useful in appraising the various components of the income statement. In Figure 24–6, for example, we see that nursing service expenses increased from $4,269 in 19X4 to $4,460 in 19X5. But we also see that nursing service expenses, as a percentage of total operating revenues, decreased from 32.8 percent in 19X4 to 31.8 percent in 19X5. On the other hand, general services expenses increased both absolutely and in relation to total operating revenues. Observations such as these give perspective to the evaluation of financial statement figures and tend to pinpoint areas for further investigation.

What Vertical Analysis Reveals

The results of vertical analysis can be viewed in another way. In Figure 24–6, the 19X5 operating expenses may be appraised in terms of "cents per dollar of operating revenue." In other words, of each $1 of operating revenue, 31.8 cents went for nursing services, 24.0 cents was expended for other professional services, 16.2 cents was employed for general services, and 22.5 cents was taken by fiscal and administrative services. Thus, out of each dollar of 19X5 operating revenues, Handy Hospital was able to "bring down" only 5.5 cents into operating income.

In the Handy Hospital balance sheets illustrated in Figure 24–7, the base figure for asset analysis is total assets, and all other asset figures in the statements are expressed as percentages of total assets. The December 31, 19X5, cash balance of $296, for example, is 3.0 percent of total assets ($296 ÷ $9,900).

Total Assets as Base Figure

The base figure for the analysis of liabilities and fund balance is their total (the same as total assets), and each component item is converted to a percentage of that base. It can be said, for example, that December 31, 19X5, accounts payable composes 3.7 percent of total assets (or of total liabilities and fund balance). This type of analysis is helpful in evaluating the balance sheet in terms of man-

Figure 24–8 Handy Hospital
Component Percentage Analysis
of Current Assets, December 31,
19X5 and 19X4

	December 31, 19X5		December 31, 19X4	
Cash	Amount	Percent	Amount	Percent
Cash	$ 296	9.5%	$ 230	8.5%
Temporary investments	110	3.5	80	3.0
Receivables (net)	2,450	79.0	2,145	79.4
Inventories	220	7.1	234	8.7
Prepaid expenses	24	0.9	11	0.4
Total current assets	$3,100	100.0%	$2,700	100.0%

agement's allocation of resources and in terms of the sources from which the assets have been financed.

For certain analytical purposes, however, it may be more useful to develop component percentages for current assets, using total current assets as the 100 percent figure. This is illustrated in Figure 24–8, where it can be seen, for example, that the cash balance is 9.5 percent of total current assets at December 31, 19X5. Similar analyses could be made, of course, of current liabilities or total liabilities.

Regardless of whether the horizontal or vertical analytical method is used for comparing items on the financial statement, these methods merely serve as tools to assist in determining where problems may exist and where a more thorough examination of underlying financial data may be desirable. The key question is why unusual relationships appear between various amounts in the financial statements. Later on in this chapter, techniques for finding the answers to such questions will be described.

Ratio Analysis

A ratio is the quotient that results when one number is divided by another. It is one number expressed in terms of another; the ratio expresses the quantitative relationship between two numbers. A ratio may be stated as a common fraction, decimally, or in percentage form. If, for example, we divided Handy Hospital's December 31, 19X5, current assets of $3,100 by its December 31, 19X5, current liabilities of $1,206, we obtain a ratio known as the *current ratio*. This ratio may be expressed as 3100 ÷ 1206, as 2.57, or as 257 percent. It may be said, then, that the current ratio is 257 percent or 2.57 to 1, or that the hospital has $2.57 of current assets for each dollar of current liabilities.

Uses of Ratios

Ratios are used in financial analysis to expedite comparisons and make relationships more understandable. Many different ratios can be computed from the data in financial statements. One does

Preparing Component Percentages for Current Assets

not, however, compute all possible ratios. Many, such as the ratio of prepaid expenses to nonoperating revenues, would be totally meaningless for analytical purposes. We must select those ratios that have significance and relevance for the purpose of the analysis. Our discussion here is directed toward the selection, computation, and interpretation of a number of ratios commonly employed in hospital financial analysis.

The management of a hospital is charged with the task of maintaining a satisfactory relationship between revenues and expenses. Opinions differ as to precisely what this relationship should be. Some have argued that a nonproprietary hospital's financial operating objective should be to break even, that is, to maintain an equality between revenues and expenses. Given the pressures of demand for more and better services, advancing technology, inflation, inadequate reimbursement systems, and other socioeconomic forces, however, others (including this writer) are convinced that a reasonable "profit" objective is both necessary and justifiable. In view of current and emerging conditions in the hospital industry, a "no-profit" fiscal objective seems totally unrealistic if the individual hospital is to avoid the erosion of its real capital and its ability to continue to provide the volume and quality of services desired by the community it serves.

Because a profit should be regarded as necessary and desirable for a particular hospital, a judgment must be made about what that profit should be. A hospital management is likely to have in mind an absolute dollar amount of profit as a financial operating objective. This amount is determined to be the figure required to produce the cash flow needed to meet specific financial requirements, such as the payment of bond interest charges, the retirement of long-term debt, the acquisition of new plant assets, the development of new healthcare programs, and the generation of additional necessary working capital. In addition, a percentage relationship between operating income and operating revenues or between operating income and total assets, for example, could be established as a goal or standard against which actual operating results might be measured. For this purpose, the ratios described here are managerially useful.

Operating Income Ratio. One frequently used measure of profitability is the *operating income ratio,* sometimes called the

Analysis of Operating Results

Evaluation of Profitability

profit margin. A computation of this ratio for Handy Hospital follows:

	19X5	19X4
1. Operating income	$ 766	$ 482
2. Total operating revenues	14,000	13,000
3. Operating income ratio (1 divided by 2)	5.47%	3.71%

Thus, in terms of the ratio of operating income to operating revenues, Handy Hospital was more profitable in 19X5 than in 19X4. In 19X5, the hospital was able to earn an operating income that was 5.47 percent of operating revenues; in 19X4, the operating income ratio was only 3.71 percent. To put it another way, Handy Hospital's 19X5 operating income was about 5.5 cents per dollar of operating revenues; the 19X4 operating income was only 3.7 cents per dollar of operating revenues. This improved operating performance may be attributable to such factors as an increase in service rates, better management of operating expenses, an increased volume of service, and a more favorable service mix (in other words, relatively greater use of those patient services that generate revenues in excess of costs). Whatever the reasons for the improved ratio, they should be identified and evaluated by the hospital's management.

Looking at the Operating Expense Ratio

Emphasis sometimes is given to the *operating expense ratio,* the mathematical complement of the operating income ratio. If the operating income ratio is 5.5 percent, for example, the operating expense ratio must be 94.5 percent; that is, operating expenses consume 94.5 cents of each dollar of operating revenue. Naturally, the lower the operating expense ratio, the greater the operating income ratio.

Return on Investment. A weakness of the operating income ratio as a measure of profitability is that it does not take into account the amount of resources invested in the hospital enterprise. Consider, for example, an investor-owned hospital having a 19X5 operating income of $100,000 and an operating income ratio of 10 percent that, by most standards, would indicate a high degree of profitability. Suppose, however, that the investor-owned hospital's average owners' equity and average total assets were $5 million and $10 million respectively, during 19X5. The rate of return (profit) on the owners' investment, then, is only 2 percent ($100,000 ÷ $5 million), and the rate of return on average total assets is only 1 percent ($100,000 ÷ $10 million).

In most types of business enterprises, such rates of return would be regarded as grossly inadequate to satisfy creditors, pay reasonable dividends to stockholders, attract new investment capital, obtain new long-term debt, or even justify a continuation of the business. Thus, the best and most useful indicator of profitability is the rate of return on the amount of assets invested and employed in an enterprise.

The rates of return on Handy Hospital's average equity and average total assets for 19X5 are computed as follows:

Computing the Rates of Return

1. Net income for the year	$ 894
2. Average equity [($6,000 + $6,894) ÷ 2]	6,447
3. Average total assets [($9,100 + $9,900) ÷ 2]	9,500
4. Rate of return on equity (1 divided by 2)	13.9%
5. Rate of return on total assets (1 divided by 3)	9.4%

In other words, Handy Hospital earned a 19X5 net income that was about 14 cents per dollar of equity and 9.4 cents per dollar of assets. These rates of return probably would be regarded as quite satisfactory by a majority of profit-seeking businesses.

Although Handy Hospital is a not-for-profit corporation, these ratios are not at all without significance or managerial usefulness. Although there are no stockholder-owners interested in cash dividends and appreciation in the value of their stock holdings, Handy Hospital does have constituents: the people of the community it serves. These people presumably are interested in the continuation of the hospital as a financially sound and efficient provider of healthcare services. The hospital's employees are interested in adequate compensation. Banks, hospital bondholders, and other creditors are concerned with the hospital's ability to meet its financial obligations. Management must find the means to finance the acquisition of expensive equipment demanded by an advancing medical technology. If philanthropy and government subsidies can be ruled out as important sources of new capital funds, the future of the voluntary not-for-profit hospital is likely to be dependent on the earning and reinvestment of adequate amounts of profit. It is for this reason that the rate-of-return concept cannot be ignored by the management of any hospital enterprise.

Significance of the Rate of Return

Times Interest Earned. A profitability ratio of particular concern to current and potential investors in hospital bond issues is the times interest earned ratio. The computation of the ratio for Handy Hospital is as follows:

	19X5	19X4
1. Net income for the year[1]	$ 894	$602
2. Bond interest expense (assumed)	108	108
3. Total (1 + 2)	1,002	710
4. Times interest earned (3 divided by 2)	9.3	6.6

Thus, the hospital earned its bond interest charges 9.3 times in 19X5 and 6.6 times in 19X4. This is an indicator of the ability of the hospital to pay the annual interest charges on its outstanding bonds. The higher the ratio, the more favorably will investors regard the hospital's bonds as investment opportunities.

Internal Analysis of Revenues and Expenses

In addition to the ratios just explained that may be used by groups external to the hospital as well as by management, certain other analytical techniques can be applied by management to evaluate various revenue and expense items. The discussion here will be limited to actual versus budget comparisons and variance analysis.

Analysis of Revenues. Assume that Handy Hospital's 19X5 patient service revenues of $14.517 million include $487,275 of daily patient service (routine service) revenues earned in a 20-bed nursing unit referred to as "Three South." The 19X5 revenue budget for this unit was $439,600. A management report may present these facts as follows:

			Variance	
	Actual	Budget	Amount	Percent
Daily patient service revenues:				
Three South	$487,275	$439,600	$47,675	10.8%

[1]Operating income may be used instead of net income.

As can be seen, the revenues of this nursing unit were $47,675, or 10.8 percent, in excess of budgeted revenues. The management question is, why? What were the factors that caused this favorable revenue variance? How much of the variance is attributable to each factor?

To answer these questions, let us assume that 6,280 patients days of service were budgeted and that actual patient days in this unit were 6,497. Knowledge of the statistical units of service permits the following computation of actual and budgeted average revenue per patient day:

	Actual	Budget
1. Revenues	$487,275	$439,600
2. Patient days	6,497	6,280
3. Average revenue per day (1 divided by 2)	75	70

Assuming this nursing unit offers private accommodations only, it is clear that service rates were increased during the year. So, we become aware that the budget variance is due to two factors: (1) an increase in service rates and (2) a higher volume of service than budgeted. The dollar amount of revenues attributable to each of these factors is computed in Figure 24-9. A similar analysis could be made, of course, in a comparison of 19X5 actual with 19X4 actual.

Factors Causing the Budget Variance

Analysis of Expenses. Assume that Handy Hospital's 19X5 general services expenses of $2,263,000 includes $484,106 of dietary department expense. The 19X5 expense budget for the dietary department was $492,750. A management report may present these facts as follows:

			Variance	
	Actual	Budget	Amount	Percent
Operating expenses:				
Dietary department	$484,106	$492,750	$8,644	1.75%

Thus, dietary department expenses for 19X5 are seen to be $8,644, or 1.75 percent, less than was budgeted. Why? What were the

Budget Volume Variance:		
Patient days of service		
19X5 actual	6,497	
19X5 budget	6,280	
Excess of actual days over budgeted days	217	
Budgeted revenue per patient day	× $70	
Budget volume variance (favorable)		$15,190
Budget Rate Variance:		
Average revenue per patient day		
19X5 actual	$ 75	
19X5 budget	70	
Excess of actual average revenue over budgeted		
average revenue	$ 5	
Actual patient days for 19X5	×6,497	
Budget rate variance (favorable)		32,485
Total budget variance (favorable)		$47,675

factors that caused this favorable budget variance? How much of
the variance is attributable to each factor?

The statistical unit of service for this department is a served
meal. So, let us assume that 328,500 served meals were budgeted
and that the actual number of meals served during the year was
336,185. This information permits the following computation of
the actual and budgeted average cost per meal served:

	Actual	Budgeted
1. Total expense	$484,106	$492,750
2. Number of meals served	336,185	328,500
3. Average cost per meal served (1 divided by 2)	$1.44	$1.50

Offsetting Volume with
Lower Cost per Meal

Now we can see that, although the volume of service was
7,685 meals higher than was budgeted (336,185 − 328,500), the
average cost per meal was six cents less than budgeted ($1.50 −
$1.44). The effects of these factors on 19X5 dietary department
expenses are shown in Figure 24–10. Note that the unfavorable
effect of a higher-than-budgeted volume was more than offset by
the favorable effect of the lower-than-budgeted cost per meal.

Budget Cost Variance:		
Average cost per meal		
19X5 budget	$ 1.50	
19X5 actual	1.44	
Excess of budgeted cost over actual cost	$ 0.06	
Actual number of meals served	×336,185	
Budget cost variance (favorable)		$ 20,171
Budget Volume Variance:		
Number of meals served		
19X5 actual		336,185
19X5 budget		328,500
Excess of actual over budget	7,685	
Budgeted cost per meal served	× $1.50	
Budget volume variance (unfavorable)		(11,527)
Net budget variance (favorable)		$ 8,644

Figure 24–10 Handy Hospital Analysis of Budget Variance Dietary Department Expenses, Year Ended December 31, 19X5

Analysis of Financial Position

While operating results and financial position are treated separately here, both are important considerations, regardless of one's point of view. The information in the balance sheet cannot be ignored when appraising operating results; neither should the income statement be bypassed entirely in evaluating the financial strength of a hospital. Careful attention also should be given the data provided in statements of changes in fund balances and in statements of cash flows.

Evaluation of Current Financial Position

The current financial strength of a hospital is a matter of great importance not only to its management but also to various external groups. If the hospital is to be able to repay bank loans and meet its short-term obligations to other creditors, it must maintain a sound current financial position. The hospital must have an adequate amount of working capital; it must maintain a satisfactory degree of liquidity; and it must not overinvest in receivables or inventories. Some of the ratios usually applied to obtain insights into the presence or absence of these desired conditions are presented here, using the financial statements of Handy Hospital as a basis for illustration.

Current Ratio. One of the most widely used measures of current financial strength is the current ratio that indicates the number of dollars of current assets per dollar of current liabilities. It shows the number of times the current assets will "pay off" the current debts of the hospital. Following is a computation of Handy Hospital's current ratio:

	December 31	
	19X5	19X4
1. Current assets	$3,100	$2,700
2. Current liabilities	1,206	1,300
3. Current ratio (1 divided by 2)	2.57	2.08

Thus, in terms of the current ratio, Handy Hospital's current debt paying ability appears somewhat stronger at the end of 19X5 than at the end of 19X4. There is, however, no one value for the current ratio that is applicable to, or desirable for, all hospitals. What may be an adequate current ratio for one hospital may be dangerously low for another. It also is worth noting that although a particular current ratio may be satisfactory at the end of one year, it may not be satisfactory for the same hospital at the end of the next year.

Quick Ratio. A weakness of the current ratio is that it does not take into account the composition of either current assets or current liabilities. The quick ratio (sometimes called the "acid test") is a more valid test of current debt-paying ability than the current ratio in that it gives some consideration to the composition of the hospital's current assets. The computation is as follows:

	December 31	
	19X5	19X4
1. Cash	$ 296	$ 230
2. Temporary investments	110	80
3. Receivables (net)	2,450	2,145
4. Quick assets (1 + 2 + 3)	2,856	2,455
5. Current liabilities	1,206	1,300
6. Quick ratio (4 divided by 5)	2.37	1.89

Difference Between Quick Ratio and Current Ratio

The basic difference between the quick ratio and the current ratio is simply that the computation of the quick ratio excludes inventories and prepaid expense items. An extreme modification of the quick ratio is the division of cash, or the total of cash and temporary investments, by current liabilities.

Current Asset Turnover. The current asset turnover is said to be an indicator of how "hard" the management of the hospital "works" the current assets—that is, the intensity of current assets usage. Handy Hospital's turnovers for 19X5 and 19X4 are computed as follows:

	19X5	19X4
1. Total operating revenues	$14,000	$13,000
2. Current assets, December 31	3,100	2,700
3. Current asset turnover (1 divided by 2)	4.52	4.81

Some analysts make the computation using total operating expenses rather than revenues as the numerator; others prefer to use working capital (current assets minus current liabilities) as the denominator (that is, a working capital turnover). In any event, a high turnover generally is indicative of efficient and productive employment of current resources.

What the Turnover Indicates

Analysis of Receivables. The amount of receivables from patient services in a hospital's balance sheet should not exceed a reasonable proportion of the charges made to patients' accounts during the same period of time. This relationship may be illuminated by computation of the accounts receivable turnover:

	19X5	19X4
1. Net patient service revenues[2]	$12,775	$12,045
2. Average receivables (net)[3]	2,298	1,983
3. Receivables turnover (1 divided by 2)	5.56	6.07

This ratio indicates roughly the number of times during the year the receivables from patients were "turned over," or collected. An increase in the turnover generally may be regarded as favorable with respect to the effectiveness of the credit and collection functions.

What Ratio Reveals About Collections

A more widely used ratio employed by hospitals in the analysis of accounts receivable involves the number of days' charges uncol-

---

[2]Excluding revenues from services rendered on a cash basis and not recorded through accounts receivable.

[3]January 1 receivables from patients plus December 31 receivables from patients, divided by 2.

lected and in receivables. This ratio is computed for Handy Hospital as follows:

	19X5	19X4
1. Net patient service revenues	$12,775	$12,045
2. Average daily charges (line 1 divided by 365 days)	35	33
3. Receivables (net), December 31	2,450	2,145
4. Number of days' charges uncollected (3 divided by 2)	70	65

One may tentatively conclude that on the average, the quality of receivables management may have declined somewhat between 19X4 and 19X5. Yet it must be recognized that this ratio is an average; some patients' accounts may be 200 days old and others may be only a few days old. It also is extremely informative to compute by major categories of patients and third-party payers (where the necessary information is available) both the receivables turnover and the number of days' charges uncollected.

Analysis of Inventories.   As is true of receivables, a hospital can have an excessive investment in inventories. A reasonable relationship should be maintained between inventories and total current assets. In addition, the relationship between inventories and total cost of supplies used may be computed as the inventory turnover:

	19X5	19X4
1. Total cost of supplies used	$1,606	$1,423
2. Average inventories[4]	227	209
3. Inventory turnover (1 divided by 2)	7.07	6.81

What Inventory Turnover Reveals

The fact that Handy Hospital "turned over" its inventories a greater number of times in 19X5 than in 19X4 generally is a favorable indication about the quality of inventory management.

In addition to inventory turnover, the average number of days' supply in inventories may be calculated as follows:

[4]January 1 inventories plus December 31 inventories, divided by 2.

	19X5	19X4
1. Total cost of supplies used	$1,606	$1,423
2. Average daily usage (line 1 divided by 365 days)	4.4	3.9
3. Inventories, December 31	220	234
4. Number of days' supply in inventories (3 divided by 2)	50	60

In evaluating inventories, it must be understood that a hospital can be understocked as well as overstocked. Either extreme is undesirable. Note also that, where the information is available, both the inventory turnover and the number of days' supply should be computed by major categories of inventory to take into account the differing characteristics of various types of supplies.

Many external users of hospital financial statements are interested in the hospital's long-run financial strength as well as in its current financial position. Hospital bondholders and mortgagees, for example, are concerned not only with the ability of the hospital to pay current interest charges but also with the long-run safety of their investments. An intelligent appraisal of a hospital's long-term financial position is also essential to sound long-term financing decisions and long-range planning on either an individual-hospital or an area-wide basis. Such an analysis is helpful as well in evaluating the consequences of long-term commitment decisions (bond issues and plant asset acquisitions, for example) that have previously been made and implemented.

Evaluation of Long-Term Financial Position

In studying a hospital's long-run financial position, an analysis is usually made of (1) changes in the absolute and relative amounts invested by the hospital in the various categories of assets and (2) changes in the absolute and relative amounts of the sources (debt and equity) of its assets. This analysis may take the form of a 5- or 10-year study of the hospital's common-size balance sheets and statements of changes in financial position. Particular attention is given to detecting substantial shifts in the allocation of resources between the current and noncurrent classifications.

A study of the hospital's asset structure should also include an examination of assets held in the restricted funds. This is particularly true with respect to the plant replacement and expansion fund, where material amounts might be available for the financing of

Plant Replacement and Expansion Fund

future construction and equipment needs. Should the hospital have term endowments, their amounts and termination dates should also be considered in evaluating the hospital's long-run financial strength.

An appraisal of a hospital's long-run financial position must necessarily include the detection and investigation of substantial shifts noted in the capital structure, that is, the relative amounts of debt and equity. For this purpose, debt ratios and equity ratios may be computed as shown here:

		December 31	
		19X5	19X4
1.	Total liabilities	$3,006	$3,100
2.	Hospital equity	6,894	6,000
3.	Total liabilities and equity (assets)	9,900	9,100
4.	Debt ratio (1 divided by 3)	30.4%	34.1%
5.	Equity ratio (2 divided by 3)	69.6%	65.9%

At the end of 19X5, we see that 30.4 percent of Handy Hospital's assets were financed by debt and 69.6 percent through equity. This position is more conservative (less risky) than that which existed at the end of 19X4, when a somewhat greater percentage of the assets was being supplied by creditors.

Debt/Equity Ratio

In some cases, the above ratios are combined into a single debt/equity ratio (total liabilities divided by total equity). The debt/equity ratio at the end of 19X5, for example, is 43.6 percent ($3,006 ÷ $6,894), meaning that the hospital has about 44 cents of debt for each dollar of equity.

The hospital's asset and capital structure as reflected in its balance sheet should always be viewed in conjunction with its statement of cash flows. This statement should preferably be presented in comparative form covering several prior periods so that trends in the sources and uses of cash resources may be clearly discerned. This permits an appraisal of the effectiveness of management's past operating, investing, and financing policies in bringing the hospital to its present financial position.

Above all, it must be recognized by all external groups that a successful hospital seldom remains the same. It either changes and grows, or it stagnates and declines. It moves in new directions, developing new programs and services in response to changes in demand and improved technology. This requires adequate financing, satisfactory operating results, and a sound financial position.

Questions

Q24-1. What are "common-size" financial statements?

Q24-2. Niceplace Hospital's nursing service expenses were $957,400 in 19X2 and $898,300 in 19X1. Prepare a horizontal analysis of the Niceplace Hospital data.

[handwritten margin: 19X2 19X1 amt % 957,400 898,300 59,100 6.6%]

Q24-3. What is meant by a vertical analysis of the balance sheet? The income statement?

Q24-4. "A hospital with a current ratio of 4 to 1 has greater current financial strength than does a hospital with a current ratio of only 2 to 1." Do you agree? Explain.

[handwritten margin: Look at comp position no]

Q24-5. State how each of the following is computed and explain what might be indicated by the results of the computation:
 a. Operating income ratio.
 b. Operating expense ratio.
 c. Return on investment.
 d. Times interest earned.

Q24-6. State how each of the following is computed and explain what might be indicated by the results of the computation:
 a. Current ratio.
 b. Quick ratio.
 c. Current asset turnover.

Q24-7. State how each of the following is computed and explain what might be indicated by the results of the computation:
 a. Accounts receivable turnover.
 b. Number of days' charges uncollected.
 c. Ratio of accounts receivable to total current assets.

Q24-8. State how each of the following is computed and explain what might be indicated by the results of the computation:
 a. Inventory turnover.
 b. Average number of days' supply in inventories.
 c. Ratio of inventory to total current assets.

Q24-9. How is the debt/equity ratio computed? Explain what might be indicated by the results of the computation.

Exercises

E24-1. Fineplace Hospital provides you with the following information:

Handwritten notes:

10,000 unfav
average rev
8400
80.00

4375 - Actual
4500 - Budget
Exces 125
x80
Exes 4.00
x 4.375
17,500
Total $7,500
favorable

Budget 500
Ac 550
Exes 0.50
#Zexp x 114,200
unfavorly 57,100

Bud 100,000
Act 114,200
Ex 14,200
Bud x 5.00
71,000
unfav 128,100

current will decrease
quick is undesirable
WKaip's unchanged

Current A 432,000 - 294,000 = 138,000
C/lay 92,000 (138,000 ÷ 1.5)
equit is 340,000 (432,000 - 92,000)
Tot LD 80% of Hos equit

A - L = HE
432,000 - 0.8 HE = HE
1.8 HE = 432,000
HE = $240,000

	Actual	Budget
Daily patient service revenues	$367,500	$360,000
Patient days of service	4,375	4,500

Required: Prepare an analysis of the budget variance in the manner illustrated in Figure 24–9.

E24–2. Highplace Hospital provides you with the following information:

	Actual	Budget
Laboratory expense	$628,100	$500,000
Number of examinations	114,200	100,000

Required: Prepare an analysis of the budget variance in the manner illustrated in Figure 24–10.

E24–3. Goodplace Hospital has a current ratio of 2 to 1 on June 30, 19X1. On July 1, 19X1, the hospital obtains a $150,000 short-term loan from a local bank.

Required: What is the effect of the loan on the current ratio, quick ratio, and working capital?

E24–4. The 12/31/X1 balance sheet of Goodwork Hospital follows. These are the only accounts in Goodwork's balance sheet. Amounts indicated by a question mark (?) can be calculated from the information given.

Cash	$ 25,000
Receivables (net)	?
Inventory	?
Plant assets (net)	294,000
	$432,000
Accounts payable	$?
Other current payables	25,000
Long-term debt	?
Hospital equity	?
	$432,000

The following additional information is available:

Current ratio	1.5 to 1
Total liabilities divided by hospital equity	0.8
Inventory turnover based on cost of supplies used and ending inventory	15 times

Required: What was Goodwork Hospital's long-term debt as of 12/31/X1?

E24–5. Verygood Hospital collected a $3,000 account receivable that had previously been written off as a bad debt against the allowance for uncollectible accounts.

Required: Compare the current ratio before this collection (X) with the current ratio after this collection (Y):
a. X greater than Y.
b. X equals Y.
c. X less than Y.
d. The answer cannot be determined from the information given.

E24–6. Getwell Hospital has a current ratio of 3 to 1. An account payable recorded last month is paid this month.

Required: What is the effect of this payment on the current ratio and working capital, respectively?
a. Rise and decline.
b. Rise and no effect.
c. Decline and no effect.
d. No effect on either.

E24–7. Gotwell Hospital has a current ratio of 4 to 1. A transaction reduces the current ratio.

Required: Compare the working capital before this transaction (X) and the working capital after this transaction (Y).
a. X greater than Y.
b. X equals Y.
c. X less than Y.
d. The answer cannot be determined from the information given.

Problems

P24–1. Greatplace Hospital provides you with the following financial statements for 19X2 and 19X1:

	December 31	
	19X2	19X1
Cash	$ 240	$ 120
Temporary investments	210	180
Receivables (net)	1,400	1,150
Inventories	300	370
Prepaid expenses	50	80
Total current assets	2,200	1,900

Plant assets (net)	$5,800	$5,100
Total	$8,000	$7,000
Current liabilities	$ 740	$ 475
Long-term debt	3,530	3,205
Fund balance	3,730	3,320
Total	$8,000	$7,000

	Year Ended 12/31	
	19X2	19X1
Gross patient service revenues	$6,600	$6,000
Deductions from revenues	790	500
Net patient service revenues	5,810	5,500
Other operating revenues	700	500
Total operating revenues	6,510	6,000
Less operating expenses:		
Nursing services	2,100	1,900
Other professional services	1,600	1,500
General services	1,300	1,100
Fiscal and administrative services	1,100	1,400
Total operating expenses	6,100	5,900
Net income for the year	$ 410	$ 100

Operating expenses include the $900 cost of supplies used, $400 of depreciation, and $240 of bond interest expense.

Required: (1) Develop a horizontal analysis of these statements. (2) Convert the above financial statements to common size. (3) Prepare a ratio analysis of 19X2 operating results. (4) Prepare a ratio analysis of the December 31, 19X2, financial position.

P24–2. Careplace Hospital supplies you with the following information relating to the 19X1 operations of its radiology department:

	Actual	Budget
Revenues	$966,400	$930,000
Expenses	393,600	372,000
Number of examinations	60,400	62,000

Required: Prepare an analysis of the budget variances for the radiology department's revenues and expenses for 19X1.

P24–3. Wellplace Hospital provides you with the following financial statements for 19X2 and 19X1:

	December 31	
	19X2	19X1
Cash	$ 168	$ 211
Temporary investments	126	34
Receivables—patients (net)	969	854
Other receivables	42	39
Inventories	296	315
Prepaid expenses	25	29
Total current assets	1,626	1,482
Long-term investments	466	442
Plant assets (net)	8,126	8,185
Other assets	167	88
Total	$10,385	$10,197
Current portion of long-term debt	$ 180	$ 180
Notes payable	125	75
Accounts payable	196	202
Accrued expenses payable	238	217
Payroll taxes withheld	81	63
Advances from third-party payers	75	55
Other	42	29
Total current liabilities	937	821
Long-term debt	1,718	1,865
Total liabilities	2,655	2,686
Fund balance	7,730	7,511
Total	$10,385	$10,197

	Year Ended 12/31	
	19X2	19X1
Gross patient service revenues	$ 8,830	$ 7,326
Deductions from patient service revenues	1,430	1,465
Net patient services revenues	7,400	5,861
Other operating revenues	505	407
Total operating revenues	7,905	6,268
Less operating expenses:		
Nursing services	2,560	2,197
Other professional services	2,050	1,615
General services	1,350	1,033

Fiscal and administrative services	$ 1,925	$ 1,614
Total operating expenses	7,885	6,459
Net operating income (loss)	20	(191)
Nonoperating revenues	224	176
Net income (loss) for the year	$ 244	$ (15)

The operating expenses include $520 of depreciation, $110 of interest expense, and $790 of supplies used.

Required: (1) Develop a horizontal analysis of these statements. (2) Convert the above financial statements to common size. (3) Prepare a ratio analysis of 19X2 operating results. (4) Prepare a ratio analysis of the 12/31/X2 financial position.

P24–4. Starplace Hospital provides you with the following information:

	December 31	
	19X2	19X1
Cash	$ 50,000	$ 35,000
Temporary investments	80,000	50,000
Receivables (net)	140,000	110,000
Inventories	35,000	28,000
Prepaid expenses	12,000	16,000
Long-term investments	230,000	190,000
Plant assets (net)	420,000	421,000
	$967,000	$850,000
Notes payable	$ 75,000	$ 25,000
Accounts payable	21,000	19,000
Accrued expenses payable	33,000	28,000
Other current liabilities	7,000	22,000
Long-term debt	500,000	450,000
Fund balance	331,000	306,000
	$967,000	$850,000

	Year Ended 12/31	
	19X2	19X1
Total operating revenues	$840,000	$780,000
Cost of supplies used	210,000	186,000
Depreciation expense	90,000	90,000
Bond interest expense	30,000	27,000
Net patient service revenues	960,000	890,000
Net income	25,000	16,000

Required: (1) Prepare a ratio analysis of operating results for 19X2. (2) Prepare a ratio analysis of the hospital's financial position at December 31, 19X2.

P24–5. Rightplace Hospital supplies you with the following information relating to the 19X1 operations of one of its nursing units:

	Actual	Budget
Revenues	$753,300	$750,000
Expenses	502,200	500,000
Patient days of service	9,300	10,000

Required: Prepare an analysis of the budget variances for revenues and expenses for 19X1.

Glossary

This glossary includes selected general accounting terms and certain special terms encountered in hospital financial management. Many of the definitions provided are adapted from a variety of sources, including the following:

Berman, Howard J., and Weeks, Lewis E., *The Financial Management of Hospitals*. Ann Arbor, Michigan: Health Administration Press, School of Public Health, The University of Michigan, 1979.

Chart of Accounts for Hospitals. Chicago: American Hospital Association, 1976.

Kohler, Eric L. *A Dictionary for Accountants.* Englewood Cliffs, N.J.: Prentice-Hall, Inc., 1983.

Accounting Standards—Original Pronouncements. Financial Accounting Standards Board, Stamford, Connecticut, 1989.

Audits of Providers of Health Care Services. New York: American Institute of Certified Public Accountants, 1990.

Hospital Statistics. Chicago: American Hospital Association, 1988.

A

Accelerated depreciation. Depreciation by a method such as sum-of-years'-digits or double-declining balance, which results in the writeoff of the cost of a depreciable asset at a more rapid rate than would occur by the straight-line method.

Accounting. The accumulation and communication of historical and projected economic data relating to the financial position of an enterprise and the results of its operations, including interpretation of the results thereof for decision-making purposes of internal management as well as groups external to the enterprise.

Accounting cycle. The procedures involved in maintaining a set of accounting records throughout an accounting period.

Accounting equation. An equation that is both the basic formula for the balance sheet and the foundation of double-entry accounting. Usually written: Assets = Liabilities + Fund balances.

Accounting period. The period of time covered by an income statement. This period generally is not less than one month or longer than one year.

Accounting principles. A body of rules, standards, and conventions that determines the manner in which transactions are recorded and in which data are presented in financial statements.

Accounts payable. Liabilities arising from the purchase of goods and services from suppliers on credit.

Accounts receivable. Assets arising from the provision of services or the sale of goods on credit to patients.

Accounts receivable aging schedule. An analysis of accounts receivable according to the length of time the accounts have been outstanding.

Accounts receivable turnover. The amount of charges to patients' accounts, during a given period, divided by the amount of accounts receivable.

Accrual basis of accounting. A method of accounting by which revenues are recognized when earned and expenses are recognized when incurred, regardless of the timing of the related cash flows.

Accrued expenses. Expenses that have been incurred but not yet paid.

Accrued income. Income that has been earned but not yet received in cash.

Accumulated depreciation. The accumulation to date of depreciation expense—that is, the total portion of the original cost of depreciable assets that already has been allocated to expense in prior and current periods.

Acute care. Inpatient general care provided to patients who are in a phase of illness that does not require the continuous observation and treatment provided in intensive-care units.

Adjusted average daily census. Average number of patients (inpatients plus an equivalent figure for outpatients) receiving care each day during the reporting period, which is usually 12 months. Derived by dividing the number of inpatient day equivalents (also called *adjusted inpatient days*) by the number of days in the reporting period.

Adjusted expenses per admission. Average expense to the hospital in providing care for one inpatient day. Adjusted expenses are derived by subtracting outpatient expenses from total expenses. Inpatient expenses are divided by total admissions to obtain the average expense per hospital stay.

Adjusted expenses per inpatient day. Expenses incurred for inpatient care only, and derived by dividing total expenses by inpatient day equivalents (adjusted inpatient days). The formula is the following:

$$\frac{\text{Total Expenses} \times \dfrac{\text{Inpatient Revenue}}{\text{Total Patient Revenue}}}{\text{Inpatient Days}}$$

Adjusted inpatient days. An aggregate figure reflecting the number of days of inpatient care, plus an estimate of the volume of outpatient services, expressed in units equivalent to an inpatient day in terms of level of effort. Derived by multiplying the number of outpatient visits by the ratio of outpatient revenue per outpatient visit to inpatient revenue per inpatient day, and adding the product (which represents the number of patient days attributable to outpatient services) to the number of inpatient days.

Adjusting entry. An entry that is necessary for adjustment of account balances to conform with the accrual basis at the end of the accounting period.

Admission. (1) An inpatient admission is the formal acceptance by a hospital of a patient who is to receive physician's, dentist's, or allied services while lodged in the hospital. (2) An outpatient admission is the formal acceptance by the hospital of a patient who is not to be lodged in the hospital while receiving physician's, dentist's, or allied services at the hospital.

Admissions. Number of patients, excluding newborns, accepted for inpatient service during the reporting period.

Allowance. The difference between gross revenue from services rendered and amounts received, or to be received, from patients or third-party payers.

Allowance for uncollectible accounts. A balance sheet valuation account reflecting the estimated amount of accounts and notes receivable that will prove to be uncollectible by reason of charity care, contractual adjustments, courtesy discounts, and bad debt losses.

Amortization. (1) The systematic allocation of an item to revenue or expense over a number of accounting periods. (2) The repayment of a loan on an installment basis.

Ancillary services. Those diagnostic and therapeutic services for which charges are customarily made, in addition to routine service charges, that include laboratory, radiology, surgical, and other services.

Assets. The economic resources of a hospital enterprise that are recognized and measured in conformity with generally accepted accounting principles.

Average daily census. The average number of inpatients, excluding newborns, receiving care each day during the reporting period.

Average length of stay. Average stay of inpatients during the reporting period. Derived by dividing the number of inpatient days by the number of admissions.

B

Bad debt. An account receivable that, although the patient has the ability to pay, is regarded as uncollectible and is recorded as a credit loss. See also *Uncompensated services*.

Balance sheet. A statement of financial position showing the hospital's assets, liabilities, and fund balances at a given date.

Beds. Average number of beds, cribs, and pediatric bassinets regularly maintained (set up and staffed for use) for inpatients during the reporting period. Derived by adding the total number of beds available each day during the reporting period and dividing this figure by the total number of days in the reporting period.

Births. Total number of infants born in the hospital during the reporting period.

Board-designated funds. Unrestricted resources set aside by action of the hospital's governing board for specific purposes or projects.

Board-designated investment funds. Unrestricted resources that, at the discretion of the governing board, have been designated for investment to produce income as if they were endowment funds.

Bond. A written promise under seal to pay a sum of money at some definite future time.

Bond discount or premium. The difference between the par or face value of a bond and the amount received (by the issuer) or paid (by the investor) when a bond is issued or purchased.

Bond indenture. The contract between the bondholders and the hospital issuing the bonds.

Bond sinking fund. A fund in which assets are accumulated in order to liquidate bonds at their maturity date or earlier.

Book value. The amount at which an asset or liability item is carried in accounting records of the hospital.

Budget. A financial plan for future operations.

C

Capital expenditure. An expenditure chargeable to an asset account when the asset acquired has an estimated life in excess of one year and is not intended for sale in the ordinary course of operations. The opposite of *revenue expenditure*.

Capital expenditure budgeting. The process of planning and controlling expenditures for property, plant, and equipment items.

Cash basis of accounting. A method of accounting by which revenues are recognized only when cash is received and expenses are recorded only when cash is disbursed.

Cash budget. A projection of cash receipts, disbursements, and balances for a given future period of time.

Cash-flow statement. A statement of actual or projected cash receipts and disbursements for a given period of time. Also referred to as a *statement of cash receipts and cash disbursements*.

Chart of accounts. A listing of account titles with account numbers that indicates the manner in which transaction data should be classified in the accounting records.

Clinic. A freestanding facility or part of another healthcare entity used for diagnosis and treatment of outpatients.

Closing the books. The process of transferring the balances in the revenue and expense accounts, including revenue deductions, to the fund balance account at the end of the fiscal year.

Community hospitals. All nonfederal short-term general and other special hospitals, excluding hospital units of institutions, whose facilities and services are available to the public. See also *Noncommunity hospitals*.

Composite depreciation. Depreciation of a number of similar assets as a group rather than on a unit-by-unit basis.

Compound interest. Interest that is computed on the principal amount invested or borrowed and on any interest earned (on such principal) that has not been paid.

Contingent liabilities. Possible liabilities that may arise on the occurrence or nonoccurrence of some future event.

Contractual adjustments. Differences between revenue at established rates and amounts realizable from third-party payers under contractual agreements.

Contractual patient. One of a group of patients for whom the hospital has agreed to provide specific inpatient or outpatient facilities and services, payment for which is made to the hospital on the basis of a contract between an outside agency and the hospital.

Control. (1) The process of ensuring insofar as possible that the objectives of an entity are realized. Its principal elements are (a) communication of plans, (b) performance appraisal, (c) corrective action, and (d) follow-up. (2) The types of organizations responsible for establishing policy for the overall operation of hospitals. The four major categories are (a) government, nonfederal, (b) nongovernment, not-for-profit, (c) investor-owned, for-profit, and (d) government, federal.

Control account. A general ledger account, the detail of which is contained in a subsidiary ledger (accounts receivable, for example).

Controllable cost. In the short run, a cost whose amount is controllable by someone in the organization. It is usually a variable cost.

Controller. The title sometimes given to the executive responsible for the accounting and finance functions in an enterprise. In large organizations, this individual may be referred to as the *director of fiscal affairs.*

Cost. The present value surrendered, or promised to be surrendered in the future, in exchange for goods and services received. Expired costs are expenses; unexpired costs are assets.

Cost basis of accounting. The use of historical, objectively determined cost as the basis of accounting for most assets.

Cost center. An organizational unit whose costs are separately accumulated in the accounts.

Cost control. The attempt to maintain actual costs at, or below, budgeted levels.

Cost finding. The segregation of direct costs by cost centers; the allocation of overhead costs to revenue-producing and other centers by inpatient, outpatient, and other classifications.

Cost or market, lower of. A valuation basis for inventories and temporary investments.

Courtesy and policy discounts. Differences between revenue recorded at established rates and amounts realizable for services provided to specific individuals such as employees, medical staff, and clergy.

Credit. As a noun, an entry or balance on the right-hand side of an account. As a verb, to make an entry on the right-hand side of an account.

Current assets. Those assets that are cash and will be converted into cash or consumed in the normal operations of the hospital within one year from the balance sheet date.

Current liabilities. Those liabilities that will be discharged with current assets in the normal course of business within one year from the balance sheet date.

Current ratio. The ratio of current assets to current liabilities.

D

Daily inpatient census. The number of inpatients present at the census-taking time each day. Generally, the inpatient census is taken each night. The census is adjusted for any inpatients who were both admitted and discharged after the census-taking time the previous day.

Days' revenue in receivables. The average number of days of billings in accounts receivable that remain uncollected at a given point in time.

Debenture bond. A bond secured, not by specific assets but only by the general credit standing of the issuer.

Debit. As a noun, an entry or balance on the left-hand side of an account. As a transitive verb, to make an entry on the left-hand side of an account.

Deductions from revenues. Revenues uncollectible by reason of charity care, contractual adjustments, courtesy discounts, and bad debts.

Default. Failure to fulfill the requirements of a contract, such as the nonpayment of interest or principal on a debt.

Deferred revenue. Future revenue that has been collected or billed but not yet earned (a liability).

Depreciation expense. That portion of the original cost of a tangible plant asset allocated to a particular accounting period.

Diagnosis-related group (DRG). A patient classification scheme that categorizes patients who are medically related with respect to primary and secondary diagnosis, age, and complications.

Discounting of receivables. A method of short-term financing in which patient receivables are used to secure a loan from a financial institution.

Dishonor. To refuse to honor (pay) a promissory note at maturity.

Donated services. The estimated monetary value of service of personnel who receive no monetary compensation, or only partial compensation, for their services. The term is usually applied to services rendered by members of religious orders, societies, or similar groups to hospitals operated by, or affiliated with, such organizations.

E

ECF. Extended care facility (for example, a nursing home).

Endowment funds. Funds with stipulations by the donors that the principal amount be maintained inviolate and in perpetuity and that only the income from investments of the funds be expended. See also *Term endowment funds.*

Equities. Rights in assets (for example, fund balances).

Expenses. Costs that have been consumed in carrying on some activity and from which no measurable benefit will extend beyond the present. Expenses are expired costs that ordinarily are accompanied by the surrendering of an asset or the incurring of a liability.

F

FICA. Federal Insurance Contributions Act, commonly known as social security.

FIFO. First-in, first-out method of inventory costing.

Fixed costs. Costs that remain substantially the same in total amount within a given range of production and period of time.

Flexible budget. A budget prepared so that it can be adjusted by interpolation to reflect what expenses should be at any level of activity within a relevant range.

Full-time equivalent (FTE) personnel. Calculated by adding the number of full-time personnel to one-half the number of part-time personnel, excluding medical and dental residents, interns, and other trainees.

Functional classification. The grouping of expenses according to the operating purposes (patient care, education, research, and so on) for which costs are incurred. Revenues also may be classified functionally.

Fund. A self-contained accounting entity set up to account for a specific activity or project.

Fund accounting. A system of accounting in which the hospital's resources, obligations, and fund balances are segregated into logical groups of accounts according to legal restrictions and administrative requirements. Each account group, or fund, constitutes a subordinate accounting entity.

Fund balance. The excess of assets over liabilities (net equity). An excess of liabilities over assets is known as a *deficit in fund balance.*

Funded debt. Long-term debt.

Funds functioning as endowment. See *Board-designated investment funds.*

Funds held in trust by others. Funds held and administered, at the direction of the donor, by an outside trustee for the benefit of an institution or institutions.

G

General fund. The name sometimes given to the unrestricted fund.

Governing board. The policy-making body of the hospital. Some of the responsibilities usually attributed to the governing board may be assumed by appropriate committees.

Gross revenues. The value, at the hospital's full established rates, of services rendered and goods sold to patients during a given time period.

H

Health Maintenance Organization (HMO). A generic set of medical care entities organized to deliver and finance healthcare services. An HMO provides comprehensive healthcare services to enrolled members for fixed, prepaid fees (premiums).

I

Imprest cash fund. See *Petty cash fund.*

Income statement. A financial statement indicating the results of operations of an enterprise in terms of revenues earned and expenses incurred for a given period of time. Also referred to as an operating statement, a statement of income and expense, or a profit-and-loss statement.

Indenture. An agreement between two or more parties specifying the reciprocal rights and duties of the parties under a contract such as a lease, mortgage, or contract between bondholders and the bond issuer.

Inpatient. A patient who is provided with room, board, and general nursing service, and who is expected to remain at least overnight and occupy a bed.

Inpatient days. Number of adult and pediatric days of care, excluding newborn days of care, rendered during the reporting period. See also *Adjusted inpatient days.*

Insolvency. The inability to meet mature obligations.

Interest. A charge for the use of money.

Interim financial statements. Financial statements—for example, monthly balance sheets and income statements—prepared at a date other than the end of the fiscal year.

Internal auditing. The work performed by a hospital's internal auditors.

Internal control. The plan of organization and all the coordinate methods and measures adopted within a hospital to safeguard its assets, check the accuracy and reliability of its accounting data, promote operational efficiency, and encourage adherence to prescribed managerial policies.

Inventory. The aggregate of those items of tangible personal property that are (1) held for sale in the ordinary course of business, (2) in process of production for sale, or (3) to be consumed currently in the production of goods or services to be available for sale.

Inventory control. The process of regulating the amount and types of supplies in inventory.

Inventory turnover. Cost of supplies used divided by the average inventory for the period.

J

Journal. A book of original entry in which transactions are recorded in chronological sequence.

L

Land improvements. Improvements made to land, including sidewalks, parking lots, driveways, fencing, and shrubbery. Land improvements are depreciable.

Ledger. The group of accounts used in recording the transactions of the hospital. A book of secondary entry.

Liability. The economic obligations of the hospital, as recognized and measured in conformity with generally accepted accounting principles.

LIFO. Last-in, first-out method of inventory costing.

Line of credit. An arrangement whereby a financial institution commits itself to lending up to a specified maximum amount during a specified period.

Liquidity. A hospital's financial position and its ability to meet currently maturing obligations.

Long-term hospital. One in which the average length of stay is 30 days or more.

Long-term investments. Investments, generally in securities, that the hospital intends to hold for longer than one year from the balance sheet date.

Long-term liabilities. Liabilities that are not payable within one year from the balance sheet (that is, all liabilities except current ones).

M

Management. The direction of resources to the attainment of desired objectives through planning and control.

Marketable security. Short-term financial instruments that can be readily purchased or sold without loss in principal.

Matching. An accounting principle that requires the recognition of related revenues and expenses in the same period.

Mortgage. A pledge of designated property as security for a loan—for example, mortgage bonds.

N

Net assets. The excess of assets over liabilities (that is, a fund balance).

Net income. The excess of revenues over expenses for a given period of time as presented in the income statements.

Net loss. The excess of expenses over revenues for a given period of time as presented in the income statements.

Net revenues. The excess of gross revenues from patient services over revenue deductions. Also called *net earnings from patient services.*

Net worth. An unsatisfactory term for net assets or fund balance.

Noncommunity hospitals. Includes federal hospitals, long-term hospitals, hospital units of institutions, psychiatric hospitals, hospitals for tuberculosis and other respiratory diseases, chronic disease hospitals, institutions for the mentally retarded, and alcoholism and chemical-dependency hospitals.

Nonexpendable funds. See *Endowment funds.*

Notes receivable discounted. Notes receivable that have been discounted with recourse at a financial institution.

Nursing-home-type unit. A hospital-managed unit offering primarily only the following types of service to the majority of all admissions: (1) skilled nursing care, (2) intermediate care, (3) personal care, and (4) sheltered/residential care.

O

Object of expenditure classification. A method of classifying expenditures—such as salaries and wages, employee benefits, supplies, and purchased services—according to their natural classification.

Objective evidence. A requirement in accounting that all transaction entries be supported, insofar as possible, by properly executed documents.

Occupancy. Ratio of average daily census to the average number of beds maintained during the reporting period.

Operating ratio. Total operating expenses divided by total operating revenues.

Opportunity cost. The measurable advantage forgone in the past or likely to be sacrificed as a result of a decision involving alternatives.

Organization chart. A diagrammatic illustration of the manner in which a hospital is organized internally.

Outpatient. A patient who is not confined overnight in a health-care institution.

Outpatient visits. Visits by patients who are not lodged in the hospital to receive medical, dental, or other services. Each appearance by an outpatient to each unit of the hospital counts as one outpatient visit. A visit consists of one or more *occasions of service.* Each examination, test, treatment, or procedure rendered to an outpatient counts as one occasion of service.

Overstocked. A condition in which inventory stocks exceed demand.

P

Patient day. The unit of measure denoting lodging facilities provided and services rendered to one inpatient between the census-taking hour on two successive days.

Percentage of occupancy. The ratio of actual patient days to maximum patient days as determined by bed capacity during any given period of time.

Periodic inventory system. A system of accounting for purchased goods and supplies by which items purchased are charged to expense accounts rather than to inventory.

Permanent funds. See *Endowment funds.*

Perpetual inventory system. A system of accounting for inventories under which a continuous, day-to-day record is kept of inventory levels.

Petty cash fund. A small fund of cash maintained for the purpose of making minor disbursements for which the issuance of a check would be inconvenient or impractical.

Physical inventory. The actual inventory as determined by physical count, usually at the end of a reporting period.

Planning. The process of establishing programs for the achievement of objectives.

Plant. Physical properties used for hospital purposes (that is, land, land improvements, buildings, and equipment). The term does not include real estate or properties or restricted or unrestricted funds not used for hospital operations.

Plant replacement and expansion funds. Funds donated for renewal or replacement of the hospital plant.

Pooled investments. Assets of two or more funds consolidated for investment purposes.

Position control plan. A management tool for controlling the number of employees on the hospital payroll and for ensuring the utilization of each employee to the point of maximum effectiveness.

Posting. Transferral of information in the journals to the ledger.

Preferred stock. A type of stock that has preference over common stock with respect to dividends, or to assets in case of liquidation, or both.

Prepaid expense. An expense-type outlay that benefits (is applicable to) subsequent accounting periods and therefore is an asset.

Prepaid income. See *Deferred revenue.*

Present value. The value today of a future receipt or payment, or successive receipts or payments, discounted at the appropriate discount rate.

Profit-and-loss statement. A less than satisfactory term for income statement.

Prospective payment system (PPS). Medicare payment made at a predetermined, specific rate based on a patient's diagnosis.

Provider. A person or other entity that undertakes to provide healthcare services.

PSRO. Professional Standards Review Organization.

Purchase order. A business document used in purchasing.

Q

Qualified audit report. An audit report that includes one or more qualifications or exceptions.

Quantity discount. A reduction in unit purchase cost received by those who purchase supplies in a quantity in excess of a set amount.

Quick assets. Cash, temporary investments, and receivables.

Quick ratio. The ratio of quick assets to current liabilities.

R

Ratio. The quotient that results when one number is divided by another.

Receiving report. A business document in which a record is made of incoming quantities of supplies.

Record date. The date on which a list of stockholders is prepared to determine those who are entitled to receive a declared dividend.

Referred outpatient. One who is admitted exclusively to a special diagnostic or therapeutic facility or service of the hospital for diagnosis or treatment on an ambulatory basis.

Refunding. The process of replacing one debt with another, usually one having a lower interest cost.

Registered bond. A type of bond whose principal (and usually interest) is payable only to the owner as recorded by the issuer.

Relative value units. Index numbers assigned to various procedures based on the relative amounts of labor, supplies, and capital required to perform the procedure.

Reserve. A term generally undesirable in accounting usage but sometimes employed in reserve for bad debts and reserve for depreciation.

Responsibility accounting. A system of accounting that accumulates and communicates historical and projected monetary and statistical data relating to revenues and controllable expenses classified according to the organizational units that produce the revenues and are responsible for incurring the expenses.

Restricted funds. Funds restricted by donors for specific purposes. The term refers to specific-purpose and endowment funds.

Retirement of indebtedness funds. Funds required by external sources to be used to meet debt service charges and the retirement of indebtedness on plant assets. The term *sinking funds* is sometimes used to describe these funds.

Revenue. Income that results from the sale of goods and the rendering of services and is measured by the charge made to patients, clients, or tenants for goods and services furnished to them. Revenue also includes gains from the sale or exchange of assets, interest, and dividends earned on investments and unrestricted donations of resources to the hospital.

Revenue expenditure. An expenditure charged against operations.

S

Salvage value. The estimated amount for which a plant asset can be sold at the end of its useful life. Also called *scrap value*.

Self-responsible patient. A patient who pays either all or part of the hospital bill from his or her own resources, as opposed to one whose bill a third party pays.

Semivariable costs. Costs that are partly variable and partly fixed in behavior, in response to changes in volume.

Short-term hospital. One in which the average length of stay is less than 30 days.

Short-term investments. See *Temporary investments.*

Sinking fund. See *Retirement of indebtedness funds.*

Specific-identification method. A system of inventory costing. Also applied in the determination of the costs of securities sold.

Specific-purpose fund. Funds restricted by donors for a specific purpose or project. Board-designated funds do not constitute specific-purpose funds.

Statement of cash flows. A statement that summarizes the cash inflows and outflows from an entity's operating, investing, and financing activities, as required by FASB Statement No. 95 (1987).

Statement of changes in fund balances. A financial statement setting forth the changes that have occurred in the amount of the fund balances during a given period of time.

Stock dividend. A dividend paid in the form of additional shares of stock.

Stockout. A demand for inventory items currently unavailable.

Straight-line method. A method of depreciation. Also a method of amortizing bond premium and discount.

Subsidiary ledger. A group of accounts that is contained in a separate ledger and that supports a single account (a control account) in the general ledger.

SYD. Sum-of-the-years'-digits method of depreciation.

T

Tangible asset. An asset—such as equipment—having physical existence.

Temporary fund. Name formerly given to specific-purpose fund.

Temporary investments. Investments, generally in marketable securities, that a hospital does not intend to hold for more than one year from the balance sheet date.

Term endowment funds. Donated funds that by the terms of the agreement become available either for any legitimate purpose designated by the governing board or for a specific purpose, designated by the donor, on the happening of an event, or on the passage of a stated period of time.

Term loan. A loan, generally obtained from a bank or insurance company, with a maturity period of more than one year. Term loans are generally amortized.

Third-party payer. Any agency (such as Blue Cross, the Medicare program, or commercial insurance companies) that contracts with healthcare providers and patients to pay for patient care.

Trade credit. Debt arising from transactions in which supplies and services are purchased on credit from suppliers.

Trial balance. A list of the accounts in a ledger, with their balances, as a given date.

U

Unamortized bond discount (or premium). That portion of bond discount (or premium) that has not yet been amortized.

Uncompensated services. Charity care and services that result in bad debts. Charity care reflects an inability to pay for all or part of services rendered that is known to exist by the provider when the services are rendered. Bad debts reflect an inability or unwillingness to pay for services that becomes known to the provider after the services are rendered and billed.

Unemployment taxes. Taxes levied by federal and state governments to finance payments to the unemployed.

Unexpended plant funds. See *Plant replacement and expansion funds.*

Unexpired cost. An asset. See also *Cost.*

Unrestricted funds. Funds that bear no external restrictions as to use or purpose (funds that can be used for any legitimate purpose designated by the governing board, as distinguished from funds restricted externally for specific operating purposes, for plant replacement and expansion, and for endowment).

Useful life. An estimate made of the number of years an item of plant equipment will be used by a hospital.

V

Variable cost. A cost that varies directly in total with changes in the level of activity.

Voucher system. A system for the processing and control of cash disbursements.

W

Weighted-average costing. A method of determining the cost of supplies used and the valuation of inventory.

Working capital. Generally, the excess of current assets over current liabilities. Sometimes called *net working capital*.

Worksheet. A device used in accounting to facilitate the preparation of financial statements.

Y

Yield. The actual rate of return on an investment, as opposed to the nominal rate of return.

Index